SWAT
Fitness

Matt Brzycki and Stuart A. Meyers

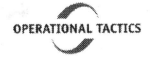

OPERATIONAL TACTICS

Gaithersburg, Maryland

Printed in the United States of America
10 9 8 7 6 5 4 3 2 1

Inquiries and orders may be directed to:
Operational Tactics, Inc.
Post Office Box 7525
Gaithersburg, Maryland 20898
www.operationaltactics.com

LCCN: 2003104017

Cover designed by Surface2, Inc.
Cover photography: Joseph V. Meyers and Stuart A. Meyers

Distributed in the United States and Mexico by Operational Tactics, Inc.

DEDICATIONS

MATT BRZYCKI dedicates this book to his lovely wife, Alicia, and their darling son, Ryan.

STUART A. MEYERS dedicates this book to his wife, Dellanira Meyers. Without her love and enduring support, neither this book nor his achievements would have been possible. Joe and Brian, their children, are a constant joy in their lives and an unwavering source of pride.

ACKNOWLEDGEMENTS

A sincere thanks goes to Tony Alexander, Ryan Bonfiglio, Troy Wilson, and Joede Vanek for volunteering their time to pose for the pictures in this book. Peter Silletti provided all exercise photographs. Operational Tactics, Inc. provided all SWAT fitness and SWAT action photographs.

TABLE OF CONTENTS

FOREWORD

For the courageous men and women who serve in law enforcement and the armed forces, physical fitness can frequently mean the difference between life and death — for themselves as well as for the public they are sworn to protect.

Matt Brzycki and Stuart Meyers have written a book which effectively focuses attention on the importance of physical fitness in the law enforcement and military fields. *SWAT Fitness* provides a thoughtful, comprehensive guide to proper conditioning, nutrition, and healthy lifestyles.

As President Kennedy said when he created the President's Council on Physical Fitness in 1960: "Physical fitness is not only one of the most important keys to a healthy body, it is the basis of dynamic and creative intellectual activity. Intelligence and skill can only function at the peak of their capacity when the body is healthy and strong."

As you read this book, it will become increasingly clear that the President's words still ring true today - for those in law enforcement and the military — and for all of us as well.

Once again, congratulations to Matt and Stuart for writing a book that may very well end up saving someone's life.

James E. McGreevey
Governor, State of New Jersey

During the past several years it has been my privilege to train military fitness leaders, especially those serving the United States Navy and Marines, as well as law enforcement conditioning specialists. I have learned a great deal from these training experiences, not the least of which is the serious need for safe, effective, and efficient exercise programs for servicemen and servicewomen.

Contrary to the general misconception, the majority of military and law enforcement personnel are not in top physical shape. They may have completed a basic training or boot camp program at one time, but few continue a comprehensive conditioning program. This is unfortunate because physical fitness requires regular exercise for maintenance and relatively hard training for improvement.

Although automation affects everyone, men and women in protection agencies are frequently called upon to perform at high levels of physical prowess. If they are unable to do so, the unfortunate consequence may be injury to others or to themselves. Fitness is essential to effectively handle most emergency situations, and poor physical performance is not an acceptable option for military, police, and firefighters.

For those who really want to do their best, look their best, and feel their best, there is good news. Matt Brzycki and Stuart Meyers have written a comprehensive conditioning book that specifically address the fitness needs of law enforcement and military individuals. Their personal and professional backgrounds make them perfectly suited to design practical and productive exercise programs that will dramatically elevate your fitness level. The authors know that physical fitness is necessary for both optimum job performance and personal health, and have therefore developed training programs that provide both short-term and life-long benefits. I am sure that you will be highly satisfied with both the exercise process and the training results as you perform the quality workouts presented in these pages. My thanks to Matt and Stuart for providing this important fitness information, and my thanks to you for putting it into practice.

Wayne L. Westcott, Ph.D.
Fitness Research Director
South Shore YMCA, Quincy, Massachusetts
Fitness Consultant, United States Navy

INTRODUCTION

Physical fitness is an integral part of all tactical operations, as well as daily life. Tactical officers perform duties ranging from carrying a 90-pound ram up 10 flights of stairs in order to breach a door, to sprinting to the scene of a suspect preparing to execute hostages. A high level of fitness is not only required to accomplish these tasks, but also to perform life-saving skills once the tasks have been completed. A tactical operation is not over once the ram arrives at the door. The door must be breached, entry must be made, suspects inside must be controlled, and all required duties of a SWAT officer must be completed. SWAT officers require an extraordinary level of physical fitness.

Whether you are a SWAT team member, someone striving to join a SWAT team, an athlete, or are seeking additional knowledge, being physically fit allows you to achieve improved physical performance. Better physical fitness can also translate into improved mental alertness. With an improved level of physical and mental fitness, a sense of well-being is created. Exercising the body also strengthens the mind. Developing a comprehensive training program will enable you to accomplish these goals.

SWAT Fitness is an educational resource designed to present critical information on how to develop and enhance the human body through exercise, proper nutrition, and weight management. Essential information on basic anatomy, muscular function, and nutrition illustrates how the human body functions. Information on flexibility, aerobic, anaerobic, strength, metabolic, and skill training provides a complete understanding of diverse exercises that must be incorporated in a comprehensive training program.

Exercise physiology, utilization of free weights, machines, and manual resistance are described in detail. A wide variety of training concepts and routines offer the opportunity to create a customized training program for every individual to obtain maximum results. In addition, the benefits of varying your training routine are presented in order to maintain these results.

Most people encounter some type of debilitating or persistent injury during their lifetimes. Under most circumstances, physical training can and should continue with certain limitations. Information on rehabilitative training sets guidelines and training methods that allow you to adapt your training program to the nature of your injury. This provides for a quicker recovery time, and still offers an increased level of physical and mental fitness.

Each person is different in physical structure, metabolic system and genetics, as well as mental constitution. Individual characteristics and goals should be reflected in the development and implementation of any training program. Sample workout cards for aerobic, anaerobic, single-set strength, and multiple-set strength training are included in order to create a reference to measure progress.

SWAT Fitness also contains important administrative and managerial topics for SWAT officers, supervisors, and law enforcement agencies. Judicial decisions relating to negligent retention, failure to train to standard, and fitness requirements for the selection of SWAT team members outline law enforcement agency liability and productivity concerns. The results of our SWAT team operational fitness standards research and development provide solutions for the application of job-related standards and reduced liability for SWAT commanders, team leaders, administrators, and operators. In addition, this book can serve as a guide to employ these contemporary standards during the selection and prolongation of SWAT team personnel.

There are many publications available presenting information on a wide variety of fitness-related topics. *SWAT Fitness* is the first book of its kind designed to take its readers down a comprehensive path to achieve the ultimate level of fitness required by elite SWAT officers to complete their exciting and dangerous life-saving missions. Proper preparation is the key to success in any endeavor. As we start down the path toward improved fitness, an understanding of the importance of physical fitness, basic anatomy, and muscular function/body mechanics should first be attained.

Chapter 1
The Importance of Physical Fitness

Physical fitness is a necessity in daily life, in order to look and feel good. It is instrumental in attaining a healthy body and can have a direct impact in your personal and professional life. Physical fitness consists of achieving a high level of flexibility, strength, power, endurance, aerobic and anaerobic capacity, nutrition, and an overall healthy body. In addition, a balance must occur in these areas to accomplish a peak level of fitness.

If most people recognize the importance of fitness, then why are so many people unfit? Generally speaking, the answer is that most people do not feel they have time in their busy schedules to exercise or to follow proper nutritional guidelines. Technology also plays a role in making our lives more comfortable and less physically demanding. Genetics, improper weight management, and physical ailments are also a part of the answer and will be discussed in detail throughout the book.

For elite SWAT officers, physical fitness and nutrition must be a lifestyle; part of everyday life. Training should not be an ordeal of "having" to go to the gym or following a fad diet. Poor physical fitness can cost someone his or her life on a tactical operation. For everyone, regardless of occupation, poor physical fitness will eventually cost a life as well: YOURS.

Why is physical fitness important? To answer this question, the importance of physical fitness in Daily Life and for SWAT Officers are presented. The following are direct or indirect benefits of improved fitness levels:

DAILY LIFE

- *Longevity* – The more physically fit you are, the longer you will live. Obviously, disease, accidents, and occupational hazards are all factors in longevity as well. However, barring an untimely occurrence, physically fit people live longer than unfit people.

- *Quality of life* – Anyone who has suffered an injury or illness has experienced a lower quality of life during that time period. When you are physically fit, you are able to be more active, tire less frequently, and generally enjoy life to a greater extent.

- *Mental and physical well-being* – There is a direct correlation between physical and mental well-being. Improved circulation, aerobic capacity, flexibility, muscular strength, and nutrition will make you feel better both mentally and physically.

- *Overall health* – An improved level of physical fitness can increase your overall health by making you more resistant to disease and illness. Generally, more physically fit people get sick less frequently and can better combat disease than less physically fit people.

- *Injury prevention* – Stronger muscles and tendons assist in reducing the likelihood of injury. The human body is like a complex machine. Oftentimes, one bodypart or muscle group can take over the workload when another part fatigues, thus maintaining structural integrity and preventing injury.

- *Shorter recovery time from injuries* – If you become injured and are physically fit, you will have a shorter recovery time than if you are not fit. In addition, if you have a muscular injury, other muscle groups can adapt to handle the workload, allowing for the injured muscle to begin repair. Note: If surgery is required to repair an injury, physical therapy is recommended both prior to, and after surgery. By performing as many of the post-surgical physical-therapy exercises as possible prior to surgery, the muscles and tendons around the injured area will get stronger and adapt, thereby facilitating a shorter recovery period.

- *Work performance* – Obviously, if your job requires physical exertion, you will be able to perform it more efficiently and effectively if you maintain a high level of fitness. However, regardless of your occupation, being more physically fit will increase your work performance by enhancing your alertness and ability to focus on required tasks.

- *Stress release* – Exercise is a great way to relieve stress. It allows you to release anxieties, frustrations, and other causes of stress in a positive, beneficial manner. Aerobic training can reduce blood pressure and cause fatigue, thereby releasing stress. In many cases, this will also result in a sense of well-being.

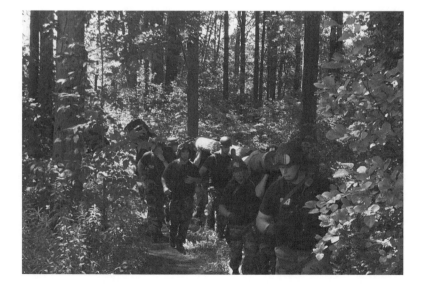

Whether you are hiking through the woods or conducting SWAT training, increased stamina is beneficial in daily life, as well as work performance.

- *Stamina* – Vince Lombardi, the legendary coach of the Green Bay Packers, once said, "Fatigue makes cowards of us all." A direct result of improved physical fitness is increased stamina. Work performance, family life, and personal fulfillment are all affected when you tire. Increased stamina will allow you to be more attentive throughout your personal and professional life.

- *Motivation* – Improved physical fitness increases your alertness, focus, and stamina, which in turn boosts motivation throughout your daily life. When you are more motivated you will train harder, increasing your fitness level. This cycle will also increase your overall productivity.

- *Physical appearance* – Most people care about their physical appearance. Billions of dollars are spent annually on clothes, cosmetics, plastic surgeries, sports supplements, low-fat foods, and other amenities designed to make them look better and younger. People are always searching for the "fountain of youth" which is within reach at all times, but requires hard work and dedication in the gym. An improved level of physical fitness can result in improved physical appearance. However, beauty is still an individual determination.

- *Sexual performance* – A poor level of fitness can result in fatigue during sexual activity. Improved physical fitness increases stamina for both males and females, causing less susceptibility to fatigue. And in many cases, improved physical fitness will enhance sexual desire and performance.

SWAT OFFICERS

- *Ability to save lives* – A SWAT team is called when a life-threatening situation exceeds the normal capabilities of a law enforcement agency. The primary mission of SWAT officers is to save lives. You, as a SWAT officer, are the bottom line. When you are called on an emergency response operation, someone is already dead, is dying, or getting ready to be killed. You must be prepared physically and mentally.

- *Adversaries are prepared* – Everyday you do not train, someone else is training to defeat you. Many criminals in prison train on a daily basis. They work out in groups, assist-

Every day you do not train, someone else is training to defeat you. Prisoners work together to obtain maximum results.

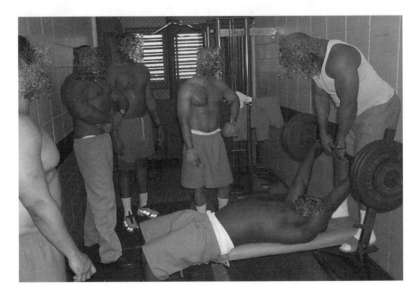

ing and competing with each other to obtain a very high level of fitness. Their dedication and commitment is reflected in their motivation for results and oftentimes, a desire for success in criminal endeavors.

- *Work performance* – Physical fitness is an integral part of all tactical operations. There are no excuses for poor performance, including an inadequate level of physical fitness. If you have a high-risk search or arrest warrant to serve on the 15th floor of an apartment building, the elevator may not be available. In this case, all team members must be able to run up the stairs, 15 floors, carrying all operational equipment including a heavy ram, and then be able to perform upon arrival. An improved level of physical fitness consisting of stronger muscles and tendons, reduced fatigue, and increased aerobic capacity can increase work performance.

- *Officer safety* – Your safety and the safety of your fellow officers is paramount. You have an obligation to your family, your SWAT team, and the families of fellow SWAT team members to place safety as a top priority. Your level of physical fitness will affect your ability to follow safety measures when you are fatigued. If SWAT officers on a critical incident are injured or die, there are no replacements to ensure mission success, or for the families of injured or dead officers.

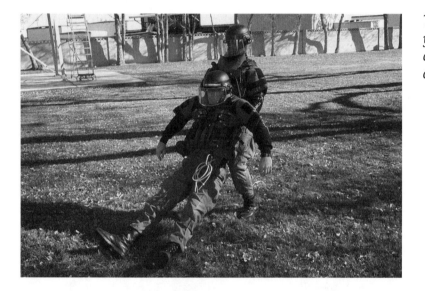

Your level of physical fitness can affect your ability to successfully rescue a critically injured officer on a tactical operation.

- *Officer rescue capabilities* – Nothing more important can occur on a tactical operation than having to rescue an injured or dying officer. The faster you can move and the more strength you possess, the more effective you will be in removing a critically injured officer from a hostile area.

- *Reduced department liability* – Physically fit officers oftentimes need to use less force on the use-of-force continuum to restrain or arrest an individual, thereby reducing department liability. In addition, departments implementing operationally-related physical fitness standards will have reduced liability with regard to officers filing civil lawsuits or union grievences when they are rejected during the selection process of tactical team members.

- *Extended operations* – SWAT operations can last minutes, hours, or days. Your ability to remain effective on a tactical operation is directly related to your level of physical fitness. In North Carolina, a bank robbery where a suspect held multiple hostages lasted three days. SWAT team members that responded to the scene received little rest throughout the incident. During the rescue attempt, a hostage was killed by an entry team member due to improper target identification; a direct result of fatigue.

- *Reduced injuries/susceptibility to illness* – Most law enforcement agencies have a minimum number of officers assigned to their SWAT teams. An injury or illness will reduce the number of personnel available for tactical operations. Physically fit officers are less prone to injury and illness, ensuring that a maximum number of officers are available at all times.

- *Decision-making* – SWAT officers are called upon to make many crucial decisions that can determine the outcome of a critical incident. The most serious of which are life-and-death decisions. Physical fitness plays a very important role in enhancing a SWAT officer's decision-making capability by aiding in the attainment of equanimity — composure under stress.

- *Stressful situations* – Tactical operations by their very nature can be very stressful. An entry team may be required to search a structure for an armed suspect waiting for the opportunity to ambush the team. In Louisiana, two SWAT team members were shot and killed, and other team members were wounded when they attempted to enter the house of a suspect. The possibility of death exists on every tactical operation. You must be able to control your emotions, adrenaline flow, breathing, and heart rate in order to be effective in your actions. A high level of physical fitness will allow you to more easily adapt and handle the stress.

- *Weapon proficiency* – Whether you are a SWAT sniper required to take a life-saving shot from an extended distance on a suspect holding hostages, or an entry team member reacting instinctively to shoot a suspect in close proximity, weapon proficiency is critical. In Pennsylvania, a suspect was preparing to execute a hostage. He was holding a gun to the hostage's head when a SWAT sniper was able to save the life of the hostage, by taking a shot from a distance of almost 200 yards away. Making this shot even more difficult was the fact that the only area the sniper could shoot was a small portion of the suspect's head, because the hostage was in front of the suspect. In addition, both the suspect and hostage were moving when the shot was taken. Muscle relaxation, proper bone support, and breath control are all very important elements of marksmanship skill. An improved level of physical fitness consisting of stronger muscles and tendons, and increased aerobic capacity can increase weapon proficiency. An ability to attain proper bone support in a shooting position is directly related to flexibility and weight management. Increased flexibility and a reduced waist size will allow you to adapt your body into preferred, more stable positions, also increasing your weapon proficiency.

- *Breaching* – If you are a door breacher, your SWAT team is depending on you to open the door to make a tactical entry. Whether you are using a ram, hydraulic pump, or sledge hammer, improved muscular strength will allow you to breach a door faster.

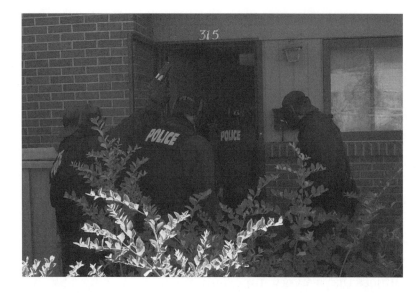

Opening a locked and/or barricaded door is critical to the success of a tactical operation. SWAT breachers will benefit from improved physical fitness.

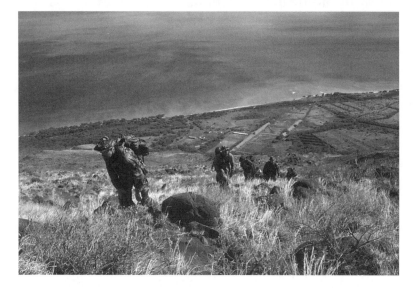

The ability to carry all mission-essential equipment, even up a mountain, may be necessary for SWAT officers.

In the event the door is fortified, improved muscular endurance and anaerobic capacity will enhance your breaching effectiveness by delaying the onset of fatigue.

- *Ability to carry tactical equipment* – Oftentimes, SWAT officers are required to carry an inordinate amount of equipment. Tactical vests, helmets, weapon systems, extra bullets/magazines, knives, chemical munitions, gas masks, diversionary devices, flashlights, and other essential equipment must be carried on a tactical operation. The weight of this equipment can easily exceed 40 pounds. Increased muscular strength and endurance will make it easier to carry these items and additional items, such as a ram or ballistic-resistant shield, for a longer period of time.

- *Increased energy* – High energy levels are essential during training and on tactical operations. Increased energy allows you to be more active and to be able to perform while carrying heavy loads of equipment. Improved physical fitness in conjunction with proper nutrition will directly affect your ability to sustain high energy levels.

Moving into position undetected is an essential skill for all SWAT officers and requires a high level of physical fitness.

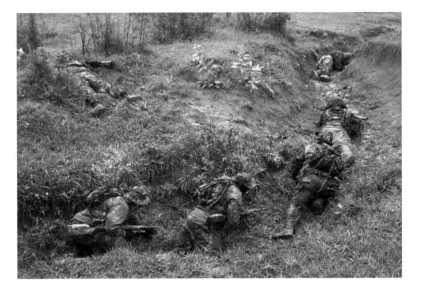

- *Movement/stalking techniques* – SWAT officers may be required to move quickly or very slowly into position on a tactical operation. You may have to sprint into position to save someone's life or slow stalk into position in order to avoid detection by the suspect. Both types of movement require a high level of physical fitness, especially when you may be required to take immediate action upon arrival at your final operational position.

- *Reliability* – Physically fit officers are generally more reliable in their work performance than officers in poor condition. The sense of well-being created through physical fitness can increase reliability in many areas. Officers are also less prone to illness or injury, making them more reliable to attend training sessions and to be available for deployment on tactical operations.

- *Mental preparation and focus* – As previously stated, physical fitness is an integral part of all tactical operations. However, mental preparation and focus are equally important. Officers with high levels of physical fitness are usually able to focus better on their responsibilities, have improved concentration, and are able to perform better on SWAT operations. The moment you lose focus in training, time is being wasted, and injuries or accidents can occur. When you lose focus on a tactical operation, the results can be catastrophic.

The benefits of physical fitness can be found in your personal and professional life. From improved work performance to reduced stress, fitness can make you feel better about yourself and your quality of life. Prior to determining your specific goals and objectives, you should obtain additional knowledge of how the human body works. This will provide a basis to design or enhance your fitness program. Understanding basic anatomy and muscular function will provide you with a solid foundation to take the next step for improved fitness.

Chapter 2
Basic Anatomy and Muscular Function

As a SWAT officer, athlete, or fitness enthusiast interested in improving fitness, understanding basic anatomy and muscular function is necessary. Essentially, any physical activity is a series of movements made by your muscles acting upon your skeleton. (Their collective efforts are reflected in the term "musculoskeletal system.")

More specifically, your body is basically a system of levers. Movement of these levers — your bones — is produced by your muscles, which are anchored to your bones by tendons. (Tendons link muscle to bone; ligaments link bone to bone.) Perhaps the most well-known and noticeable tendon in your body is the Achilles tendon which fastens the calf muscles to the heel bone.

MUSCLE: TYPES AND STRUCTURE

There are three different types of muscle tissue: cardiac, smooth, and skeletal. Cardiac muscle makes up most of the heart wall, smooth muscle is found in the walls of blood vessels, and skeletal muscle acts across your joints to produce movement.

Muscles are made up of numerous muscle fibers which are made up of many myofibrils. (To get an idea of this arrangement, picture a telephone cable containing hundreds of wires.) Myofibrils contain two contractile protein filaments — the thinner actin and the thicker myosin — that run parallel to one another. Muscular contractions occur at this level.

MUSCULAR CONTRACTIONS

"Contraction" refers to the process in which a muscle generates force. The force exerted by a muscle on the weight of an object is known as the "tension"; the force exerted by the weight of an object on a muscle is known as the "load." So, tension and load are opposing forces.

There are three types of muscular contractions: concentric, eccentric, and isometric. Concentric and eccentric contractions are more common than isometric contractions in physical training, SWAT operations, and competitive events. But isometric contractions do occur and, therefore, must be considered.

A concentric muscular contraction is one in which a muscle shortens against a load. The movement of the resistance is done in a direction away from the earth or opposite the direction of gravity. Examples of concentric contractions are raising a weight, rising from a squat position, and running up a hill. In a concentric contraction, muscular tension is more than the external load. Since the mechanical work is positive, a concentric muscular contraction is sometimes referred to as the "positive phase" of a movement.

An eccentric muscular contraction occurs when a muscle lengthens against a load. The movement of the resistance is done in a direction toward the earth or in the direction of gravity. Examples of eccentric contractions are lowering a weight, descending into a squat position, and running down a hill. In an eccentric contraction, muscular tension is less than the external load. Because the mechanical work is negative, an eccentric muscular contraction is typically referred to as the "negative phase" of a movement.

Finally, an isometric (or static) contraction is one in which the contractile component of a muscle shortens while the elastic connective tissue lengthens by the same amount, thereby producing no change in the overall muscle-tendon length. An example of an isometric contraction would be holding a weight in a static position, maintaining a squat position, and staying motionless in a tactical shooting position. Since there is no joint movement during an isometric muscular contraction, the mechanical work is zero. (Of course, energy must be provided in order to produce an isometric contraction. Although there is no mechanical work performed, there is metabolic work.)

THE SLIDING FILAMENT THEORY

As noted previously, movement of the skeletal system is produced by contraction of your muscles. The most widely accepted theory of explaining muscular contraction is the Sliding Filament Theory. As the name of this theory implies, one set of proteinous filaments is thought to slide over the other and overlap (like pistons in a sleeve), thereby shortening the muscle. Here's how: The myosin filaments have tiny protein projections in the shape of globular heads which extend toward the actin filaments. During a concentric muscular contraction these projections (or "crossbridges") are believed to bind to the actin filament, and then swivel in a ratchet-like fashion — much like oars in a boat — in such a way that it pulls the actin over the myosin filament. The crossbridges then uncouple from the actin filament, pivot, reattach, and repeat the cycle. Thus, this process can be summed up as "attach-rotate-detach-rotate." A single myosin crossbridge may attach and detach with an actin filament hundreds of times in the course of a single muscular contraction (such as during one repetition of an exercise). This process occurs along the entire myofibril and among all the myofibrils of a muscle fiber. However, the crossbridges do not attach-rotate-detach-rotate at the same time, since this would result in a series of jerks rather than a smooth movement.

COMMON JOINT MOVEMENTS

Several terms are frequently used in the jargon of physical training to describe various joint movements. Familiarity with these terms will assist in understanding the function of most muscles.

"Flexion" is a decrease in the angle between two bones and "extension" is an increase in the angle between two bones. "Abduction" refers to movement of a limb away from the mid-line of the body and "adduction" is movement of a limb toward the mid-line of the body. Finally, "rotation" is turning about the vertical axis of a bone.

THE MAJOR MUSCLES

Incredible as it may seem, there are more than 600 muscles in the human body — and about six billion muscle fibers. In fact, each one of your forearms consists of 19 separate muscles with such exotic-sounding names as "extensor carpi radialis brevis" and "flexor digitorum superficialis." Discussing muscles in such great detail is well beyond the scope and purpose of this book. Instead, the focus will be on your major muscles.

The major muscles can be grouped in the following main areas: the hips, upper legs, lower legs, torso, upper arms, lower arms, abdominals, lower back, and neck. Brief notes on the location and primary functions of each muscle are given along with anatomical terminology that is generally accepted in discussions of physical training. (Anterior and posterior views of the muscles of the body are illustrated in Figures 2.1 and 2.2, respectively.)

HIPS

Your hip region is made up of three main muscle groups: the gluteals, adductors, and iliopsoas.

Gluteals. The gluteals (or "glutes") are located on the back of the hips. They are composed of three primary muscles: the gluteus maximus, gluteus medius, and gluteus minimus. The largest and strongest muscle in the body is the gluteus maximus (which forms your buttocks). The main function of this muscle is hip extension (driving your upper legs backward). The gluteus medius and gluteus minimus cause hip abduction (spreading your legs apart). The gluteal muscles are involved significantly in walking, running, jumping, crawling, and various climbing movements (such as up stairs, over fences, and through windows).

Adductors. The adductor group is composed of five muscles that are located throughout the inner thigh: the gracilis, pectineus, adductor longus, adductor brevis, and adductor magnus (which is the largest of the five). The muscles of the inner thigh are used during hip adduction (bringing your legs together).

Iliopsoas. The "iliopsoas" is actually a collective term for the primary muscles on the front of your hips: the iliacus, psoas major, and psoas minor. The main function of the iliopsoas is hip flexion (bringing your knees to your chest). The iliopsoas has a major role in many activities — especially those that involve lifting your knees, such as when walking, running, crawling, and climbing. The iliopsoas is sometimes considered with the muscles of the abdomen.

UPPER LEGS

The two main muscle groups of your upper legs (or thighs) are the hamstrings and quadriceps.

Hamstrings. The hamstrings (or "hams") are located on the back of your upper legs and actually include three muscles: the semimembranosus, semitendinosus, and biceps femoris. Together, these muscles are involved in knee flexion (bringing your heels toward your buttocks) and hip extension. The hamstrings are used extensively in running, jumping, and climbing. One of the best reasons to strengthen the hamstrings is that they are quite susceptible to pulls and tears. Clearly, strong hamstrings are necessary to counterbalance the effects of the powerful quadriceps muscles.

Quadriceps. The quadriceps (or "quads") are the most important muscles on the front of your upper legs. As the name suggests, the quadriceps are made up of four muscles. The vastus lateralis is located on the outside of the thigh; the vastus medialis resides on the medial (inner) side of the thigh above the patella (the kneecap); between these two thigh

11

muscles is the vastus intermedius; and finally, laying on top of the vastus intermedius is the rectus femoris. The main function of the quadriceps is knee extension (straightening your legs). The quadriceps are involved in walking, running, cycling, kicking, jumping, and climbing.

LOWER LEGS

The calves and the "dorsi flexors" are the two major muscle groups in your lower legs.

Calves. The calves are made up of two important muscles — the gastrocnemius (or "gastroc") and soleus — that are located on the back of your lower legs. These two muscles have a common tendon of insertion (the Achilles tendon) and are jointly referred to as the "triceps surae" or, more simply, the "gastroc-soleus." The soleus actually resides underneath the gastrocnemius and is used primarily when your knees are bent at 90 degrees or more (such as in the seated position). The calves are involved in plantar flexion (extending your ankles or rising up on your toes). The calves have a major part in running, jumping, and climbing (especially stairs).

Dorsi Flexors. The front of your lower leg contains four muscles that are sometimes simply referred to as the "dorsi flexors." The largest of these muscles is the tibialis anterior. The dorsi flexors are primarily used in dorsi flexion (flexing your ankles) and are involved when cycling with toe clips. Strengthening the dorsi flexors is critical to safeguard against shin splints.

TORSO

The three major muscle groups in your torso are the chest, upper back, and shoulders.

Chest. The major muscle surrounding the chest area is the pectoralis major. It is thick, flat, and fan-shaped, and the most superficial muscle of the chest wall. The pectoralis minor is a thin, flat, and triangular muscle that is positioned beneath your pectoralis major. The "pecs" pull your upper arms across your body. Like most of the muscles in the torso, the chest is involved in throwing and pushing.

Upper Back. The latissimus dorsi is the long, broad muscle that comprises most of the upper back. As a matter of fact, the "lats" are the largest muscle in your upper body. Its primary function is to pull your upper arms backward and downward. The muscle is particularly important in assorted pulling and climbing movements as well as crawling. In addition, developing the latissimus dorsi is necessary to provide muscular balance between your upper back and chest.

Shoulders. The shoulders are made up of 11 muscles of which the deltoids are the most important. The "delts" are actually composed of three separate parts (or "heads"). The anterior deltoid is found on the front of the shoulder and is used when raising your upper arm forward; the middle deltoid is located on the side of the shoulder and is involved when lifting your upper arm sideways; the posterior deltoid resides on the back of the shoulder and is used to draw your upper arm backward. Several other deep muscles of the shoulder are sometimes referred to as the "internal rotators" (the subscapularis and teres major) and the "external rotators" (the infraspinatus and teres minor). In addition to performing rotation, these muscles are also largely responsible for maintaining the integrity of the shoulder joint and in preventing shoulder impingement. The shoulders play a vital role in throwing, pushing, carrying, crawling, and climbing.

UPPER ARMS

The two main muscles of your upper arms are the biceps and triceps.

Biceps. The prominent muscle on the front of your upper arm is technically known as the "biceps brachii." The biceps are involved in elbow flexion (bending your arms). As the name suggests, the biceps have two separate heads. The separation can sometimes be seen as a groove on a well-developed upper arm when the biceps are fully flexed. The biceps assist the torso muscles — especially the lats — in pulling, carrying, and climbing.

Triceps. The horseshoe-shaped muscle located on the back of your upper arm is formally known as the "triceps brachii." This muscle has three distinct heads: the long, lateral, and medial. The primary function of the triceps is elbow extension (straightening your arms). The triceps assist the torso muscles in throwing and pushing.

LOWER ARMS

Your forearms (or lower arms) contain muscles that are numerous and diverse.

Forearms. As stated earlier, each forearm consists of 19 different muscles. These muscles may be divided into two groups on the basis of their position and functions. The anterior group on the front of the forearm causes wrist flexion (bending your wrist) and pronation (turning your palm downward); the posterior group on the back of your forearm causes wrist extension (straightening your wrist) and supination (turning your palm upward). Since the muscles of the forearms affect the wrists, hands, and fingers, they are extremely important in pulling, carrying, climbing, and gripping.

ABDOMINALS

The three main muscles that comprise your abdominals are the rectus abdominis, obliques, and transversus abdominis.

Rectus Abdominis. This long, narrow muscle extends vertically across the front of the abdomen from the lower rim of the rib cage to the pelvis. Its main function is torso flexion (pulling your torso toward your lower body). The fibers of this muscle are interrupted along their course by three horizontal fibrous bands which gives rise to the term "washboard abs" when describing an especially well-developed abdomen. The rectus abdominis helps to control breathing when preparing to take a shot, and plays a major role in forced expiration during intense physical training.

Obliques. The external and internal obliques reside on both sides of the mid-section. The external oblique is a broad muscle whose fibers form a V across the front of the abdominal area, extending diagonally downward from the lower ribs to the pubic bone. The external oblique has two main functions: torso lateral flexion (bending your torso to the same side) and torso rotation (turning your torso to the opposite side). The internal oblique is located immediately under the external oblique on both sides of the abdomen. The fibers of the internal oblique form an inverted V along the front of the abdominal wall, extending diagonally upward from the pubic bone to the ribs. The internal oblique has two functions: torso lateral flexion (bending your torso to the same side) and torso rotation (turning your torso to the same side). In short, the obliques are used during movements in which your torso bends laterally or twists. These muscles are also active during expiration and inspiration, respectively.

Transversus Abdominis. The transversus abdominis is the innermost layer of your abdominal musculature. The fibers of this muscle run horizontally across the abdomen. The primary function of the transversus abdominis is to constrict the abdomen. This muscle is also involved in forced expiration and helps to control breathing.

LOWER BACK

Your lower back contains several muscles of which the erector spinae are the most important.

Erector Spinae. The main muscles in the lower back are the erector spinae (or "spinal erectors"). Their primary purpose is torso extension (straightening your torso from a bent-over position). However, the erector spinae also assist in torso lateral flexion (bending your torso to the side) and torso rotation (turning your torso). Low-back pain is one of the most common and costly medical problems today. It has been estimated that 80% of the world's population will experience low-back pain sometime in their lives with annual costs of more than $50 billion. Insufficient strength seems to be a factor related to low-back pain.

NECK

The major muscles of your neck include the neck flexors, neck extensors, and trapezius.

Neck Flexors. The muscles on the front of the neck can be collectively referred to as the "neck flexors." A major neck flexor is the sternocleidomastoideus. This muscle has two parts — one located on each side of the neck — that start behind the ears and run down to the sternum (breastbone) and clavicles (collarbones). When both sides of the sternocleidomastoideus contract at the same time, it causes neck flexion (bringing your head toward your chest); when one side acts singly, it results in neck lateral flexion (bending your neck to the side) or neck rotation (turning your head). Like the other muscles of the neck, the neck flexors help to maintain the head motionless in a tactical shooting position.

Neck Extensors. The back of the neck contains several muscles that can simply be grouped as the "neck extensors." These muscles are mainly used in neck extension (bringing your head backward).

Trapezius. The trapezius is a kite-shaped (or trapezoid-shaped) muscle that covers the uppermost region of the back and the posterior section of the neck. The primary functions of the "traps" are shoulder elevation (shrugging your shoulders as if to say, "I don't know"), scapulae adduction (pinching your shoulder blades together), and neck extension. The trapezius is often considered part of the shoulder musculature.

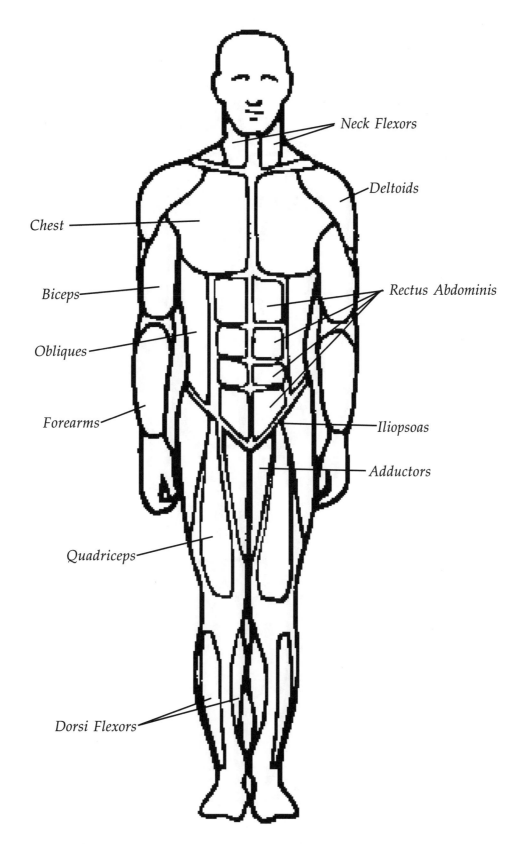

Figure 2.1: ANTERIOR VIEW OF THE MUSCLES OF THE BODY (artwork courtesy of Cybex International, Inc.)

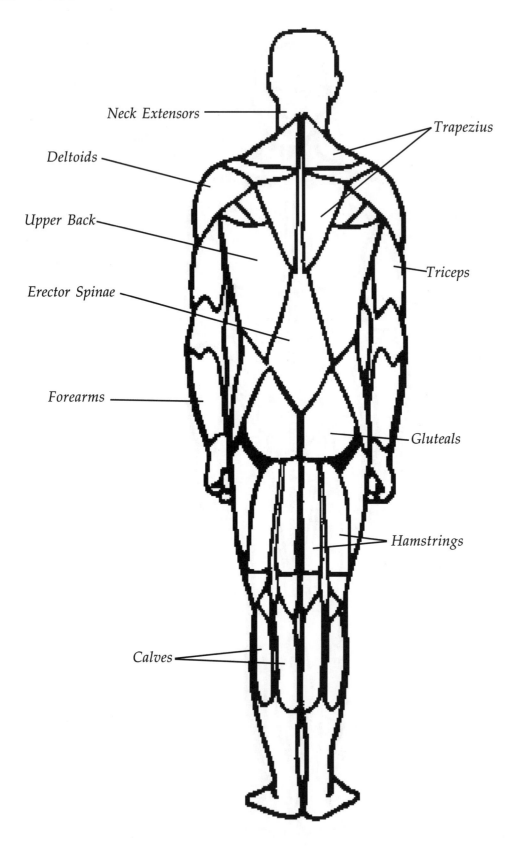

Figure 2.2: POSTERIOR VIEW OF THE MUSCLES OF THE BODY (artwork courtesy of Cybex International, Inc.)

Chapter 3
Flexibility Training

Flexibility can be defined as "the range of motion (ROM) throughout which your joints can move." The best way to maintain — or improve — the ROM of your joints is to perform specific flexibility movements to stretch the surrounding muscles. Flexibility training is undoubtedly the simplest and most effortless physical activity that can be performed — the exertion level is quite low and relaxation is an absolute requirement. Nevertheless, many individuals often overlook or underemphasize their flexibility training.

Increasing flexibility serves several purposes for SWAT officers. First, becoming more flexible may reduce susceptibility to injury. Secondly, improving flexibility allows the movement of your joints through a greater ROM which makes it easier to assume body positions that are difficult (if not impossible). Thirdly, being more flexible enables you to exert strength over a greater ROM. Finally, stretching your muscles may relieve and/or reduce the general muscular soreness that can result from doing unfamiliar activities or intense physical training (although this has yet to be corroborated by research).

FACTORS AFFECTING FLEXIBILITY

The most significant contributor to decreased flexibility seems to be a lack of physical activity. Obviously, you can avoid a loss of flexibility by simply participating in physical training on a regular basis. However, there are many other factors that also affect your ROM — some over which you have little or no control.

There is a distinct relationship between age and the degree of flexibility. The greatest increase in flexibility usually occurs up to and between the ages of 7 and 12. During early adolescence, flexibility tends to level off and thereafter begins to decline with increasing age. Therefore, one of the goals of flexibility training is to slow or perhaps reverse this decline.

To a degree, flexibility is also related to gender. Some men are more flexible than some women but, in general, women are more flexible than men. (Women retain this advantage throughout life.)

In addition, understanding that flexibility is affected by several genetic (or inherited) characteristics, such as the insertion points of your tendons as well as your percentage of body fat (especially that which is around your mid-section) is important. Your ROM also has genetic limitations that are structural which includes your bones, tendons, ligaments, and skin along with the extensibility of your muscles.

As you may already be painfully aware, previous injury to a muscle or connective tissue may also affect your ROM. Furthermore, immobilizing a joint during rehabilitation may cause the connective tissue to adapt to its shortest functional length thereby reducing the ROM of the joint.

Finally, body temperature is another factor that influences the flexibility of your joints. Muscles and connective tissue that are warmed up will be more flexible and extensible than muscles and connective tissue that are not.

ASSESSING FLEXIBILITY

Because ROM is affected by the aforementioned factors, assessing flexibility in a fair manner is difficult. In addition, some measurements of flexibility can be misleading. A perfect example of this is the traditional sit-and-reach test in which a person sits on the floor with straight legs and reaches forward, as far as possible. This test is often used to measure the flexibility of the lower back and hamstrings. A sit-and-reach test, however, does not take into consideration limb lengths. Everything else being equal, those with long arms and/or short legs have a distinct anatomical advantage in a sit-and-reach test. These individuals may appear to be quite flexible, but may actually be quite inflexible. Conversely, those with short arms and/or long legs have a distinct anatomical disadvantage in a sit-and-reach test. These individuals may appear to be quite inflexible, but may really be quite flexible. In the case of a sit-and-reach test, using a goniometer to measure the angle of flexion between the lumbar spine and the upper legs yields an appraisal of flexibility that is more impartial. (A goniometer is a protractor-like instrument with two movable arms that enable you to measure joint angles.)

Lastly, it should be noted that flexibility is joint-specific — a high degree of flexibility in one joint does not necessarily indicate high flexibility in other joints. Along these lines, it would not be uncommon for flexibility to vary from one side of your body to the other.

In conclusion, the purpose of assessing flexibility should not be to compare your performance to that of someone else. Flexibility assessments are much more meaningful when your present flexibility is compared to your past flexibility.

WARMING UP

The research regarding the need for a warm-up seems to be inconclusive. Some studies have shown that performances with a prior warm-up are better than those without a warm-up; other studies have shown that performances with a prior warm-up are no different than those without a warm-up. Nevertheless, a warm-up has both physiological and psychological importance.

For years, warming up was synonymous with stretching. However, warming up and stretching are two separate entities and must be treated as such. A warm-up is meant to prepare you for an upcoming session of physical training; on the other hand, stretching is meant to induce a more long-term change in your ROM.

A warm-up should precede flexibility training. Warm-up activities usually consist of low-

Regardless of athletic activity, a light jog as a warm-up is meant to prepare you for upcoming physical training while stretching is meant to increase your range of motion.

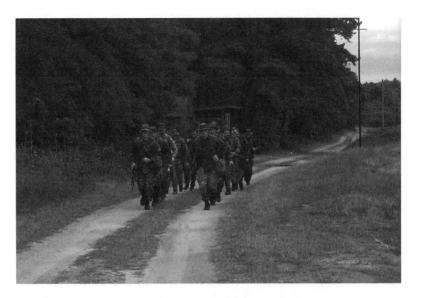

intensity movements such as light jogging or calisthenics. Regardless of the warm-up activity chosen, the idea is to systematically increase your body temperature and the blood flow to your muscles. Breaking a light sweat during the warm-up indicates that your body temperature has been raised sufficiently and that you are ready to begin stretching your muscles. As noted previously, muscles and connective tissue that are warmed up have increased flexibility and extensibility. (When the environmental temperature is high, it is likely that your body temperature is already elevated enough to start stretching your muscles.)

Biological tissue is most extensible at the end of physical training when the body temperature is elevated. Because of this, some authorities recommend that stretching should be performed *after* completing physical training. Doing so may also reduce the general muscular soreness that sometimes follows intense physical training.

By the way, there is no need to warm-up or stretch prior to strength training — provided that you perform a relatively high number of repetitions and lift the weight in a deliberate, controlled manner. But warming up prior to a physical activity that involves rapid muscular contractions — such as sprinting — is highly advisable to reduce the risk of injury.

SEVEN STRETCHING STRATEGIES

Though ROM may be limited by the factors that were mentioned previously, it can be improved through flexibility training. Like all other forms of physical training, flexibility training has certain guidelines that must be followed in order to make the stretches safe and effective. Adopting these guidelines permits you to maintain or improve your current ROM. Additionally, you will be less likely to injure yourself and perform closer to your physical potential.

Seven stretching strategies are as follows:

1. STRETCH under control without bouncing, bobbing, or jerking movements. Bouncing during the stretch actually makes the movement more painful, and increases your risk of muscular soreness and tissue damage.

2. INHALE and EXHALE normally during the stretch without holding your breath. When you hold your breath, it elevates your blood pressure which disrupts your balance and breathing mechanisms.

3. STRETCH comfortably in a pain-free manner. Since pain is an indication that you are stretching at or near your structural limits, you should only stretch to a point of mild discomfort.

4. RELAX during the stretch. Relaxing mentally and physically allows you to stretch your muscles throughout a greater ROM.

5. HOLD the stretched position for about 30 - 60 seconds. Gradually stretching your muscles to a point of mild discomfort, holding that position, and then gradually returning them to their pre-stretched state enables you to stretch farther with little risk of pain or injury.

6. ATTEMPT to stretch slightly farther than the last time. Progressively increasing your ROM — and the time that you hold each stretch — improves your flexibility.

7. PERFORM flexibility movements on a regular basis. You should stretch at least once a day, especially before physical training, fitness testing, tactical deployments, or any other activity that may involve explosive, ballistic movements.

FLEXIBILITY MOVEMENTS

Although the human body has roughly 200 joints, performing a flexibility movement (or a "stretch") for each one is not necessary. The joints range from those that are relatively immovable (such as the sutures of your skull) to those that are freely movable (such as your hips and your elbows). You can stretch the muscles of major joints in a comprehensive manner by performing the 14 flexibility movements that are described on the following pages. Included in the discussions of each movement are the muscle(s) stretched, starting position, performance description, and training tips for making the movement safer and more effective. (If you need help to identify the muscles, you can refer to the anatomy charts that are shown in Chapter 2.) The flexibility movements that are described in this chapter are as follows: neck forward, neck backward, lateral neck, scratch back, handcuff, standing calf, tibia stretch, sit-and-reach, V-sit, lateral reach, butterfly, spinal twist, quad stretch, and knee pull. There are many variations of these stretches that involve the same muscle groups. Because of this, flexibility training can be individualized to meet your personal preferences.

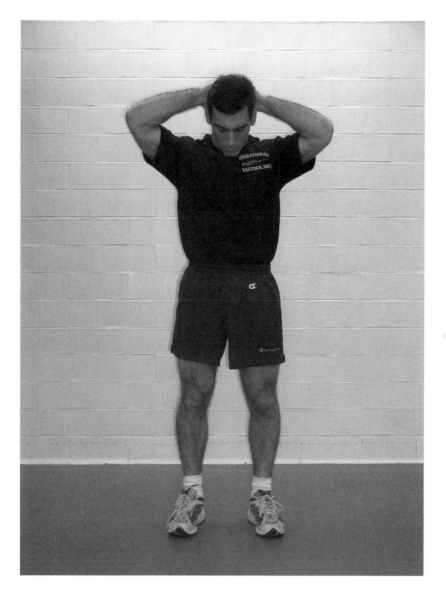

NECK FORWARD

Muscles Stretched: neck extensors and trapezius

Starting Position: While standing, interlock your fingers behind your head.

Performance Description: Slowly pull your chin to your chest.

Training Tips:

- Be especially careful when doing this movement since your cervical area is involved.
- This movement may also be performed sitting.

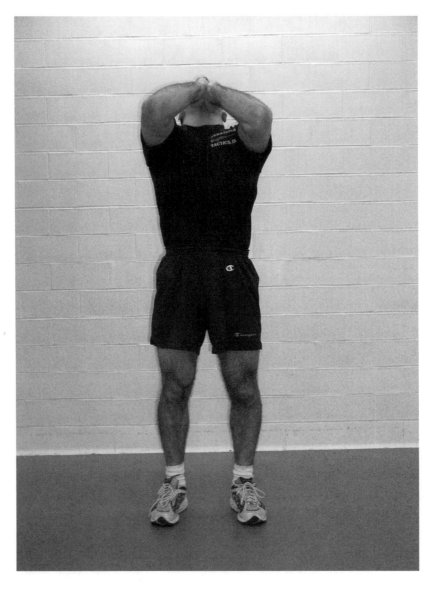

NECK BACKWARD

Muscle Stretched: sternocleidomastoideus (both sides)

Starting Position: While standing, place your hands underneath your chin.

Performance Description: Slowly push your head backward.

Training Tips:

- Be especially careful when doing this movement since your cervical area is involved.
- This movement may also be performed sitting.

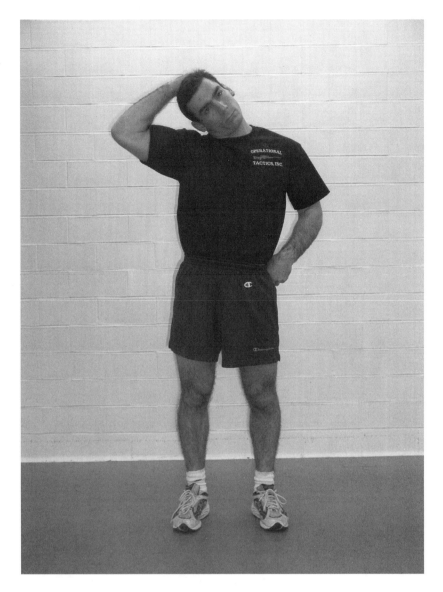

LATERAL NECK

Muscle Stretched: sternocleidomastoideus (one side)

Starting Position: While standing, place your right hand on the left side of your head.

Performance Description: Slowly pull your head to your right shoulder. Repeat the stretch for the other side of your neck.

Training Tips:

- Be especially careful when doing this movement since your cervical area is involved.
- This movement may also be performed sitting.

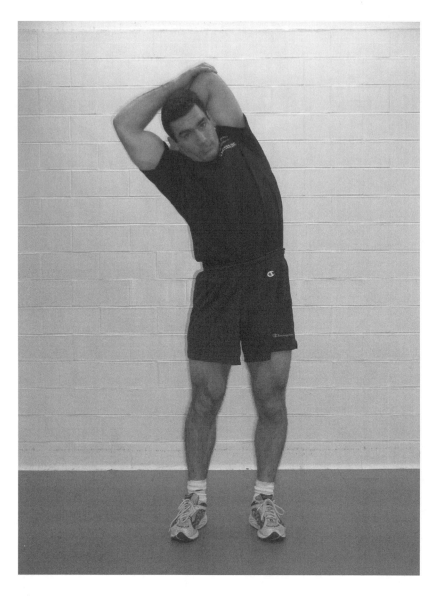

SCRATCH BACK

Muscles Stretched: upper back ("lats"), triceps, and obliques

Starting Position: While standing, place your left hand on the upper part of your back (behind your head) and grab your left elbow with your right hand.

Performance Description: Slowly pull your upper torso to the right. Repeat the stretch for the other side of your body.

Training Tips:

- For this movement to be most effective, your hips should not move and your feet should remain flat on the ground.

- You should try to gradually reach farther down your back during the stretch.

- This movement may also be performed sitting.

- This movement may be contraindicated if you have shoulder-impingement syndrome.

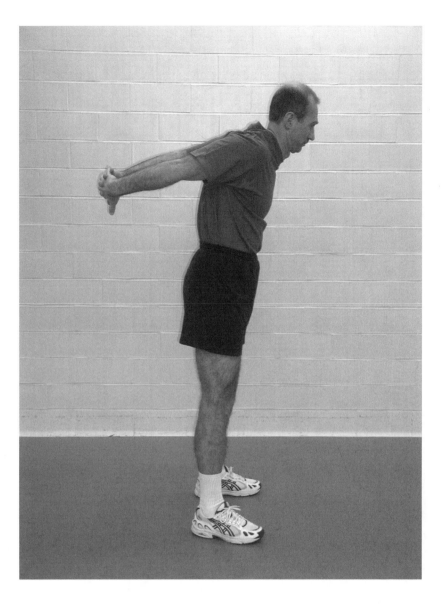

HANDCUFF

Muscles Stretched: chest, anterior deltoid, and biceps

Starting Position: While standing, place your hands behind your back and interlock your fingers.

Performance Description: Slowly lift your hands up as high as possible.

Training Tips:

- A partner may assist you in obtaining a greater stretch by carefully lifting up your hands as you do the stretch.

- This movement may also be performed sitting.

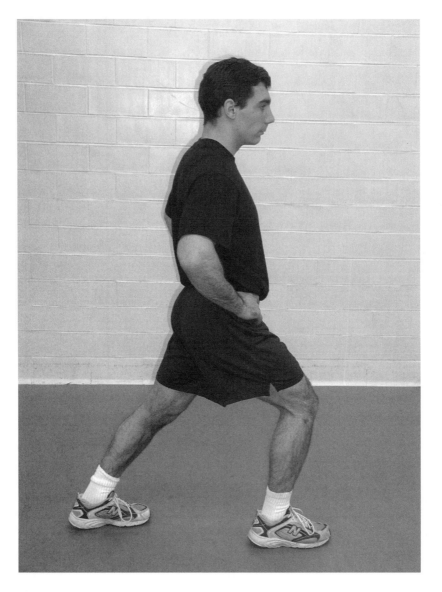

STANDING CALF

Muscles Stretched: calves and iliopsoas

Starting Position: While standing, step forward with your right foot.

Performance Description: Bend your right leg at the knee but keep your left leg straight and your left foot flat on the ground. Repeat the stretch for your other leg.

Training Tips:

- For this movement to be most effective, the heel of your back foot should remain flat on the ground and both of your feet should be pointed forward.

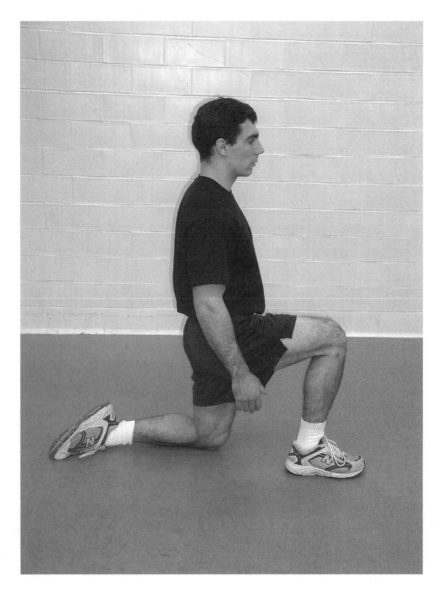

TIBIA STRETCH

Muscles Stretched: dorsi flexors

Starting Position: Kneel down on your left knee so that your upper leg is perpendicular to the ground. Position your right leg so that your upper leg is parallel to the ground, your lower leg is perpendicular to the ground, and your foot is flat on the ground.

Performance Description: Press your left lower leg and the top part of your left foot flat on the ground. Repeat the stretch for your other leg.

Training Tips:

* For this movement to be most effective, the top part of the foot being stretched should be flat on the ground.

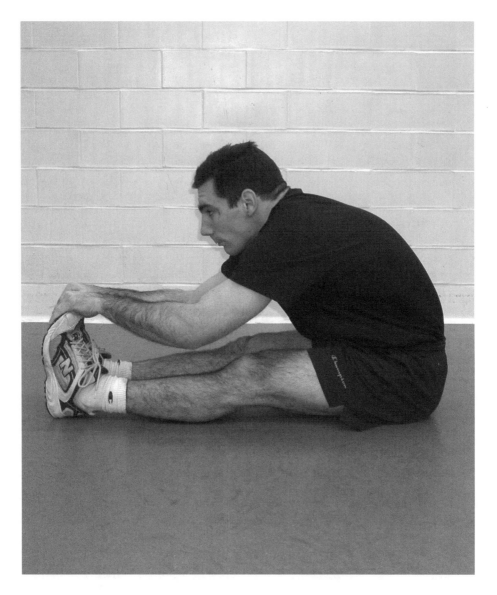

SIT-AND-REACH

Muscles Stretched: gluteus maximus (buttocks), hamstrings, calves, upper back ("lats"), and lower back

Starting Position: While sitting, straighten your legs, put them together and point your toes upward.

Performance Description: Slowly reach forward as far as possible without bending your legs.

Training Tips:

- For this movement to be most effective, your legs should remain straight and your toes should be pointed upward. You can progressively stretch farther by reaching for your ankles, your toes, and finally your insteps.

- A partner may assist you in obtaining a greater stretch by carefully pushing on your upper back as you do the stretch.

- This movement may also be performed standing (with your legs straight and your arms hanging straight down).

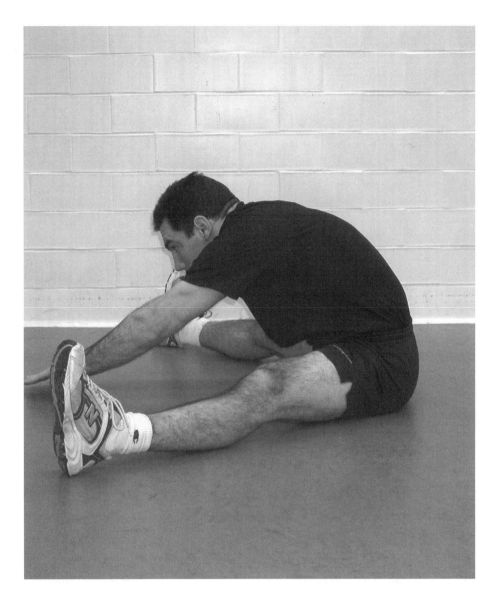

V-SIT

Muscles Stretched: gluteus maximus (buttocks), hip adductors (inner thigh), hamstrings, calves, upper back ("lats"), and lower back

Starting Position: While sitting, straighten your legs, spread them apart as far as possible and point your toes upward.

Performance Description: Slowly reach forward as far as possible without bending your legs.

Training Tips:

- For this movement to be most effective, your legs should remain straight and your toes should be pointed upward. You can progressively stretch farther by "walking" your fingers forward.

- A partner may assist you in obtaining a greater stretch by carefully pushing on your upper back as you do the stretch.

- This movement may also be performed standing (with your legs spread apart and your arms hanging straight down).

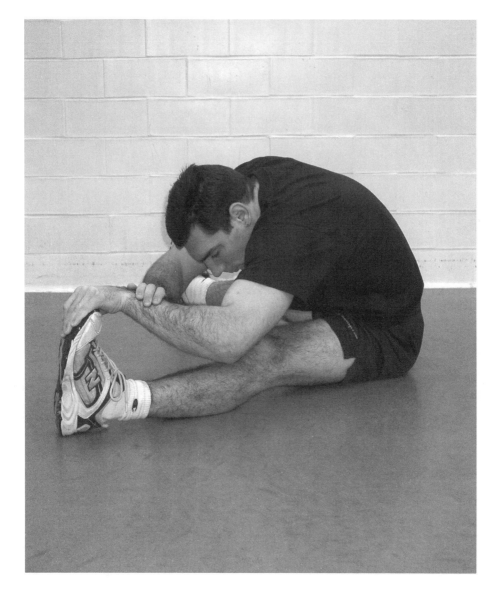

LATERAL REACH

Muscles Stretched: gluteus maximus (buttocks), hip adductors (inner thigh), hamstrings, calves, upper back ("lats"), obliques, and lower back

Starting Position: While sitting, straighten your legs, spread them apart as far as possible and point your toes upward.

Performance Description: Slowly reach down your left leg as far as possible without bending your legs. Repeat the stretch for the other side of your body.

Training Tips:

• For this movement to be most effective, your legs should remain straight and your toes should be pointed upward. You can progressively stretch farther by "walking" your fingers forward.

• A partner may assist you in obtaining a greater stretch by carefully pushing on your upper back as you do the stretch.

• This movement may also be performed standing (with your legs spread apart and your arms reaching down your leg).

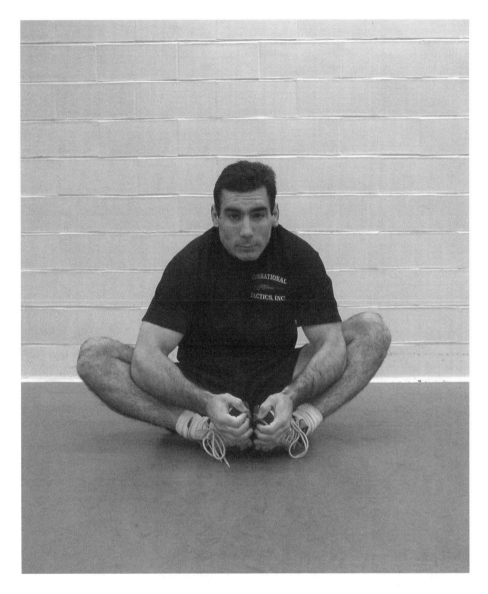

BUTTERFLY

Muscles Stretched: hip adductors (inner thigh) and lower back

Starting Position: While sitting, place the soles of your feet together, draw your heels as close to your body as possible, and place your elbows on the insides of your knees.

Performance Description: Bend your torso forward while slowly pushing down with your elbows against your knees.

Training Tips:

- A partner may assist you in obtaining a greater stretch by carefully pushing on the insides of your knees as you do the stretch.

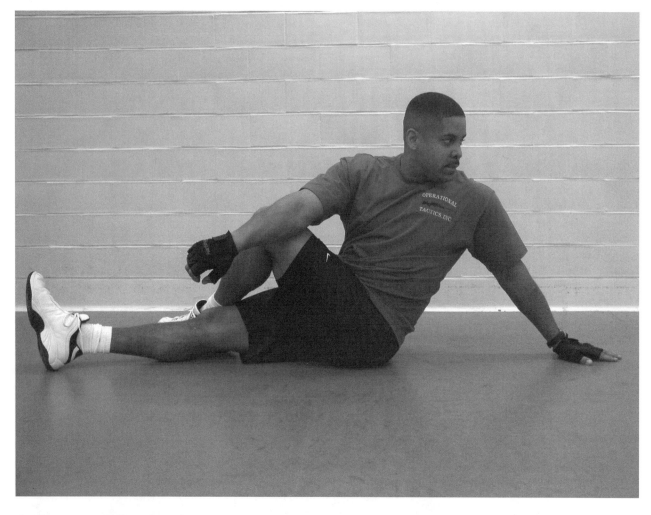

SPINAL TWIST

Muscles Stretched: hip abductors (gluteus medius), obliques, and lower back

Starting Position: While sitting, keep your right leg straight, place your left foot on the outside of your right knee, and place your right elbow against the outside of your left knee.

Performance Description: Look to your left as far as possible while slowly pushing with your right elbow against the outside of your left knee. Repeat the stretch for the other side of your body.

Training Tips:

• This movement may also be performed lying supine (by keeping your shoulders flat on the ground and crossing one leg over your body).

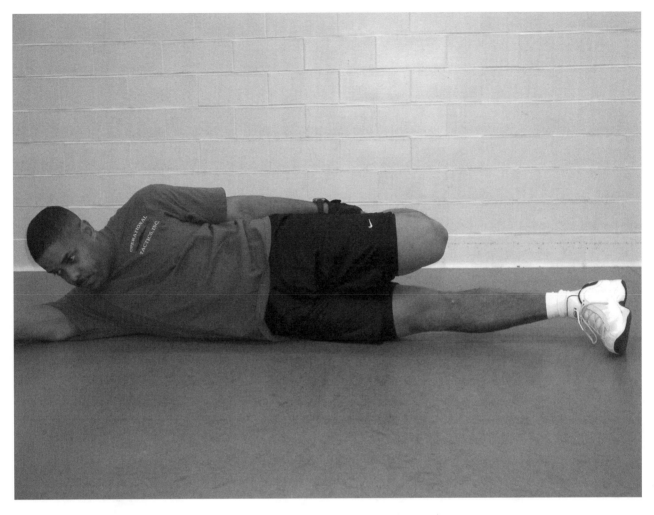

QUAD STRETCH

Muscles Stretched: quadriceps, iliopsoas, and abdominals

Starting Position: Lie on your right side and grab your left instep with your left hand.

Performance Description: Pull your left heel toward your buttocks. Repeat the stretch for the other side of your body.

Training Tips:

* This movement may also be performed lying prone.

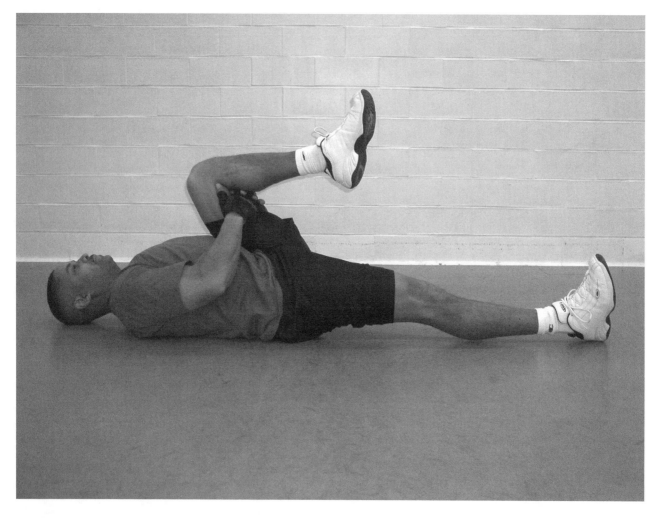

KNEE PULL

Muscles Stretched: gluteus maximus (buttocks), hamstrings, and lower back

Starting Position: While lying supine on the ground, straighten your right leg, point your toes upward and grasp your left leg behind your knee.

Performance Description: Pull your left leg toward your chest. Repeat the stretch for the other side of your body.

Training Tips:

• Using your arms to pull your leg toward your chest will permit a better stretch.

Chapter 4
Exercise Physiology

Insight into how the human body produces and utilizes energy during physical training is very important. Familiarity with various energy (or metabolic) systems will also help understand how the physiological processes affect physical performance.

ADENOSINE TRIPHOSPHATE

The energy liberated during the breakdown of food is used to make a chemical compound called "adenosine triphosphate" (ATP). This compound is stored in most living cells — particularly muscle cells — and has an extremely high-energy yield. The structure of ATP consists of an adenosine component that is bonded to three chemically important phosphate groups. The energy from ATP is not necessarily in its chemical make-up, but in the so-called high-energy phosphate bonds that hold the compound together. When one of the phosphate bonds is broken — meaning that it is removed from the rest of the molecule — energy is released and adenosine diphosphate (ADP) plus inorganic phosphate are formed. The energy liberated during the breakdown of ATP is the primary — and immediate — source of energy used to perform muscular work.

ENERGY SYSTEMS

In order to perform physically for prolonged periods of time, a constant supply of ATP must be made available to your muscle cells. Unfortunately, they can only store a limited amount of ATP. As such, your muscle cells must be capable of resynthesizing (or rebuilding) ATP from ADP and inorganic phosphate.

A typical ATP molecule may exist for only a few seconds before its bonds are broken and energy is released. The ADP formed by this chemical event is rapidly remade into ATP. Interestingly, energy is also required to remake ATP. In fact, all of your energy systems have one common and primary purpose: to reconstruct ATP in order to supply energy so that your muscles can perform physical activity.

The process by which ATP is reassembled involves the interaction of three different series of chemical reactions. Two of these can operate in the absence of oxygen and are termed "anaerobic"; the other series of reactions can only operate in the presence of oxygen and is labeled "aerobic." The two anaerobic pathways are the ATP-PC System and Anaerobic Glycolysis; the aerobic pathway is the Aerobic System.

The ATP-PC System

In the ATP-PC (or Phosphagen) System, the energy used to rebuild ATP comes from the breakdown of a chemical compound known as "phosphocreatine" (PC). Like ATP, PC is stored in your muscle cells and has a rather high-energy yield. Since ATP and PC both contain phosphate groups, they are collectively referred to as "phosphagens." Similar to ATP, PC releases a large amount of energy when its phosphate group is removed. (The end-products of this breakdown are creatine and inorganic phosphate.) The energy yielded by this process is immediately available and is used to reconstruct ATP. In fact, as quickly as ATP is broken down during muscular efforts, it is continuously remanufactured by the energy released from the breakdown of PC. Ironically, PC can only be rebuilt from the energy released by the breakdown of ATP.

The phosphagen stores in your working muscles — that is, your ATP and PC pools — would probably be spent after an all-out exertion lasting about a handful of seconds. If you are in reasonably good condition, this equates to sprinting roughly 40 yards or running up several flights of stairs at breakneck speed. So, the total amount of ATP energy available from this metabolic system is very limited. Obviously, the usefulness of your stored phosphagens is in their rapid availability rather than in their total quantity. Fast, powerful movements — such as sprinting and jumping — could not be performed without this energy system. It is no surprise, then, that your ATP-PC System is the predominant energy pathway for physical efforts of very high intensity and brief duration — less than about 30 seconds.

Anaerobic Glycolysis

In your body, carbohydrates are converted into glucose (or "blood sugar") which can either be instantly utilized in that form or stored as glycogen in the liver and muscles for later use. The term "glycolysis" means "to break down glycogen" and, as noted earlier, "anaerobic" basically means "in the absence of oxygen." Therefore, "Anaerobic Glycolysis" literally means "to break down glycogen in the absence of oxygen." When glycogen is broken down, energy is released and is used to reassemble ATP. A complete breakdown of glycogen, however, requires oxygen. Since the presence of oxygen is not necessary during Anaerobic Glycolysis, the breakdown of glycogen is only partial and pyruvic acid is formed as a by-product. Pyruvic acid is subsequently converted into a substance called "lactic acid" (or "lactate") — which is why Anaerobic Glycolysis is often referred to as the "Lactic Acid System."

When a log is burned, ash is always left as a waste product. In a way, lactic acid is the glycolytic ash of this anaerobic pathway. The point at which lactic acid first begins to appear in your blood is known as your "anaerobic threshold." When lactic acid enters your blood at a greater rate than it leaves, there is a rise in the concentration of lactic acid in your blood. High concentrations of lactic acid can irritate your nerve endings and cause pain. The accumulation of lactate is also believed to cause excessive breathing, feelings of fatigue, and heaviness in the muscles. Because it is a fatiguing by-product, lactic acid essentially acts as a performance inhibitor during Anaerobic Glycolysis. In fact, your muscles and blood can only

For the most part, your Aerobic System becomes the principal energy pathway after roughly three minutes of continuous exertion.

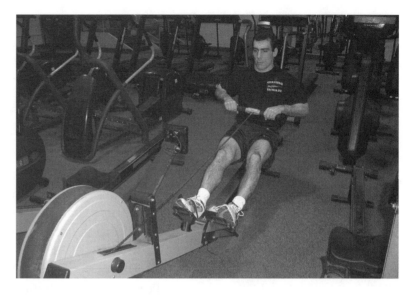

tolerate about *2.0 - 2.5 ounces* of lactic acid before fatigue occurs. (Some lactic acid is formed under resting conditions, but it does not accumulate because the rate of production equals the rate of removal.)

Anaerobic Glycolysis — with a helping hand from your ATP-PC System — is responsible for supplying ATP for all maximal efforts that last between approximately 30 - 90 seconds. If you are in reasonably good condition, this window of time correlates to sprinting a distance of about 220 - 440 yards. Therefore, the first minute or so of physical training depends upon your ability to replenish ATP without the use of oxygen. The resynthesis of ATP is quite rapid, but — in the absence of oxygen — is somewhat limited.

The Aerobic System

There is an unlimited supply of oxygen available to meet your physiological needs. Think about it: Oxygen is literally everywhere around you. But the amount of energy that you can produce with oxygen is determined by the efficiency of your Aerobic System.

During prolonged physical efforts, your Aerobic System is the last process in your chemical chain-of-command for energy production. In the Aerobic System, glycogen is once again broken down to release energy that is used to rebuild ATP — which is why this system is sometimes known as "Aerobic Glycolysis." Because oxygen is used in this process, the breakdown of glycogen is complete. Relative to your anaerobic pathways, your Aerobic System can operate for a longer duration because no fatiguing by-products — such as lactic acid — are produced in the presence of oxygen. Rather than form lactic acid from pyruvic acid, this particular system converts pyruvic acid into two end-products: carbon dioxide and water. However, carbon dioxide is continually removed by the blood and transported to the lungs where it is exhaled; water is either used in the cell or excreted in the urine. So, glycolytic reactions occur in both the anaerobic and aerobic domains — the difference is that lactic acid is not formed when sufficient oxygen is available. Another feature of your Aerobic System is that it can also break down both carbohydrates and fat to liberate energy for the reconstruction of ATP while your anaerobic pathways can only use carbohydrates. (Energy can also be provided by a third macronutrient: protein. Nonetheless, it is not normally used as a source of energy.)

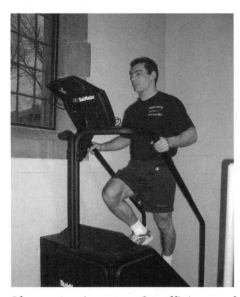

If you can improve the efficiency of your energy systems through physical training, then you can also improve your performance potential.

The process of rebuilding ATP aerobically occurs in specialized areas of your muscle cells called "mitochondria." These areas produce such a large amount of energy that the mitochondria are often referred to as the "powerhouse" of the cell. Muscle cells are usually very rich in mitochondria. In particular, an abundance of mitochondria is found in cardiac muscle (your heart) and slow-twitch muscle fibers.

Your Aerobic System becomes the primary energy pathway once your anaerobic systems are unable to keep up with the metabolic demands of an activity and lactic acid begins to accumulate. Physical efforts that are between about 1.5 - 3.0 minutes in duration are the shared responsibility of Anaerobic Glycolysis and the Aerobic System. For the most part, your Aerobic System becomes the principal energy pathway after roughly three minutes of continuous exertion which would correlate to running a distance that is beyond about one-half mile. (Research suggests that at least 10 - 15 minutes of continuous activity is usually needed for you to obtain aerobic benefits. If you are in reasonably good condition, this time frame equates to a distance of roughly 1.5 miles.) The longer the duration of an activity, the greater the importance of your Aerobic System. Interestingly, your Aerobic System is also the preferred energy pathway under resting conditions.

A major advantage of your Aerobic System is that it produces relatively large amounts of energy. But due to the transport and delivery of oxygen, the Aerobic System is a time-consuming process. Therefore, this system cannot produce energy rapidly enough to meet the demands of short-term, high-intensity movements such as pulling/knocking down a suspect or running 10 yards with a one-person ram.

THE ENERGY CONTINUUM

The need for a particular energy system is determined by the time and intensity requirements of a specific activity. At one end of the so-called energy continuum is your ATP-PC System which is the dominant energy pathway for short-term, high-intensity efforts; at the other end of the scale is your Aerobic System which is the dominant energy pathway for long-term, low-intensity efforts. In between these two extremes of the continuum, the vast majority of energy is supplied by Anaerobic Glycolysis with some assistance from your ATP-PC System. Also in the middle of the continuum are many tasks and activities which require a mixture of both your anaerobic and aerobic pathways such as running 440 - 880 yards, rowing 400 - 800 yards, swimming 100 - 200 yards, wrestling 2- or 3-minute periods, and boxing 3-minute rounds.

Your body does not exclusively choose one metabolic pathway over another — your exercising muscles simply use whatever energy source is readily available to meet the existing physiological demands. Generally, your body selects the most efficient metabolic pathway to maximize the resynthesis of ATP and to minimize the accumulation of lactic acid.

Your level of blood lactate is an excellent indicator of which energy system is mainly relied upon during your effort. A high level of blood lactate indicates that Anaerobic Glycolysis was your primary energy system; conversely, a low level of blood lactate means that your Aerobic System was your primary energy system.

Although one of your metabolic pathways may serve as the principal source of energy for a given activity, all three pathways contribute to the supply of ATP that is required to perform most activities. Stated otherwise, both anaerobic and aerobic pathways contribute some ATP during physical training with one system generally contributing more. For example, negotiating an obstacle course is primarily anaerobic because it consists largely of a series of brief, all-out efforts such as sprinting short distances, climbing a rope or cargo net, crawling under wires, going across a horizontal ladder (or "monkey bars"), and so on. But the obstacle course also has an aerobic component since the anaerobic efforts are required over an extended period of time. This would also apply to completing a fitness course that involves sprinting short distances and performing sets of push-ups, pull-ups, sit-ups, and other callisthenic-type movements. In both of these examples, energy is needed from the anaerobic pathways as well as the aerobic pathway. In fact, a blend of all energy systems is the most likely scenario for the majority of tasks and activities that you might perform.

Remember that as the time of an activity increases, the continuum shifts away from anaerobic work toward aerobic work. Note that your energy systems operate in phases on a progressive scale. Moreover, your body does not shift abruptly from one source of energy to another — the transition from one energy pathway to another is very subtle. In a sense, all three metabolic processes overlap each other. So if you can improve the efficiency of your energy systems through physical training, then you can also improve your performance potential.

To summarize: The predominant energy pathway used during activities that require 30 seconds or less is your ATP-PC System. Activities requiring between 30 - 90 seconds use a blend of your ATP-PC System and Anaerobic Glycolysis. For activities that are between 1.5 - 3.0 minutes in duration, energy is provided by the collective efforts of Anaerobic Glycolysis and your Aerobic System. And after three minutes of continuous activity, your Aerobic System predominates.

THE "ULTIMATE PUMP"

The most important muscle in your body is the heart — a large, hollow, cone-shaped organ that is located just behind the sternum (or breastbone). Your heart is the primary driving force behind your three energy systems. The human heart is about 5.0 inches long, 3.5 inches wide and 2.5 inches thick — roughly the size of a man's clenched fist. The average adult male heart weighs about 10 ounces while its female counterpart weighs about 8 ounces.

Your heart is the ultimate endurance muscle or "pump" — it contracts about 100,000 times each day, pausing only briefly after a contraction to fill with more blood for its next contraction. This muscular pump is comprised of left and right halves. Each half of your heart consists of two chambers: an atrium and a ventricle. The atria are the recovery chambers of your heart and the ventricles are the pumping chambers.

Your blood has two routes or circuits: the Systemic Circuit and the Pulmonary Circuit. In the Systemic Circuit, the powerful left ventricle of your heart pumps oxygen-enriched blood to your body tissues (such as your skeletal muscles). The blood collects carbon dioxide and other metabolic wastes and returns to the right atrium of your heart. In the Pulmonary Circuit, the right ventricle of your heart sends oxygen-depleted blood that is laden with carbon dioxide to your lungs. The blood drops off carbon dioxide, picks up oxygenated blood and returns to the left atrium of your heart.

Normally, the right half of your heart pumps the same amount of blood as the left half of your heart. However, the left half of your heart is much stronger and better developed than the right half. The reason for this is because the left half of your heart must pump blood throughout your entire body (the Systemic Circuit) while the right half only has to pump blood to your lungs (the Pulmonary Circuit).

Blood Pressure

When your heart forces blood through the blood vessels, the fluid is under pressure. Your blood pressure is a measure of the force exerted by your blood against the arterial walls. Blood pressure actually has two measures: systolic and diastolic. Your systolic blood pressure is the maximum pressure in your arteries during ventricular contraction; your diastolic blood pressure is the maximum pressure during ventricular relaxation — that is, when your heart relaxes between beats as the atria and ventricles fill with blood.

Blood pressure is measured in millimeters of mercury (mmHg). An example of a blood-pressure reading would be 124/82 in which the upper number (124) is the systolic pressure and the lower number (82) is the diastolic pressure. An "optimal" resting blood pressure is a systolic reading of less than 120 *and* a diastolic reading of less than 80; a "normal" resting blood pressure is a systolic reading of 120 – 129 *and* a diastolic reading of 80 – 84. From a clinical standpoint, high blood pressure (or hypertension) is when the resting blood pressure exceeds either a systolic reading of 140 *or* a diastolic reading of 90. Individuals who have chronic high blood pressure should seek medical consultation. The same holds true for those who have chronic low blood pressure (or hypotension).

During physical activity, your systolic pressure changes more than your diastolic. Your systolic pressure increases in proportion to your effort and can rise to 200 mmHg or more. During intense training, the diastolic pressure of healthy individuals remains the same or drops slightly. (During physical activity, an increase in diastolic pressure is considered abnormal and cause for alarm.) Maximum blood pressure usually occurs at maximum heart rate.

Heart Rate

As the blood surges out of the ventricles, it pounds the arterial wall. This impact is transmitted along the length of the artery and can be felt as a throb or a "pulse" at those points where an artery is just under your skin. The beat of your pulse is synchronous with the beat of your heart. To a degree, the rate of the heartbeat is dependent upon the size of the organism. A good rule of thumb is the smaller the size of the organism, the faster the beat of the heart. A normal resting heart rate for humans is about 60 - 80 beats per minute (bpm). Women's hearts beat about 6 - 8 times per minute faster than those of men. Children's hearts beat even more rapidly — as high as 130 bpm at birth. Animals larger than humans have slower heart rates — an elephant has one of only 20 bpm. In contrast, a shrew's heart beats 1,000 times per minute.

Active individuals usually have lower resting heart rates than inactive individuals. As a matter of fact, some highly fit people have resting heart rates of less than 40 bpm. A lower resting heart rate would be especially important if the heart is limited to a certain number of beats over the course of a lifetime. For instance, suppose that the human heart can only beat about 2.5 billion times before it simply wears out from the labors of continual usage. In this scenario, a person with an average resting heart rate of 70 bpm could expect to live a little less than 68 years; on the other hand, someone with an average resting heart rate of 60 bpm could expect to live a little more than 79 years. If there is a limit to the number of times that a heart can beat in a lifetime, a decrease in the resting heart rate of just 10 bpm would translate into more than 11 additional years of life. While this notion has yet to be proven scientifically, it is still quite intriguing. And it does generate an added importance of having a lower resting heart rate.

The Training Effect

Like other muscle tissue, physical training can cause your heart to increase in size or "hypertrophy." (Its inverse — a decrease in muscular size — is known as "atrophy.") Specifically, its ventricular wall becomes thicker from anaerobic training (that is, activities of high intensity and short duration such as strength training) and its ventricular cavity becomes larger from aerobic training (that is, activities of low intensity and long duration such as long-distance running). This adaptation permits your heart to accept more blood and to expel it more powerfully. As your heart becomes a better-conditioned muscle, its ability to circulate blood also improves.

"Stroke volume" refers to the amount of blood pumped by your heart per beat. If you are a male, each beat of your heart may pump anywhere from 0.07 - 0.12 liters of blood while you are at rest. During intense activity, stroke volume may increase to 0.2 liters of blood per beat or more. Generally speaking, women have lower values for stroke volume than men under all conditions (which is probably due to the fact that the size of the female heart is, on average, smaller than that of her male counterpart). Finally, someone with a high level of fitness has a greater stroke volume than someone with a low level of fitness.

"Cardiac output" refers to the amount of blood pumped by your heart per minute. It is the product of your stroke volume and your heart rate. At rest, the volume of blood pumped by your heart is about 5.0 liters per minute (L/min). During intense activity, the amount of blood that is pumped may increase to more than 25.0 L/min. When exercising with the same level of intensity, women tend to have a slightly higher cardiac output than men.

During physical training, your stroke volume increases progressively up to a certain point and then it levels off. In other words, there is a physiological limit to the amount of blood that your heart can pump per beat. Once your stroke volume is maximal, further increases in your cardiac output are possible only through increases in your heart rate. As your level of fitness improves, the point at which your stroke volume reaches a steady-state value becomes higher.

As mentioned previously, your resting heart rate will be lower as a direct result of physical training — especially from aerobic training. A slower heart rate coupled with a larger stroke volume — that is, the ejection of a larger volume of blood — indicates an efficient circulatory system. This is true because your heart will not beat as often for a given cardiac output. If your heart pumps more blood per beat and needs less beats to function, you have increased the efficiency of your muscular pump. As an example, if your resting heart rate is 71 bpm and your heart ejects 0.07 liters of blood per beat then your resting cardiac output is about 5.0 L/min [71 bpm x 0.07 liters per beat = 4.97 L/min]. As a result of improved fitness, suppose that you have increased your stroke volume to 0.08 liters of blood per beat. In this case, you would need a resting heart rate of only 62 bpm in order to produce the same resting cardiac output of roughly 5.0 L/min [62 bpm x 0.08 liters per beat = 4.96 L/min]. So for the same resting cardiac output, your heart would pump a greater volume of blood using less beats — a characteristic of an efficient circulatory system.

THE RESPIRATORY PROCESS

Respiration is a combination of inspiration and expiration. Inspiration (or inhalation) is an active process in which your lungs inflate and air enters your body. The primary muscle of respiration is the diaphragm — a large, dome-shaped sheet of muscle located in the upper abdominal cavity. Expiration (or exhalation) is a passive process in which your lungs deflate and air is released into the environment. During intense activity, however, expiration is an active process that is facilitated by the abdominal muscles and the internal intercostal muscles (which reside between your ribs along with your external intercostal muscles).

The respiratory process is accomplished without continuous conscious effort. Actually, respiration is a rhythmic action: Inflation of your lungs during inspiration causes expiration; deflation of your lungs during expiration causes inspiration.

At rest, a healthy adult's rate of respiration is about 10 - 12 breaths per minute. During intense activity, your rate of respiration may increase to 40 - 50 breaths per minute. The volume of air entering or leaving your lungs during a single breath is known as your "tidal volume." Under resting conditions, your tidal volume is around 0.5 liters of oxygen per breath and may increase to about 3.0 liters of oxygen per breath during intense activity.

Your respiratory system has two major functions: to exchange gases (that is, to deliver oxygen and to eliminate carbon dioxide) and to maintain your acid-base balance.

The Gas Exchange

Your diaphragm — with assistance from your external intercostal muscles in conjunction with the natural changes of pressures within your body — produces an open trade of oxygen and carbon dioxide. The venous blood sent to your lungs by the right ventricle is low in oxygen and high in carbon dioxide. In the lungs, your blood unloads carbon dioxide and loads oxygen. The blood returns to the left atrium as arterial blood that is high in oxygen and low in carbon dioxide.

A second exchange of gases occurs between your blood and tissues. In this case, your thickly muscled left ventricle pumps arterial blood to your biological tissues. Once again, the blood delivers oxygen and removes carbon dioxide. Essentially, this gas exchange converts arterial blood into venous blood. The venous blood returns to your right atrium where the entire process of gas exchange and transport is repeated over and over again.

Acid-Base Balance

The respiratory process also regulates your acid-base balance — that is, the pH of your body. Recall that lactic acid is a direct end-product of anaerobic training and is the prime suspect in muscular fatigue. Without a system to remove (or "buffer") this metabolite, your body fluids would become more acidic and unsettle your delicate acid-base balance.

Your pH is a direct measure of acidity or alkalinity. The lower the pH, the greater the acidity — a pH that is less than 7.0 is considered to be acidic while a pH that is greater than 7.0 is considered to be alkaline. (A pH of 7.0 is neutral.) During intense activity, the increased production of carbon dioxide and lactic acid may briefly lower your muscle pH from a normal resting value of about 7.0 to a level of 6.4. (In human muscle, pH values as low as 6.25 have been recorded.) The lactate diffuses from your muscles into neighboring tissues and ultimately overflows into your blood. This causes your blood pH to temporarily drop from a normal resting level of about 7.4 to as low as 6.8. An environment that is too acidic may inhibit several chemical reactions that are needed for energy production or may result in pain, distress, and muscular fatigue. So, your acid-base system is essentially an alarm mechanism that alerts you to reduce your level of effort because your acid levels have become too high.

Unfortunately, blood lactate is always created during anaerobic training. What separates individuals who are highly fit from those who are not is the degree to which lactic acid can be tolerated and how quickly it can be metabolized. As you improve your fitness through physical training, you will be better suited to discard waste products, exchange gases, and neutralize the metabolically-produced acids thereby delaying muscular fatigue. Otherwise, you must abbreviate — or perhaps even terminate — your activities until you attain a more acceptable metabolic environment.

PHYSIOLOGICAL OVERLOAD

Any type of physical training — whether it is done for flexibility, aerobic, anaerobic, strength, metabolic, power, or skill improvements — must incorporate a well-known foundational concept in exercise physiology called the "Overload Principle." The term "overload" means that a targeted physiological and/or neurological system is made to work harder than it is accustomed to working. This suggests that there is a minimum threshold level that must be surpassed before a specific, long-term adaptation is produced.

Over a period of time, you will likely find that the same task or activity — which was originally difficult — can be performed with less exertion. As a result, making your physical training progressively more challenging is critical in order to provide an overload, and produce further physiological improvements in the target system (such as your musculoskeletal, circulatory, and/or respiratory system).

Because of this, keeping accurate records of your physical performances is important. Maintaining records of your key program components allows you to track progress, thereby making your workouts more productive and more meaningful.

GENETIC INFLUENCES

The most important factor that influences your anaerobic and aerobic potential is your genetic (or inherited) characteristics. For the most part, you cannot change the qualities that you have acquired from your ancestors. Stated otherwise, you have little control over what you have inherited.

The "genetic profile" of someone who has a high level of aerobic ability differs greatly from that of someone who has a high level of anaerobic ability. One of the most influential of all inherited attributes in your genetic portfolio is the composition (and distribution) of your muscle fibers. (A fiber is a single muscle cell.) Your muscle fibers can be categorized as slow twitch (ST) or Type I and fast twitch (FT) or Type II. From a functional standpoint, muscle fibers differ in a number of ways including speed of contraction, magnitude of force, and degree of fatigability. (Subsequent mention of FT fibers will encompass both subtypes.)

Relative to FT fibers, ST fibers contract more slowly and produce lower amounts of force (due to their smaller diameters), but they fatigue less readily. (Although ST fibers contract more slowly than their FT counterparts, this is not to say that they do not contract quickly. Indeed, their speed of contraction is measured in milliseconds.) Because ST fibers are highly aerobic and heavily dependent upon oxygen for energy, they are often referred to as being "oxidative"; because FT fibers are highly anaerobic and heavily dependent upon glycogen for energy, they are often referred to as being "glycolytic."

Studies of twins have shown that the composition and distribution of muscle fibers is determined almost entirely by hereditary factors. Most muscles have a blend of about 50% ST fibers and 50% FT fibers. (The fibers are intermingled throughout each muscle.) Some people, however, inherit a greater proportion of one fiber type that allows them to be successful during efforts of varying demands and durations. For example, an individual who has inherited a high percentage of ST fibers has the genetic potential to produce relatively small amounts of force for long periods of time and, therefore, will excel during low-intensity, long-term efforts; on the other hand, a person who has inherited a high percentage of FT fibers has the genetic potential to generate relatively large amounts of force for short periods of time and, therefore, will excel during high-intensity, short-term efforts. Note that an individual's fiber-type mixture will likely differ from one muscle to another and may even vary from one side of the body to the other.

Except for monozygotic (identical) twins, each person is a unique genetic entity with a different genetic potential. Some people are predisposed toward being more successful at aerobic activities while others are destined to become more successful at anaerobic activities. Regardless of your genetic destiny, your goal should be to realize your physical potential.

Chapter 5
Aerobic Training

The most important aspect of your physical profile — and the best indicator of overall health — is your aerobic fitness. Specifically, your aerobic fitness is a measure of how well your muscles consume, transport, and utilize oxygen during physical activities. The best way to improve these physiological mechanisms is through aerobic training.

The metabolic pathway that is responsible for your aerobic fitness is your Aerobic System (which is vital in efforts that are of low intensity and prolonged duration.) Therefore, the primary target of your aerobic training is your Aerobic System.

The main purpose of aerobic training is to improve the functional ability of your Aerobic System. By improving your aerobic fitness, your heart and aerobic pathway can operate more productively and more efficiently. Another purpose of aerobic training is to improve your performance potential. By reducing your resting heart rate, for example, it will be easier for you to maintain a good sight picture and trigger control, thereby improving your weapon system accuracy. Also, a SWAT officer with a high level of aerobic fitness surrenders to fatigue less quickly than someone with a low level of aerobic fitness. A final purpose of aerobic training is to establish a solid foundation of aerobic support prior to any anaerobic training. The more finely tuned your aerobic pathway becomes, the better your anaerobic pathways are able to function. Clearly, your aerobic pathway must operate as efficiently and effectively as possible to provide physiological support for your anaerobic pathways.

Besides the many physiological adaptations, aerobic training — when used in conjunction with sound nutritional practices — helps to maintain your percentage of body fat at an acceptable level.

AEROBIC GUIDELINES

Your aerobic fitness may be developed and maintained by using several easy-to-follow guidelines. These guidelines — which have been created by the American College of Sports

Medicine (ACSM) based upon the existing scientific evidence concerning exercise prescription for healthy adults — can be organized under the acronym "FITT" which stands for "Frequency, Intensity, Time, and Type." (Most of you can safely begin an exercise program of moderate intensity. However, the ACSM recommends that men at or above the age of 40, and women at or above the age of 50 receive a medical examination before beginning an intense program of physical training.)

Frequency

In order to improve your aerobic fitness, the ACSM suggests that you perform appropriate aerobic activities 3 - 5 days per week. Training less than three days per week does not appear adequate enough to promote any meaningful changes in your aerobic fitness; training more than five days per week produces a negligible amount of aerobic improvement (which usually is not worth the time spent).

Having said that, doing aerobic training more frequently is beneficial when weight (fat) loss is a goal. But beginning with too much activity too soon may very well lead to an overuse injury such as tendinitis. This is especially true of certain populations including older adults, and those who are inactive or in poor physical condition. Individuals who are susceptible to overuse injuries should initially perform aerobic training 2 - 3 days per week to reduce their potential for orthopedic problems. As these individuals adjust and adapt to the unfamiliar physical demands, their dosage of aerobic training can be increased to 3 - 5 weekly workouts.

Intensity

Other than your genetics, the most important component of your aerobic training is your level of intensity (or effort). Your heart rate increases in direct proportion to the demands of an activity. As such, your training heart rate is commonly used as an estimate of your aerobic intensity. Since there is a slight, but steady decrease in your maximal heart rate with aging, estimates of it are made on the basis of your age. The ACSM recommends that you maintain a level of 60 - 90% of your age-predicted maximum heart rate in order to receive a benefit from aerobic training. (Previously, the ACSM recommended training with 70 - 85% of the age-predicted maximum heart rate. In 1990, the ACSM expanded their guideline presum-

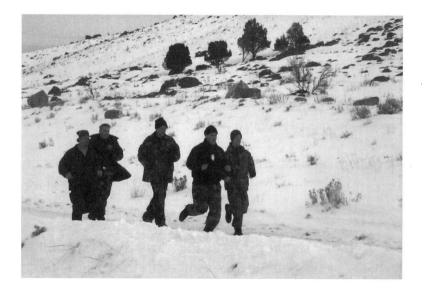

Your training heart rate is commonly used an estimate of your aerobic intensity. This is affected by environmental factors such as altitude, temperature, and humidity. Training under a variety of weather conditions will enhance your opportunity for success.

ably to encompass extremes in the population — the poorly conditioned and the highly conditioned.)

One way to find a rough estimate of your age-predicted maximum heart rate in beats per minute (bpm) is to simply subtract your age from 220. For example, the age-predicted maximum heart rate of a 30-year-old individual is 190 bpm [220 - 30 = 190]. To find the recommended heart-rate training zone, multiply 190 bpm by 0.60 and 0.90. This means that a 30-year-old individual needs to maintain a heart rate between about 114 - 171 bpm while training to elicit aerobic improvements [190 bpm x 0.60 = 114 bpm; 190 bpm x 0.90 = 171 bpm].

In the case of maximal heart rate, noting that the equation "220 minus age" has a standard deviation of about 11 bpm is important. Considering all 30-year-old individuals, this means that about 68.26% of them have maximal heart rates between 179 - 201 bpm, 95.44% between 168 - 212 bpm and 99.73% between 157 - 223 bpm.

Some people may need to maintain their heart rates above the training zone that is recommended for others of the same age. If you are highly active or have an above-average level of fitness, for example, you should train with a higher percentage of your age-predicted maximum heart rate to receive a sufficient cardiac workload; in contrast, if you are inactive or have a below-average level of fitness, you should train at a lower percentage of your age-predicted maximum heart rate to avoid potential risks. Using a lower level of intensity may also be necessary in the early stages of aerobic training to increase the likelihood of adherence to the program.

Remember, a favorable response depends upon training with an appropriate level of intensity. "Intensity" is a relative term that depends upon each individual's level of fitness. For some people, training with a lower percentage of their age-predicted maximum heart rate may actually represent a high level of intensity and an adequate cardiac workload *for them*. Stated otherwise, exercise of low intensity for an active individual may be of high intensity for an inactive individual. Depending upon the initial level of fitness, training with an intensity that is below the suggested range can actually produce some improvement in aerobic fitness.

To determine an appropriate level of intensity, you should adjust your effort based upon whether the activity feels too easy or too difficult. If it feels too easy, increase your intensity; if it feels too difficult, reduce your intensity. Also keep in mind that your intensity — and your heart rate — is influenced by many factors including the environmental conditions (such as the altitude, temperature, and humidity), your body position (such as being seated or upright), and the amount of muscle mass being trained. (Everything else being equal, training larger muscles will produce a higher heart rate than training smaller ones.)

Your heart rate can be easily measured at several different sites on your body. Numerous heart-rate monitors are available commercially that provide a reasonably accurate reading of your heart rate. But the easiest and least expensive way to determine your heart rate is to measure it yourself. This can be done by locating your pulse at either the carotid artery (in your neck) or the radial artery (in your wrist). Simply place the tips of your index and middle fingers over one of these sites. (During intense activity, your carotid and radial arteries are easy to find.) Immediately after a session of aerobic training, count your pulse for 10 seconds. Multiplying that number by six gives you a good estimate of your heart rate while training (in beats per minute). You can obtain a similar estimate by counting your pulse for 15 seconds and multiplying that number by four.

Time

The ACSM recommends that you do 20 - 60 minutes of continuous or intermittent activity in order to improve your aerobic fitness. (The ACSM defines "intermittent" as a "minimum of 10-min[ute] bouts accumulated throughout the day." So, two 15-minute workouts would equal 30 minutes of aerobic activity.) Keep in mind, too, that the time of the activity is inversely proportional to the intensity of the activity. So, the length of your effort can be relatively brief provided that your level of effort is relatively high. In fact, a review of the literature by the ACSM suggests that training for as little as 10 - 15 minutes can significantly increase your aerobic fitness. But a workout this brief would have to be extremely intense in order to obtain the desired benefit. Generally speaking, investing 20 minutes of continuous or intermittent activity with an appropriate level of effort is enough to improve your aerobic fitness.

Also note that if the length of your aerobic effort is too brief, your workout might not produce a desirable expenditure of calories. This may be an important consideration — particularly if one of your primary objectives is to lose weight. If this is your main intention, you should perform aerobic activities for at least 30 minutes but no more than 60. (Guidelines for a safe and effective weight-management program are detailed in Chapter 18.)

When your intensity is low — for whatever reason — your activities should be conducted for a longer period of time to induce an aerobic improvement. Take into account, though, that lengthy workouts may be inappropriate for some people in the initial stages of aerobic training. For one thing, performing too much activity too soon increases the risk of incurring an overuse injury. For another, some individuals may initially have such low levels of fitness that they may only be able to tolerate 5 – 10 minutes of aerobic training. In either case, the length of the aerobic workouts can be gradually increased as they improve their levels of fitness.

Type

The combined application of the aforementioned guidelines concerning the frequency, intensity, and duration of aerobic training provides a meaningful workload for your heart and aerobic pathway. If these three ingredients of aerobic training produce the same expenditure of total calories, your physiological adaptations will be similar regardless of the aerobic activity that you perform. Therefore, you can use a variety of activities to obtain aerobic improvements.

The preferred types of aerobic activities are those that require a continuous effort, are rhythmic in nature, and involve large amounts of muscle mass. Outdoor activities that can be used to meet these criteria include cross-country skiing, cycling, hiking/backpacking, ice/in-line (or roller) skating, jogging/running, rowing, and walking; indoor activities include aerobic dancing, rope jumping, swimming, and stationary exercises on specialized equipment such as rowers, cycles (upright or recumbent), motorized treadmills, and stair climbers/steppers. Most of these aerobic options are recreational activities that can be performed — and enjoyed — throughout a lifetime.

You can also obtain aerobic benefits from activities such as soccer, basketball, and racquet sports. Remember, your intensity level can vary a great deal during these activities due to their discontinuous nature. The way these activities are structured also influences your level of intensity: Playing full-court basketball is generally more demanding than half-court basketball; playing a singles match is generally more demanding than a doubles match.

To avoid boredom, changing your activities from time to time is important. Fortunately, aerobic training allows a large amount of variety in terms of your activity selections.

Each aerobic activity has its advantages and disadvantages. For instance, swimming is desirable since it is a non-weightbearing activity — the water supports your bodyweight which virtually eliminates the compressive forces on your bones and joints. On the other hand, swimming requires a fairly high degree of proficiency. If you have poor swimming skills, your heart rate may exceed your recommended training zone in a struggle just to keep yourself afloat. And if you are not skilled at swimming, you will also tire very quickly. Therefore, swimming is not a good aerobic option for anyone who has poor swimming fundamentals. But swimming represents an excellent choice if your skills are adequate.

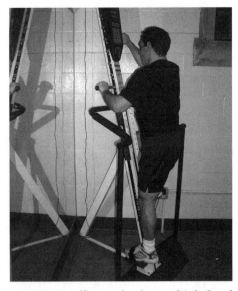

A SWAT officer who has a high level of aerobic fitness surrenders to fatigue less quickly than someone who has a low level of aerobic fitness.

In addition, some aerobic activities are not advisable if you are prone to certain injuries or are likely to complicate an existing orthopedic condition. For example, rope jumping is a high-impact, weightbearing activity that has a greater risk of orthopedic stress and overuse injuries than low-impact, non-weightbearing activities. Thus, rope jumping is not recommended if you are a larger-than-average person — larger due to either fat tissue or muscle tissue — because of the excessive stress that is placed on your ankles, knees, and lower back. Furthermore, someone who has chronic low-back pain would be more comfortable cycling in a recumbent position — which offers support for the lower back, thereby decreasing the amount of stress on the lumbar spine — instead of in the traditional upright position. So, the best advice is for you to select suitable aerobic activities that are enjoyable, compatible with your skill levels, and orthopedically safe.

If you happen to be a competitive athlete preparing for a specific event — such as running or swimming — the best activities to do are the ones that you are going to perform in competition. In one study, for example, 11 subjects in an experimental group did a 10-week program of running (intervals) and showed significantly greater improvements in their maximum oxygen intakes in running than in swimming (an average increase of 6.3% compared to 2.6%). So if you want to become a better runner, you must primarily run; if you want to become a better swimmer, you must primarily swim. This concept also applies to your fitness tests. If your test requires you to run, the best way for you to prepare is to run. This is not to say that your aerobic training should only involve running. But it should receive priority in your training. This concept is, perhaps, best summarized in the words of one researcher: "mission dictates training."

Otherwise, the best aerobic activities are the ones that you enjoy the most. As long as it is orthopedically appropriate, the type of activity that you choose to strengthen your heart and aerobic pathway is not as critical as the frequency, intensity, and duration of the activity. Your Aerobic System does not know if you pedaled on a recumbent cycle one day and ran on a motorized treadmill the next. The only thing that really matters is whether or not you applied a meaningful workload to your heart and aerobic pathway.

APPROPRIATE AEROBIC TRAINING

In a nutshell, you should perform your aerobic training at a frequency, intensity, and time that is developmentally appropriate and orthopedically safe while using suitable activities that require a sustained effort. If you are a healthy adult, your specific training prescription is to perform aerobic activities 3 - 5 times per week [frequency] at 60 - 90 percent of your age-predicted maximum heart rate [intensity] for 20 - 60 minutes [time] using appropriate activities that require a prolonged effort [type]. Bear in mind that all of these guidelines must be included in your physical training in order to improve your aerobic fitness.

MEANINGFUL AEROBIC TRAINING

Over a period of time, you will likely find that the same aerobic workout — which was originally difficult — can be performed with less effort. As you become more fit, your training heart rate will be lower for a given level of intensity. Because of this, you must increase your intensity as needed, so that you are always training with an appropriate percentage of your maximum heart rate. In addition, your ability to maintain a higher training heart rate will become easier. As a result, understanding that you need to make your aerobic training progressively more challenging to make further improvements in your aerobic fitness is important.

To ensure that you produce continued aerobic improvements, you can progressively overload your Aerobic System by (1) completing the same distance at a faster pace (that is, in a shorter amount of time); (2) covering a greater distance at the same pace; or (3) gradually increasing both the distance and the pace. As an example, suppose you cycled 4.0 miles in 20 minutes. In a future aerobic workout, you should try to either cycle 4.0 miles in less than 20 minutes, cycle more than 4.0 miles in 20 minutes, or cycle slightly more than 4.0 miles in a little less than 20 minutes. Regardless of which tactic you employ, you made your Aerobic System work harder than it was accustomed to working.

Consequently, keeping accurate records of your aerobic performances is vital. Maintaining records permits you to keep track of your progress, thereby making your aerobic workouts more productive and more meaningful. During aerobic training, the key program components to monitor include the date of your workout, the duration of your workout, the distance you completed, and the level of your intensity — that is, your training heart rate. (Appendix A contains a sample workout card for aerobic training.)

PREDICTING OXYGEN INTAKE

Oxygen intake (or oxygen consumption) is a very reliable and widely accepted indicator of your aerobic fitness. Like virtually all of your other physiological characteristics, your aerobic potential is greatly influenced by your genetics (especially as it relates to your predominant muscle-fiber type).

There are a number of ways to accurately measure oxygen intake in a laboratory. One way is to step up on and down from a bench of a standard height at a fixed rate of stepping. Another way is to pedal a cycle ergometer in an upright or recumbent position using your legs and/or arms. (An ergometer is a device that measures work.) In terms of assessing oxygen intake, the most widely used laboratory apparatus is probably the motor-driven tread-

Your heart rate can be easily measured by locating your pulse at either the carotid artery (in your neck) or the radial artery (in your wrist). Simply place the tips of your index and middle fingers over one of these sites. Immediately after a session of aerobic training, count your pulse for 10 seconds. Multiplying that number by six provides a good estimate of your heart rate while training (in beats per minute).

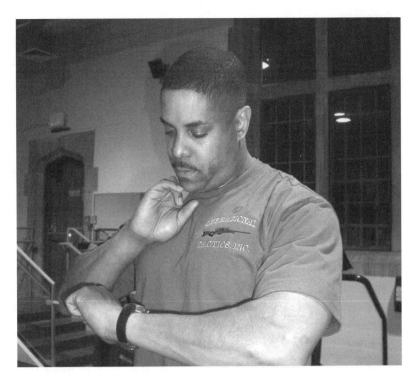

mill. Each of these devices makes it possible for you to perform at different levels of intensity while maintaining your body in a relatively stable position. This allows you to be instrumented in order to measure your various physiological responses. For instance, your expired air can be collected and analyzed to determine the exact amount of oxygen that you consumed, as well as the response of your heart rate, blood pressure, and body temperature.

Laboratory testing is an excellent means of providing you with accurate and valid data. However, laboratory testing can be expensive, time-consuming, and impractical — if it is even available. Fortunately, there is a much more practical way of assessing your oxygen intake without having the drawbacks of laboratory testing. Since these assessments are performed outside the laboratory, they are referred to as "field tests." Certain field tests have a high correlation to laboratory tests of oxygen intake. One of the most popular field tests that can be used to determine oxygen intake is the 1.5-Mile Running Test. The primary objective of this test is to run 1.5 miles in the least amount of time. For this field test to be as accurate as possible, you must run exactly 1.5 miles and it must be on a level (or horizontal) surface. Because of this, running on an indoor or outdoor track is preferred. Generally, the results of the 1.5-Mile Running Test are an excellent predictor of your oxygen intake. But realize that this particular test of aerobic fitness favors runners, since it involves running.

Table 5.1 lists predicted values of oxygen intake based upon the time you take to complete a 1.5-mile run on a level surface. Various running times are given in five-second intervals between 8:00 - 15:55. These values are a relative measure of how much oxygen you consumed in milliliters per kilogram of your bodyweight per minute (or ml/kg/min).

Oxygen Consumption: Relative

Imagine a 30-year-old man who weighs 198 pounds and can run 1.5 miles in 12:30. Note in Table 5.1 that his oxygen intake for this particular running time is 42.12 ml/kg/min — or simply 42.12. In other words, he consumed about 42.12 milliliters of oxygen for every kilo-

TIME	VALUE	TIME	VALUE	TIME	VALUE	TIME	VALUE
8:00	63.84	10:00	51.77	12:00	43.73	14:00	37.98
8:05	63.22	10:05	51.37	12:05	43.45	14:05	37.77
8:10	62.61	10:10	50.98	12:10	43.17	14:10	37.57
8:15	62.01	10:15	50.59	12:15	42.90	14:15	37.37
8:20	61.42	10:20	50.21	12:20	42.64	14:20	37.18
8:25	60.85	10:25	49.84	12:25	42.38	14:25	36.98
8:30	60.29	10:30	49.47	12:30	42.12	14:30	36.79
8:35	59.74	10:35	49.11	12:35	41.86	14:35	36.60
8:40	59.20	10:40	48.75	12:40	41.61	14:40	36.41
8:45	58.67	10:45	48.40	12:45	41.36	14:45	36.23
8:50	58.15	10:50	48.06	12:50	41.11	14:50	36.04
8:55	57.63	10:55	47.72	12:55	40.87	14:55	35.86
9:00	57.13	11:00	47.38	13:00	40.63	15:00	35.68
9:05	56.64	11:05	47.05	13:05	40.39	15:05	35.50
9:10	56.16	11:10	46.73	13:10	40.16	15:10	35.33
9:15	55.68	11:15	46.41	13:15	39.93	15:15	35.15
9:20	55.21	11:20	46.09	13:20	39.70	15:20	34.98
9:25	54.76	11:25	45.78	13:25	39.48	15:25	34.81
9:30	54.31	11:30	45.47	13:30	39.26	15:30	34.64
9:35	53.87	11:35	45.17	13:35	39.04	15:35	34.48
9:40	53.43	11:40	44.87	13:40	38.82	15:40	34.31
9:45	53.01	11:45	44.58	13:45	38.61	15:45	34.15
9:50	52.59	11:50	44.29	13:50	38.39	15:50	33.99
9:55	52.18	11:55	44.01	13:55	38.19	15:55	33.83

TABLE 5.1: PREDICTED VALUES OF OXYGEN INTAKE (in ml/kg/min) BASED UPON THE TIME TO COMPLETE A 1.5-MILE RUN ON A LEVEL SURFACE

gram that he weighed during each minute of his 1.5-mile run. (Elite male endurance athletes — such as cross-country runners and skiers — have recorded oxygen intake values as high as the low 80s.)

Table 5.1 is only valid for determining your oxygen intake during a 1.5-mile run. The ACSM offers this formula for determining oxygen intake in ml/kg/min for a run of any known distance and duration on a level surface:

oxygen intake = (speed in m/min) x (0.2 ml/kg/min per m/min) + 3.5 ml/kg/min

As an example, suppose that you just completed a 5,000-meter race in 20:00. In this case, your running speed was 250.0 meters per minute [5,000 m ÷ 20.0 min = 250.0 m/min]. Next, multiply your speed [250.0 m/min] by the oxygen cost of horizontal running [0.2 ml/kg/min per m/min] and add the oxygen cost of resting [3.5 ml/kg/min]. This calculation yields a value of 53.5 ml/kg/min [250.0 m/min x 0.2 ml/kg/min per m/min + 3.5 ml/kg/min = 53.5 ml/kg/min]. For this formula to be accurate, you must run on a level surface at a speed of at least 5.0 miles per hour (mph) or 134.0 m/min. (To convert mph to m/min, multiply the mph by 26.8; to convert miles to meters, multiply the number of miles by 1,609.)

A similar formula can be used to determine oxygen intake for walking speeds between 1.9 - 3.7 mph. At lower speeds, walking is generally a more efficient process than running. In fact, the oxygen cost of horizontal walking at a given speed is about one half that of horizontal running. Therefore, the only difference in the previously mentioned formula is that the walking speed is multiplied by 0.1 ml/kg/min per m/min (the oxygen cost of horizontal walking) and then added to 3.5 ml/kg/min (the oxygen cost at rest). So, if you walked 3,000 meters in 30 minutes, your oxygen intake would be 13.5 ml/kg/min [100.0 m/min x 0.1 ml/kg/min per m/min + 3.5 ml/kg/min = 13.5 ml/kg/min].

Oxygen Consumption: Absolute

Oxygen intake can also be expressed in absolute terms in liters per minute (L/min). To determine your oxygen intake in L/min, you must first convert your bodyweight to kilograms (kg). To do this, divide your bodyweight in pounds (lb) by 2.2. Using the earlier example of the 30-year-old male, his 198-pound bodyweight is equal to 90 kg [198 lb ÷ 2.2 kg/lb = 90 kg]. Next, multiply his bodyweight (in kilograms) by his oxygen intake (in ml/kg/min) and divide by 1,000 (to convert from milliliters to liters). Staying with the same example as before yields a value of 3,790.8 ml/min [90 kg x 42.12 ml/kg/min = 3,790.8 ml/min]. To divide by 1,000, simply move the decimal point three places to the left. This means that a 198-pound individual who ran 1.5 miles in 12:30 would consume about 3.79 liters of oxygen during every minute of his run. (Values of more than 5.0 L/min are fairly common in highly fit individuals.)

Oxygen-Intake Expectations

According to the ACSM, the following regression equations can be used to predict your expected oxygen intake (in ml/kg/min) based upon your activity level, age, and gender:

Active men: 69.7 - (0.612 x age)

Active women: 42.9 - (0.312 x age)

For instance, an active 30-year-old man would be expected to have an oxygen intake of about 51.34 ml/kg/min [0.612 x 30 = 18.36; 69.7 - 18.36 = 51.34]. Comparing your expected oxygen intake to your actual oxygen intake is helpful in determining whether you have any Functional Aerobic Impairment (FAI). Your FAI may be found by subtracting your actual oxygen intake from your expected oxygen intake. This value is divided by your expected oxygen intake and then multiplied by 100 (to convert to a percentage). If the 30-year-old man in this example was found to have an actual oxygen intake of 42.12 ml/kg/min, he would have an FAI of about 18.0% [51.34 ml/kg/min - 42.12 ml/kg/min ÷ 51.34 ml/kg/min x 100 = 17.96%]. A negative percentage indicates that your actual oxygen intake is better than expected. Once again, note that heredity plays an important role in determining your level of aerobic fitness.

Finally, the purpose of assessing your aerobic fitness should not be to compare your performance to that of another. Making comparisons between people is unfair because everyone has a different genetic potential for achieving aerobic fitness. Fitness assessments are more meaningful and fair when your performance is compared to your last performance — not to the performance of others.

ESTIMATING CALORIC EXPENDITURE

A calorie is basically a unit of energy. In scientific terms, a "calorie" is defined as "the amount of heat required to raise the temperature of one gram of water by one degree Celsius." In practical terms, a calorie is a measure of your energy intake (eating) as well as your energy expenditure (exercising).

The caloric equivalent of one liter of oxygen ranges from 4.7 calories when fats are used as the sole source of energy to 5.0 calories when carbohydrates are used as the sole source of energy. (The caloric equivalent of one liter of oxygen is 4.4 calories when proteins are used as the only source of energy. Under most circumstances, however, protein utilization during exercise is negligible in terms of energy production and is usually disregarded.) For all practical purposes — and with little loss in precision — you use about 5.0 calories for every liter of oxygen that you consume. To determine your rate of caloric expenditure, simply take your oxygen intake in L/min and multiply it by 5.0 calories per liter (cal/L). Recall the earlier example of the 198-pound male whose oxygen intake was 3.79 L/min. In this case, his rate of caloric expenditure would be almost 19 calories per minute [3.79 L/min x 5.0 cal/L = 18.95 cal/min].

To determine the total number of calories that he used during his 1.5-mile run, multiply his rate of caloric expenditure (in cal/min) by his running time. In this case, multiplying 18.95 cal/min by 12.5 minutes (12:30 in decimal form) indicates that he used about 237.0 calories during his run [18.95 cal/min x 12.5 min = 236.88 cal].

MET LEVELS

Another way to quantify oxygen intake (and caloric/energy expenditure) is by assigning an activity a "MET" or "Metabolic EquivalenT." A MET is a multiple of your oxygen intake while at rest. The amount of oxygen you consume while you are resting in a seated position is 1.0 MET — which is about 3.5 ml/kg/min. A level of 2.0 METs is equal to an oxygen intake of 7.0 ml/kg/min [3.5 ml/kg/min x 2.0 = 7.0 ml/kg/min]. Therefore, an activity that has a value of 2.0 METs requires twice as much oxygen (or energy) as complete rest (that is, 7.0 ml/kg/min compared to 3.5 ml/kg/min); an activity that has a value of 6.0 METs requires three times as much oxygen as an activity that requires 2.0 METs (21.0 ml/kg/min compared to 7.0 ml/kg/min).

You can easily express your oxygen intake in METs. To do so, simply divide your oxygen intake in ml/kg/min by 3.5 ml/kg/min. For instance, the 198-pound male in the ongoing example had an oxygen intake of 42.12 ml/kg/min when he ran 1.5 miles in 12:30. In this case, his oxygen intake is equal to about 12.0 METs [42.12 ml/kg/min ÷ 3.5 ml/kg/min = 12.03 METs].

ACTIVITY	cal/kg/min	MET
aerobic dancing	0.105	6.00
badminton, competitive	0.147	8.40
badminton, recreational	0.076	4.34
basketball, half-court	0.088	5.03
basketball, full-court	0.132	7.54
cycling, outdoor, at 10.00 mph	0.123	7.03
cycling (ergometer), 300 kpm	0.065	3.71
cycling (ergometer), 900 kpm	0.149	8.51
cycling (ergometer), 1,200 kpm	0.193	11.03
dancing, ballroom, rumba	0.103	5.89
dancing, ballroom, waltz	0.084	4.80
golf	0.085	4.86
handball	0.143	8.17
hiking, 3.00 mph with a 40-pound pack	0.100	5.71
judo	0.195	11.14
karate	0.195	11.14
mountain climbing	0.147	8.40
racquetball	0.143	8.17
rope jumping, 60 - 80 skips/min	0.158	9.03
rope jumping, 120 - 140 skips/min	0.193	11.03
rowing, indoor (Concept II), 2:32/500m (7.36 mph)	0.118	6.74
rowing, indoor (Concept II), 2:00/500m (9.32 mph)	0.175	10.00
running, level surface, 9:00/mi (6.67 mph)	0.196	11.20
running, level surface, 7:00/mi (8.57 mph)	0.247	14.13
running, level surface, 6:00/mi (10.00 mph)	0.286	16.32
skating, recreational	0.083	4.74
skiing, cross-country, 3.00 mph	0.132	7.54
skiing, cross-country, 10.00 mph	0.293	16.74
soccer	0.132	7.54
squash	0.143	8.17
stair climbing (StairMaster® 4000PT®), level 5	0.114	6.51
stair climbing (StairMaster® 4000PT®), level 9	0.170	9.71
swimming, back stroke, 25 yd/min	0.088	5.03
swimming, back stroke, 50 yd/min	0.183	10.46
swimming, breast stroke, 25 yd/min	0.088	5.03
swimming, breast stroke, 50 yd/min	0.183	10.46
swimming, front crawl, 25 yd/min	0.088	5.03
swimming, front crawl, 50 yd/min	0.183	10.46
swimming, side stroke, 40 yd/min	0.161	9.20
tennis, competitive	0.161	9.20
tennis, recreational	0.103	5.89
volleyball, competitive	0.117	6.69
volleyball, recreational	0.051	2.91
walking, level asphalt road, 2.50 mph	0.051	2.91
walking, level asphalt road, 3.50 mph	0.064	3.66
weight training	0.116	6.63
weight training, circuit	0.185	10.57

TABLE 5.2: ESTIMATES OF CALORIC EXPENDITURE (in cal/kg/min) AND MET LEVELS FOR SELECTED ACTIVITIES

You can also use the MET level to estimate your rate of caloric expenditure in calories per kilogram of your bodyweight per minute (cal/kg/min) and your calories per minute (cal/min). One MET is equal to about 0.0175 cal/kg/min. Therefore, your caloric expenditure can be estimated in cal/kg/min by multiplying your MET level by 0.0175 cal/kg/min. For example, the 198-pound male who recorded a MET level of 12.03 used about 0.210525 cal/min/kg [12.03 x 0.0175 cal/kg/min = 0.210525 cal/kg/min]. To estimate his cal/min, multiply his bodyweight in kilograms [90] by his cal/kg/min [0.210525]. This produces a value of about 18.95 cal/min [90 kg x 0.210525 cal/kg/min = 18.947 cal/min]. (Recall that his rate of caloric expenditure was previously estimated as 18.95 cal/min using a different series of calculations.)

Table 5.2 lists a wide range of activities along with estimates of cal/kg/min and MET levels that you can use to estimate your caloric expenditure. Remember, these are only estimates. Caloric expenditure during activities other than walking and running are difficult to predict. Your exact caloric expenditure depends heavily upon your skill at performing the activity as well as your motivation to do so. It is also influenced by the environmental conditions such as the wind, terrain, altitude, temperature, humidity, and air pollution. Nevertheless, this information still provides a reasonably accurate estimate of your caloric expenditure during various activities.

Chapter 6
Anaerobic Training

A large portion of your physical training and tactical operations is composed of brief, intense movements that rely heavily upon your anaerobic abilities. The best way to prepare for these specific physiological demands is through anaerobic training.

The main purpose of anaerobic training is to improve the functional ability of your anaerobic pathways (that is, your ATP-PC System and Anaerobic Glycolysis). A second purpose is to improve your performance potential as a SWAT officer — especially as it relates to performing short-term, high-intensity activities such as running up several flights of stairs, and carrying or dragging another individual a short distance as quickly as possible.

The most common method of anaerobic training is to perform a series of intense efforts that last for brief periods of time such as sprinting. In order for your anaerobic training to be most effective, it must be done in an organized manner. Performing anaerobic training on an informal basis can certainly provide favorable benefits, but a formal program that is structured and has a scientific foundation is more precise and more productive.

To obtain desirable improvements, your anaerobic efforts must be done in an aggressive and enthusiastic fashion. Furthermore, understanding that manipulating the time and the intensity of your efforts will emphasize different anaerobic energy systems is important.

Finally, before you begin your anaerobic training, you must first establish a solid base of aerobic support. Your anaerobic pathways cannot function at optimal levels without assistance from your aerobic pathway. (Chapter 5 details how to effectively train your aerobic pathways.)

ANAEROBIC GUIDELINES

Anaerobic training is somewhat more complex than aerobic training. Your anaerobic systems play a significant role in activities that last anywhere from a split second to roughly three minutes — assuming, of course, that your intensity of effort is great enough to elicit an anaerobic response. The complications arise because you have two energy pathways — your ATP-PC System and Anaerobic Glycolysis — that operate within this anaerobic window of time. Specifically, your ATP-PC System predominates during activities that are approximately 30 seconds or less; activities that last between about 30 - 90 seconds involve the joint efforts of your ATP-PC System and Anaerobic Glycolysis; finally, Anaerobic Glycolysis — with an important contribution from your Aerobic System — provides energy during activities that are between roughly 1.5 - 3.0 minutes. (Your Aerobic System becomes your principal energy pathway after about three minutes of continuous activity.)

To engage your anaerobic pathways, your intensity must be great enough such that you cannot train continuously for much more than about three minutes at a time. Anaerobic intensity can be measured the same way as aerobic intensity: by monitoring your training heart rate. But anaerobic training requires higher levels of intensity than aerobic training. In order to involve your anaerobic pathways, you must raise your heart rate to near-maximal levels for brief periods of time. Elevating your heart rate to 90% or more of your age-predicted maximum is usually a good indicator that you are utilizing your anaerobic pathways. (Chapter 5 describes how you can determine your age-predicted maximum heart rate.)

Here is another similarity between anaerobic training and aerobic training: If you are highly active or have an above-average level of fitness, you should train with a higher percentage of your age-predicted maximum heart rate; if you are inactive or have a below-average level of fitness, you should train with a lower percentage of your age-predicted maximum heart rate.

Remember, anaerobic training is characterized by high-intensity efforts performed over relatively short periods of time. Unlike aerobic training — where a decreased level of intensity can be sacrificed for an increased duration of activity — performing your anaerobic training with a level of effort that is as high as possible for a specific amount of time is an absolute requirement.

In determining whether or not your effort is anaerobic, the duration of the activity is more critical than the distance of the activity. As an example, suppose that two individuals who have different levels of fitness each ran 440 yards as fast as possible. The person who has the higher level of fitness may have completed the distance in one minute while the person who has the lower level of fitness may have needed two minutes. So, the distance run by the two individuals was the same, but the time taken to perform the activity was different which resulted in the use of different energy pathways: One minute of intense effort involves the ATP-PC System and Anaerobic Glycolysis while two minutes of all-out effort utilizes Anaerobic Glycolysis and the Aerobic System.

Having said that, considering distances when performing anaerobic training is often more practical. If a three-minute threshold is used as the maximum limit of time for involvement of your anaerobic pathways, you can easily determine a range of distances for your anaerobic training. For instance, in three minutes most people who are in reasonably good condition can run about one-half mile. At the other end of the energy continuum, your ATP-PC System can be effectively targeted by an all-out effort that lasts a handful of seconds or less — which correlates to running distances of up to about 40 yards. (You can determine a precise range of distances for your anaerobic efforts during rowing, running, swimming, and other physical activities based upon these time frames and your personal level of fitness.)

Because of its highly intense nature, most people should only perform anaerobic training once or twice a week. Highly conditioned individuals *may* opt for greater frequency. In this case, the number of anaerobic workouts is dependent upon the duration of your efforts. Long- and middle-duration anaerobic efforts of 1.5 - 3.0 minutes (such as running between about 440 - 880 yards) can be done 2 - 3 days per week; short-duration anaerobic efforts of less than 90 seconds (such as running roughly 440 yards or less) can be performed 3 - 4 days per week. If you reach a point where you are no longer making improvements, then you are probably performing too much anaerobic training.

MEANINGFUL ANAEROBIC TRAINING

After a period of time, you will likely notice that the same anaerobic workout — which was originally challenging — can be done with less effort. Therefore, making your anaerobic training progressively more difficult is critical so that you can produce further improvements in your anaerobic fitness.

To ensure that you derive continual anaerobic improvements, you can progressively overload your anaerobic systems by (1) covering the same distances at a faster pace (that is, in shorter amounts of time); (2) decreasing the length of your recovery between efforts; or (3) gradually increasing the distances and decreasing the length of your recovery between efforts. Consider this example: Suppose that as part of your workout, you swam a series of four 100-yard sprints in an average time of 1:30 (that is, one minute and 30 seconds) and took an average recovery time of 3:00 between your efforts. In a future anaerobic workout, you should try to (1) swim the four 100s in an average time of less than 1:30; (2) take an average recovery time of less than 3:00 between the four 100s; or (3) swim the 100s in an average time of a little less than 1:30 and take an average recovery time of slightly less than 3:00 between your efforts. Regardless, you made your anaerobic systems work harder than they were accustomed to working.

Because of this, keeping accurate records of your anaerobic performances is important. Maintaining records allows you to monitor progress, thereby making your workouts more productive and more meaningful. During anaerobic training, the main program components to document include the date of your workout, the distances of your efforts, the durations of your efforts, and the durations of your recovery between your efforts. (Appendix B contains a sample workout card for anaerobic training.)

Whenever possible, practice anaerobic activities that are sport- or tactical operation-specific. For example, a SWAT officer should practice low crawling 30 yards while wearing full SWAT gear and a gas mask.

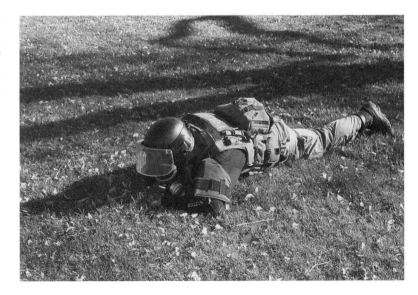

APPROPRIATE ANAEROBIC ACTIVITIES

If you are a competitive athlete training for a specific event — such as rowing or cycling — the best activities to do are the ones that you are going to perform in competition. If you want to become a better rower, you must mainly row; if you want to become a better cyclist, you must mainly cycle. Therefore, the best method of anaerobic training for sports or activities that involve running is running. You can — and should — use other activities to minimize the impact forces that are associated with running. In order to be able to run effectively, however, you must run during the majority of your workouts. An individual might be in excellent condition to perform a non-weightbearing activity (such as rowing or cycling), but not when suddenly required to do a weightbearing activity (such as running).

There is another consideration for a SWAT officer who is also a competitive athlete: Your workouts should approximate the specific nature of your sport or activity. Anaerobic training should be task-specific in the sense that the actual times and distances of your efforts should be based upon the requirements of your sport or activity. For example, if your sport or activity involves a series of intense efforts that are 30 yards or less, then these specific distances should receive the most emphasis during your anaerobic training. At least some of your efforts, however, should also consist of times and distances that are beyond those normally encountered in competition.

The concepts for task specificity also hold true for SWAT training. If your training requires you to complete a 30-yard low crawl while wearing full SWAT gear and a gas mask in 60 seconds or less, for example, then the best way to prepare is by doing a 30-yard low crawl while wearing full SWAT gear and a gas mask in 60 seconds or less. You can certainly help ready yourself for this task with other activities such as strength training. But the best way to prepare for an activity is to do the activity.

METHODS OF ANAEROBIC TRAINING

Several different methods can be used to develop your anaerobic pathways. Remember that the parameters for time and intensity (that is, your training heart rate) must be satisfied in order for an activity to be considered as anaerobic. So, doing an activity with an intense effort in about three minutes or less is necessary to develop your anaerobic pathways.

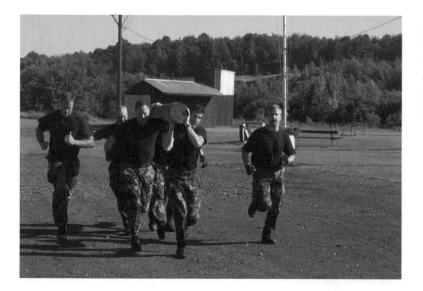

Anaerobic training can also become a SWAT team-building exercise. With the use of a telephone pole to simulate an injured officer on a stretcher, SWAT team members can compete in relay races.

For the sake of simplicity, most of the ensuing discussions of anaerobic training use running as the example. However, all of the methods used to increase your running performance can be applied to virtually any physical activity as well as any type of equipment. For instance, if your goal for a particular workout is to run six 440-yard sprints in 90 seconds per sprint, you could simply cycle, row, or do another activity with an intense effort for 90 seconds a total of six times. (Recall that the use of different activities and equipment to achieve a desired benefit also applies to aerobic training.)

Lastly, do not forget that your Aerobic System provides underlying support for your anaerobic efforts. Therefore, you should develop a strong aerobic foundation before attempting any anaerobic training.

There are three main methods of anaerobic training: interval training, fartlek training, and acceleration sprints.

Interval Training

Structured interval training has been around since the 1930s, and has been especially popular for running and swimming. Regardless, the principles of interval training can be applied to virtually any type of physical activity.

Essentially, interval training is a series of repeated segments or "intervals" of intense activity — such as sprinting — alternated with periods of recovery that can be either reduced activity or complete inactivity. An example of this technique is running a given distance at an intended pace, recovering and then repeating the run-recovery sequence until your workout is completed.

Interval training allows you to repeatedly reach and sustain a high level of intensity for a cumulative time that is greater than what you could achieve during continuous training with the same intensity. The reason for this is because the recovery periods allow your anaerobic energy systems the opportunity to partially recover, thereby permitting you to make a physiological comeback between your intense efforts. Dividing your workout into short, intense efforts with intervals of recovery interspersed between consecutive efforts permits you to perform a greater volume of work at the same intensity. So, with an appropriate amount of recovery between your anaerobic efforts, you can run a series of six 440-yard sprints at a pace that might otherwise completely exhaust you after two or three consecutive 440s without a recovery period.

An interval program consists of seven different components that can be manipulated to effectively overload your anaerobic energy systems. All seven of these elements are dependent upon your level of fitness — someone who has a low level of fitness will not be able to perform as much volume of training as someone who has a high level of fitness. These seven variables are:

1. The number of repetitions.

One variable to consider during interval training is the number of repetitions (or times) that you perform your anaerobic efforts. For instance, you might do eight repetitions of a specified distance during your workout.

2. The distance.

A second variable during interval training is the distance or the length of the high-intensity effort — such as running one-half mile or swimming 100 yards in a specified time. An interval workout usually begins with longer anaerobic efforts and tapers down to shorter ones. For instance, you would complete all of the 440-yard sprints followed by all of the 220-yard sprints and so on.

If you are an athlete interested in improving your anaerobic fitness to better prepare yourself for competition, the length of your intense efforts should approximate the requirements of your sport or activity. So, a softball player who is looking to get to first base more quickly should emphasize intense efforts of 20 yards (60 feet).

3. *The work interval.*

The intended time of your anaerobic effort is the work interval. Your goal, for example, might be to row a specified distance in a work interval of 30 seconds or less. Or to prepare for a specific part of your SWAT fitness test, you might run up eight flights of stairs in full SWAT gear while carrying a one-person ram in 30 seconds or less.

4. *The recovery interval.*

The time allotted to recuperate between your anaerobic efforts — that is, the work intervals — is the recovery (or rest) interval. Receiving a sufficient amount of recovery between your anaerobic efforts is important. This allows your depleted anaerobic energy system(s) enough time to recover so that you can make another intense effort. As an example, the recovery intervals between your work intervals might provide 90 seconds of recovery.

The duration of your recovery interval is related to the time that it takes you to complete your work interval. You can customize the duration of your recovery interval by using your heart rate to determine when you are physiologically ready to begin your next work interval. For example, you might begin your next work interval when your heart rate drops to a predetermined level such as 60% of your age-predicted maximum heart rate. An appropriate decrease in heart rate depends upon several factors including the length of the next work interval and your level of fitness.

Your recovery interval can consist of either complete inactivity or low-intensity activities such as slow walking or easy jogging. Generally speaking, the more intense the work interval, the less intense the recovery interval. (Complete inactivity allows your ATP-PC System the opportunity to recover. Performing mild work during the recovery interval inhibits or partially blocks complete restoration of your ATP-PC System. This places greater demands upon your other anaerobic energy system: Anaerobic Glycolysis.)

Incidentally, most sports and activities have built-in recovery intervals because of their intermittent nature. Though these inherent respites are unofficial, unscientific and unpredictable, they produce a fairly successful replenishment of your all-important ATP stores.

5. *The work:recovery ratio.*

The recovery interval is usually expressed in relation to the work interval. This is known as the "work:recovery ratio" and is most often designated as 1:1, 1:2, 1:3, or 1:4. These ratios state that your recovery interval should be one, two, three, or four times the duration that it took to perform your work interval. As a rule of thumb, the shorter the duration of your effort — and the higher the intensity of your effort — the greater the work:recovery ratio. Because of the high level of intensity, any anaerobic effort that you complete in less than 30 seconds requires at least a 1:3 work:recovery ratio. As an example, an all-out effort that takes you 15 seconds to perform should be followed by a recovery interval of about 45 seconds or more. Anaerobic work done in 30 - 90 seconds needs between a 1:3 and 1:2 work:recovery ratio. Finally, performing anaerobically for 90 - 180 seconds requires between a 1:2 and 1:1

WORK/TIME (sec)	DISTANCE (yds)	WORK:RECOVERY RATIO
0 - 30	0 - 220	1:4 to 1:3
30 - 90	220 - 440	1:3 to 1:2
90 - 180	440 - 880	1:2 to 1:1

TABLE 6.1: SUMMARY OF TIMES, RUNNING DISTANCES, AND WORK:RECOVERY RATIOS
Note: The ranges of time apply to both the highly and poorly conditioned; the running distances are for those who are in reasonably good condition.

work:recovery ratio. A summary of times, running distances, and their accompanying work:recovery ratios are shown in Table 6.1.

6. The workout distance.

The sum of all the distances performed in your interval workout is the workout distance. When performing work intervals that last between about 1.5 - 3.0 minutes, the total distance of your workout should not exceed about 2.0 - 2.5 miles (or 3,520 - 4,400 yards) of running; when performing work intervals that are less than about 90 seconds, the total distance of your workout should not exceed about 1.5 - 2.0 miles (or 2,640 - 3,520 yards) of running. (In general, swimming distances equate to roughly 20% of running distances.)

7. The frequency of workouts.

A final variable to consider is the frequency of your interval workouts. Except for highly conditioned individuals, interval training should not be performed more than once or twice a week because of the high level of intensity that is required.

A prescription for interval training can be written in shorthand. In the language of interval training, for example, a workout written as "8 x 110 yds (0:20/1:00)" indicates that you are to perform eight, 110-yard work intervals and that each effort should be done in 20 seconds (or less) with a recovery interval of 60 seconds between each of the eight repetitions. (Note that the work:recovery ratio is 1:3 because each effort is less than 30 seconds in duration.)

Table 6.2 is a detailed example of a nine-week interval program for running that has an anaerobic emphasis. Once again, it should be noted that interval training designed for running can be easily adapted to virtually any type of activity such as swimming, cycling, and stair climbing.

Fartlek Training

Fartlek training is thought to be the predecessor of interval training. Originally developed by the Swedes, fartlek training was introduced to the United States in the 1940s. The Swedes are famous in physical-education circles for developing systems of training that were basic in structure and used the outdoors as much as possible. As such, fartlek training is usually performed outside over natural, but varied terrain that ranges from flat surfaces to steady inclines and declines. For this reason, fartlek training was probably a precursor of the hill training that is often used by modern runners. Fartlek training can also be done indoors using a wide variety of equipment.

Sometimes referred to as "speed play," fartlek training is quite similar to interval training. In structure, fartlek training is less formal and less exact than interval training. Nonetheless, fartlek training achieves anaerobic improvements by using different combinations of effort levels such as walking, jogging, and running. The work and recovery intervals are left entirely up to the individual — you can change your pace and recover at your own discretion. So, there is definitely an emphasis on "playing" with speed. A sample fartlek workout for running that emphasizes your anaerobic systems might look as follows:

1. jog 440 yards

2. walk 220 yards

3. jog 440 yards

4. walk 220 yards

5. sprint 100 yards uphill and walk 100 yards downhill in an alternating fashion for six minutes

6. jog 440 yards

7. walk 440 yards

8. sprint 50 yards and walk 50 yards in an alternating fashion for three minutes

Acceleration Sprinting

An effective technique that is used by competitive runners to increase their running speed is acceleration sprinting. This technique, however, can also be used to increase speed in other activities such as cycling, rowing, and swimming. As the name implies, acceleration sprinting is characterized by a gradual increase in your speed until a full, all-out effort is reached. When running, for example, you would begin by jogging then increase to striding and finally accelerate to sprinting the intended distance or duration. Between work intervals, your recovery intervals can consist of either complete inactivity or reduced activity such as walking or easy jogging. Gradually increasing your speed throughout your effort allows you to concentrate on your technique which is enormously important in speed development. Acceleration sprinting also provides a smooth transition towards an all-out sprint, thereby minimizing the potential for a muscle strain or pull. A series of 100-yard acceleration sprints for running might look like this:

1. jog 20 yards, stride 30 yards, and sprint 50 yards

2. walk 50 yards and repeat the series for a total of ten times

MEASURING ANAEROBIC FITNESS

Evaluating anaerobic fitness is rather complicated. The difficulty arises because no single test serves as a reliable indicator of your anaerobic fitness. Remember, your two anaerobic energy sources — the ATP-PC System and Anaerobic Glycolysis — contribute in varying ways to a wide range of efforts that last from less than one second, up to about three minutes. To obtain a true picture of your anaerobic fitness, performing several tests across the anaerobic spectrum is necessary. (Needless to say, measuring an instantaneous effort has plenty of room for error.)

There is an inverse relationship between the duration that you can sustain an intense effort, and the power requirements of the effort — the shorter the duration of an intense effort,

WEEK	SPRINT REPS	DISTANCE (yds)	WORK: RECOVERY RATIO	WORK TIME	RECOVERY TIME	WORKOUT DISTANCE	WORK-OUTS PER WEEK
1	4	880	1:1	2:35	2:35	3,520	1
2	3	880	1:1	2:30	2:30		1
	2	440	1:2	1:15	2:30	3,520	
3	2	880	1:1	2:30	2:30		1
	4	440	1:2	1:15	2:30	3,520	
4	1	880	1:1	2:25	2:25		1
	6	440	1:2	1:15	2:30	3,520	
5	4	440	1:2	1:10	2:20	2,640	2
	4	220	1:3	0:35	1:45		
6	3	440	1:2	1:05	2:10	2,640	2
	4	220	1:3	0:34	1:42		
	4	110	1:3	0:17	0:51		
7	2	440	1:2	1:05	2:10	2,640	2
	6	220	1:3	0:34	1:42		
	4	110	1:3	0:16	0:48		
8	1	440	1:2	1:05	2:10	2,640	2
	6	220	1:3	0:33	1:39		
	8	110	1:3	0:16	0:48		
9	1	440	1:2	1:05	2:10	2,640	2
	4	220	1:3	0:33	1:39		
	8	110	1:3	0:15	0:45		
	8	55	1:4	0:07	0:28		

the greater the output of power. Therefore, you can estimate your anaerobic fitness by measuring your power output.

In scientific terms, "power" is defined as "the amount of work done per unit of time" — or, more simply, "work divided by time." In this case, "work" is "the application of a force over a distance" — or "force times distance." For example, if you moved 100 pounds [lb] a distance of 3 feet [ft], you did 300 foot-pounds [ft-lb] of work [100 lb x 3 ft = 300 ft-lb]. If you performed this effort in 0.25 seconds [sec], your power output was 1,200 ft-lb/sec [300 ft-lb ÷ 0.25 sec = 1,200 ft-lb/sec].

In a laboratory setting, one of the most popular tests of anaerobic ability is the Margaria-Kalinen Power Test. At the start of this test, you are to stand six meters in front of a staircase. Initiating movement on your own, you would run up the stairs as fast as possible, stepping on every third step (that is, taking three steps at a time).

Your power output during this test can be calculated by multiplying your bodyweight times the vertical distance between the third and the ninth step divided by the time of your effort (to the nearest hundredth of a second). For instance, suppose you weigh 198 pounds and covered a vertical distance of four feet in 0.75 seconds. In this case, your power output would be 1,056 foot-pounds per second [198 lb x 4 ft ÷ 0.75 seconds = 1,056 ft-lb/sec]. (Professional football players have recorded values that exceed 1,950 ft-lb/sec.)

Several field tests have a high correlation with your anaerobic ability. Tests evaluating all-out efforts that last a mere instant include the vertical jump, standing long jump, and medicine-ball put. A test of anaerobic ability that is a little farther up the energy continuum is running a 40-yard dash.

Of slightly longer duration is a popular laboratory test known as the "Wingate Anaerobic Test" — which is basically a 30-second all-out sprint on a stationary cycle. Finally, your overall anaerobic abilities — that is, the effectiveness of your ATP-PC System and Anaerobic Glycolysis — can be inferred from intense efforts that last about 30 - 90 seconds such as sprinting 220 - 440 yards as fast as possible or running up eight flights of stairs in full SWAT gear while carrying a one-person ram.

As noted previously, the upper end of the anaerobic spectrum is actually about three minutes. Keep in mind, your Aerobic System begins providing help for intense efforts that are beyond roughly 90 seconds in duration. Therefore, a valid measurement of your unassisted anaerobic abilities should involve efforts of less than about 1.5 minutes.

Chapter 7
Strength Training

Your physical training will not be complete without incorporating some type of strength training. While there is general consensus as to how to conduct other components of your physical training — such as your aerobic, anaerobic, and flexibility training — it is not the case with strength training. Most authorities agree that strength training can be extremely beneficial. Many, however, disagree over which approach is best for increasing muscular strength (and size). The different approaches — and the abundant amount of conflicting information — often leave people quite confused.

A common practice is to adopt the programs of successful individuals (or teams) — a custom that frequently adds to the confusion. If you were to compare the programs of individuals who are very strong, you might be in for quite a surprise: Not only is it likely that their approaches are greatly different, but in many cases, they offer contradictory information. Some do fast repetition speeds, others controlled speeds; some perform mostly multiple sets, others mostly single sets; some utilize split routines, others total-body workouts; some primarily use free weights, others primarily machines; some incorporate periodization, others do not; some favor one-repetition maximum efforts, others discourage them; some do plyometrics, others oppose them.

Yet — despite using vastly different approaches to strength training — many programs are highly effective. How, then, do you choose which program to follow if you are looking to improve your muscular strength (and size)?

CHOOSING A PROGRAM

When choosing a program, considering the scientific research is important. Interestingly, science has been unable to determine that one method of strength training is superior to others. Research has only shown that a variety of methods can be used to increase strength. For example, one researcher found no statistically significant differences in the strength increases produced by nine different training routines that consisted of various combinations of sets and repetitions. Improvements in strength can also be produced by a variety of equipment. Studies have shown that there are no significant differences in the strength increases between groups that used free weights and groups that used machines.

When choosing a program, considering anecdotal evidence is also important. Though anecdotal reports lack the same scientific scrutiny as research studies, their sheer volume is so overwhelming in this case that they cannot be overlooked. The fact is that countless individuals have obtained significant improvements in their muscular strength (and size) despite doing different programs.

So, it is possible for many types of programs (and approaches) to yield favorable results. In determining which of these programs to implement, you should ask the following five questions:

Is It Productive?

The program must be productive. For you to invest time in a strength-training program if it does not produce meaningful results makes little sense. A program will be productive as long as it is based upon scientific research, common sense, and deductive reasoning not unfounded advice, wild speculation, and wishful thinking.

Is It Comprehensive?

The program must be comprehensive. A strength-training program should address all of the major muscles in your body — not just the "showy" ones. Frequently, injury-prone muscles get ignored (such as those surrounding the knee, ankle, neck, and lower back) while cosmetic muscles get emphasized (such as the chest, biceps, triceps, and abdominals). If you happen to be a competitive athlete, a comprehensive strength-training program is one that is performed year-round — including throughout the off-season and the in-season. Training during the season is especially important since this is when athletes need to be at their best in terms of strength and conditioning.

Is It Practical?

The program must be practical. In other words, it must be relatively easy to understand. In some instances, strength-training programs are grossly overcomplicated and correspond-

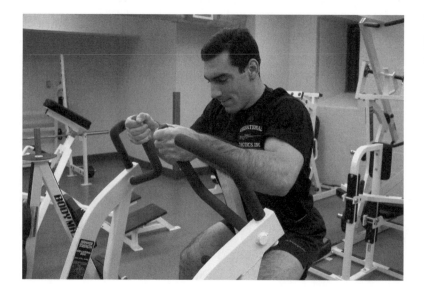

Your physical training will not be complete unless you incorporate some type of strength training.

ingly confusing. The use of pseudoscientific terminology adds to the confusion. Strength training need not be complicated.

Is It Efficient?

The program must be efficient. It should produce the *maximal* possible results in the *minimal* amount of time. A program that requires you to lift weights for lengthy periods of time or more than several workouts per week is not an efficient use of your time . . . nor is it necessary. By utilizing a program that is time-efficient, you will have a greater opportunity to pursue other professional activities such as perfecting your operational tactics, practicing your marksmanship skills, and performing other types of physical training. And do not forget about the extra time that you could dedicate toward your personal activities and interests. You should *invest* time in the weight room not *spend* time.

Is It Safe?

The program must be safe. At first glance, many programs can look quite appealing. Closer inspection, however, may reveal that the programs are highly questionable in terms of safety. There is no need whatsoever to perform potentially dangerous activities or exercises in the weight room. SWAT operations have inherent participatory risks and, as a SWAT officer, you have accepted those risks as part of the job. But this does not mean that you should accept unnecessary risks in the weight room.

In short, the program that you choose should be productive, comprehensive, practical, efficient, and safe. These are the criteria that form the underlying theme for the information that follows.

GUIDELINES FOR STRENGTH TRAINING

Unless you happen to be a competitive weightlifter or bodybuilder, there is absolutely no need for you to train like one. These athletes have different goals than SWAT officers. Essentially, the main goal of a competitive weightlifter (that is, a powerlifter or Olympic-style lifter) is to do one repetition with as much weight as possible; the main goal of a bodybuilder is to achieve the best physique possible. With no disrespect intended, neither of these goals has much relevance to a SWAT officer.

The main purpose of strength training is to reduce your risk of injury. If you can increase the strength of your muscles, connective tissues, and bones to tolerate more stress, you will reduce the likelihood of incurring an injury. Another purpose of strength training is to improve the functional ability of your musculoskeletal system. By increasing your functional strength, you will also have taken an important step toward realizing your physical potential. This will also allow you to perform your SWAT-related activities more easily. Furthermore, you will surrender less quickly to fatigue. Besides the physical and physiological benefits, strength training also provides various psychological benefits. This includes increased mental alertness as well as improved self-confidence and self-esteem.

You can increase your muscular strength (and size) in a manner that is productive, comprehensive, practical, efficient, and safe by implementing the following ten guidelines:

1. Train with an appropriate level of intensity (or effort).

The most important factor that determines your results from strength training is your genetic (or inherited) characteristics (which includes the insertion points of your tendons, your predominant muscle-fiber type, and so on). Unfortunately, you cannot control the genetic cards that you were dealt. The most important factor that you *can* control is your level of intensity. (In the weight room, "intensity" should not be confused with "a percentage of a maximum weight." Rather, "intensity" is another word for "effort.")

A high level of intensity is necessary for maximizing your response to strength training. In the weight room, a high level of intensity is characterized by performing each set to the point of concentric muscular fatigue or "failure." In simple terms, this means that you have exhausted your muscles to the extent that you literally cannot raise the weight for any additional repetitions.

If you fail to reach a desirable level of intensity — or muscular fatigue — your increases in strength (and size) will be less than optimal. Evidence for this notion is found in the Overload Principle. Coined by Dr. Arthur Steinhaus in 1933, this principle has become one of the most widely referenced in exercise physiology. According to Dr. Roger Anoka — a renowned biomechanist and author — the Overload Principle states, "To increase their size or functional ability, muscle fibers must be taxed toward their present capacity to respond." He adds: "This principle implies that there is a threshold point that must be exceeded before an adaptive response will occur."

Stated otherwise, a minimal level of muscular fatigue must be produced in order to provide a stimulus for adaptation. Your effort must be great enough to surpass this threshold so that a sufficient amount of muscular fatigue is created to trigger an adaptation. Given proper nourishment and an adequate amount of recovery between workouts, your muscles will adapt to these demands by increasing in strength (and size). The extent to which this "compensatory adaptation" occurs then becomes a function of your inherited characteristics.

POST-FATIGUE REPETITIONS

After you have reached muscular fatigue in a given exercise, you can increase your intensity even further by immediately performing several additional post-fatigue (or intensification) repetitions. But before a discussion of post-fatigue repetitions, reiterating and introducing a few basic concepts and terminology is necessary. Recall that raising a weight is sometimes referred to as the "positive phase" of a repetition and involves a concentric muscular contraction; lowering a weight is occasionally referred to as the "negative phase" of a repetition and involves an eccentric muscular contraction.

Understand that your eccentric (or negative) strength is always greater than your concentric (or positive) strength in the same exercise. Stated differently, you can always lower more weight than you can raise (again, in the same exercise). In fact, research has shown that your eccentric strength is roughly 40% greater than your concentric strength (at least in the case of a fresh muscle). So if the most weight you can raise is 100 pounds, you can probably lower about 140 pounds.

Two points can be deduced from these facts: First, when you reach muscular fatigue — that is, when you cannot do any more repetitions — it is because your concentric strength has been exhausted to such a degree that you are unable to raise the weight. Second, when you reach muscular fatigue, you cannot produce enough force to raise the weight, but you can still produce enough force to lower the weight.

This information will help you to understand — and, hopefully, to appreciate — the merits of post-fatigue repetitions. There are two main types of post-fatigue repetitions that are quite popular and productive: negatives and regressions.

In a negative-only repetition, your training partner raises the weight while you (the lifter) lower it.

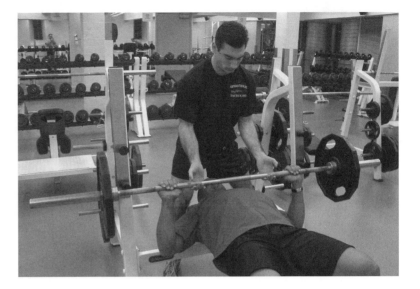

Negatives

As noted earlier, when you cannot perform the positive portion of a repetition (raising the weight), you can still do the negative portion of a repetition (lowering the weight). This is the basis — and the value — of performing post-fatigue repetitions known as "negatives" once you can no longer raise the weight at the end of a set. In a negative-only repetition, your training partner raises the weight while you (the lifter) lower it. This is repeated for 3 - 5 repetitions with each one lasting about 6 - 8 seconds (depending upon the range of motion of the particular exercise).

As an example, suppose that you reached concentric muscular fatigue in the bench press with a barbell. Your partner would help you raise the bar off your chest until your arms are almost fully extended. Then, you would lower the bar under control until it touches the middle part of your chest. (A variation of even greater intensity is to do "forced repetitions" in which your partner adds a little extra resistance by pushing down on the bar as you lower it.) In effect, these post-fatigue repetitions are positive-assisted and negative-resisted.

Performing a few negatives at the end of a set allows you to reach eccentric muscular fatigue — when your muscles have been exhausted to the point that you cannot even lower the weight. And that is why a set-to-fatigue followed immediately by several negative-only repetitions is so brutally effective: You have managed to exhaust your muscles completely — both concentrically and eccentrically.

Regressions

One of the disadvantages of negative-only repetitions is that unless you have a training partner (or competent spotter), you cannot — with very few exceptions — administer them to yourself. (For the most part, you can only give yourself negatives when doing exercises with your bodyweight such as push-ups, dips, pull-ups, chins, and sit-ups.)

If you do not have access to a training partner, you can perform post-fatigue repetitions known as "regressions." Shaun Brown, the current Strength Coach of the Boston Celtics, coined the term "regressions" in the mid 1980s. (Regressions are also called "breakdowns," "burnouts," "drop sets," and "strip sets.") When you reach concentric muscular fatigue, your muscles are still capable of producing concentric force. However, their force-produc-

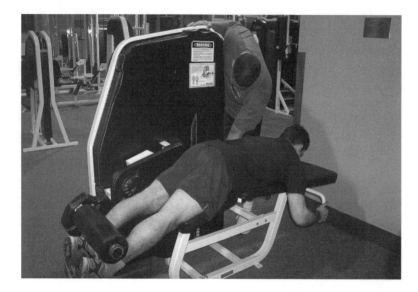

When performing regressions, you (or your training partner) quickly reduce the starting weight by about 25 - 30% and you (the lifter) do 3 - 5 regressive repetitions with the lighter load.

ing capacity is not enough to raise that particular level of resistance for any more repetitions. But you could do more repetitions with less resistance. When performing regressions, you (or your training partner) quickly reduce the starting weight by about 25 - 30% and you (the lifter) do 3 - 5 regressive repetitions with the lighter load.

For instance, say that you just reached concentric muscular fatigue after completing your 14th repetition with 100 pounds on the prone leg curl. You (or your training partner) would immediately decrease the weight to about 70 - 75 pounds. Then, you would attempt to perform a "set" of 3 - 5 repetitions with the lighter load.

If you desire, you can do a second "series" of regressions. Continuing with the previous example, you would immediately reduce the 70 - 75 pounds to about 50 - 55 pounds and try to do another "set" of 3 - 5 repetitions with that weight.

MUSCULAR FATIGUE

In order to achieve optimal improvements in muscular strength (and size), you must produce an appropriate level of muscular fatigue. If you produce too little muscular fatigue, then you may not have stimulated any compensatory adaptation. But if you produce too much muscular fatigue, then you may not have permitted any compensatory adaptation; it may even cause a loss in strength (and size). The General Adaptation Syndrome (GAS) is a three-stage process that was proposed by Dr. Hans Selye to explain the physical effects of stress. The GAS may be applied to the stress placed upon the muscles during strength training. In the first stage, the physiological stress or demands that are placed upon the muscles cause damage (or microtrauma). This is followed by the second stage during which the body defends itself against the stress-induced damage by compensatory adaptation (that is, by increasing in muscular strength and size). But stress that is too severe induces a third stage in which the demands on the muscles exceed their ability to recover and adapt.

Therefore, your level of intensity should be high . . . but it should also be appropriate. To better appreciate the concept of using an appropriate level of intensity, consider this analogy: If you used a shovel on a regular basis for short periods of time you would form calluses on your palms. Basically, the calluses are a compensatory (and protective) adaptation to frictional heat. If you shoveled for a long enough period of time, however, you would develop blisters instead. Here, the excessive demands have surpassed the adaptive ability of your tissue because the stress was too much and too frequent. In brief, you should train with a high level of intensity without overdoing it. In regards to this point, post-fatigue repetitions should be used with care.

How do you know if the demands on your muscles are too little or too much? You should monitor your performance in the weight room in terms of the resistance that you use and the repetitions that you do. If you continue to make progress in your performance, then the demands are appropriate.

The main reason why most people fail to realize their strength (and size) potential is simply because they do not train with a high enough level of intensity. Simply, a submaximal effort yields submaximal results. Keep in mind, too, that "you play like you practice." If you perform your strength training with a low level of effort, will you be able to ratchet up your intensity when you need to do so in a tactical situation or other physical activity?

That being said, you must also use your judgment in deciding what level of intensity is suitable for you. "Intensity" is a relative term that depends upon your current level of fitness. Exercise of low intensity for an active individual may be of high intensity for an inactive individual. So if you have not been training on a regular basis or are not in the best of shape, then you should adjust your effort accordingly. Remember, you can control your level of intensity when you train: Your efforts can be as easy or as difficult as you desire.

The fact that your results from strength training are directly related to your level of effort should not come as much of a surprise. Like anything else in life, how hard you work at your other physical training, your operational tactics, your marksmanship skills, and even your relationships largely determines your success at those endeavors.

2. Attempt to increase the resistance that you use or the repetitions that you perform in relation to your previous workout.

In the late 1940s, Dr. Thomas DeLorme coined the term "progressive-resistance exercise." In fact, he is often referred to as the "father of progressive-resistance exercise." Dr. DeLorme began lifting weights in 1932 at the age of 16 in an attempt to increase his muscular size and strength. During World War II, he applied the lessons that he had learned from his own experience to the rehabilitation of large numbers of wounded soldiers.

Unfortunately, little of what is done in most weight rooms can be characterized as "progressive." Hearing of someone who performs the same number of repetitions with the same amount of resistance over and over again, workout after workout is not uncommon. Suppose that today you did 10 repetitions with 150 pounds on the seated row and a month later you are still doing 10 repetitions with 150 pounds. Did you increase your strength? Probably not. On the other hand, what if you were able to do 12 repetitions with 165 pounds in that exercise a month later? In this case, you performed 20% more repetitions with 10% more resistance — excellent progress over the course of one month.

Changes in the functional and structural abilities of your muscles depend upon the continued application of the Overload Principle. This means that your muscles must be overloaded with progressively greater demands if they are to continually increase in strength (and size). For this reason, your muscles must experience a workload that is increased steadily and systematically throughout the course of your strength-training program. This is often referred to as "progressive overload." Legend has it that Milo of Croton — a renowned warrior and athlete who won numerous prizes as a wrestler in the Olympic and Pythian Games in ancient Greece — periodically lifted a baby bull on his shoulders. As the bull increased in size and weight, so did Milo's strength. This crude method of progressive overload has been credited with the improvement of his legendary strength.

In order to overload your muscles, every time you train you must attempt to increase the resistance that you use or the repetitions that you perform in comparison to your previous workout. This can be viewed as a "double-progressive" technique (that is, resistance and repetitions). Stated otherwise, you must impose demands upon your muscles that they have not previously experienced by using more resistance or performing more repetitions. Exposing your muscles to progressively greater demands stimulates compensatory adaptation in response to the unaccustomed workload. Specifically, your muscles adapt to such demands by increasing in strength (and size). The extent to which this occurs then becomes a function of your inherited characteristics.

In a nutshell, the double-progressive technique would be implemented in this manner: If you reach muscular fatigue within your prescribed repetition range — say you did 18 repetitions and your range is 15 - 20 — you should repeat the weight for your next workout and try to improve upon the number of repetitions that you did; if you attain or surpass the maximal number of prescribed repetitions in an exercise — say you did 15 repetitions and your range is 10 - 15 — you should increase the weight for your next workout.

Your progressions in resistance need not be in Herculean leaps and bounds. You should increase the resistance in an amount with which you are comfortable . . . but the resistance that you use must always be challenging. Fortunately, this may be accomplished much more systematically than the method used by Milo and his growing bull. Your muscles will respond better if the progressions in resistance are about 5% or less — depending upon the degree to which the exercise was challenging. Suppose, for example, that an exercise has a repetition range of 15 - 20. If it was extremely difficult for you to do 20 repetitions, then you should make a slightly smaller progression in resistance than if it was fairly easy for you to do 21 or 22 repetitions.

When you make smaller progressions, you will hardly notice the slightly heavier resistance and your repetitions will not decline much if at all. In other words, it is much easier for your muscles to adapt to subtle increases in resistance than larger ones. Consider this example: Imagine that an exercise has a repetition range of 15 - 20 and you did 200/20 (200 pounds/20 repetitions). If you increase the resistance by 10% the next time you do that exercise (that is, to 220 pounds), you would probably notice the heavier weight and it could result in a "loss" of several repetitions. If you managed 16 repetitions, you must improve the number of repetitions by 25% (from 16 to 20) before you can make your next progression in resistance — which may prove to be a very difficult task. If, instead, you had increased the resistance by only 2.5

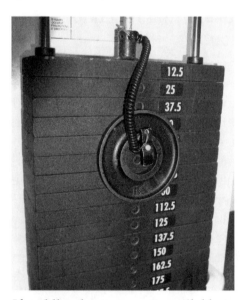

If saddle plates are not available to make progressions, you can take an Olympic plate and secure it to the weight stack of the machine by first inserting a selector pin through the hole in the Olympic plate and then into one of the selectorized plates.

pounds (that is, to 202.5 pounds), detecting the slightly heavier weight is not likely and you could probably get 202.5/20. Another 2.5-pound increase the next time you do that exercise may result in 205/20. Eventually, you might progress to the point where you were doing 220 pounds for at least 18 or 19 repetitions. So, you made the 20-pound increase in a number of small progressions instead of one large progression and, as a result, you allowed your muscles to adapt gradually to the resistance. And now, you may only need to increase your repetitions by one or two in order to make your next progression in resistance. This example is hypothetical, of course, but it would not be unusual for this to actually happen. The point is that your muscles will respond better to smaller increases in resistance rather than larger ones.

To make slight progressions in resistance, you can use smaller Olympic plates for exercises done with free weights and plate-loaded machines. Smaller plates are made that weigh as little as 1.25 and 2.5 pounds. If lighter plates are not available, you can simply hang something from the bar (or the movement arm of the machine) such as a small ankle weight. You can also use ankle weights to make progressions in dumbbell exercises. Making a five-pound progression from 25- to 30-pound dumbbells may not seem like much, but it represents an increase in resistance of 20%. Rather than increasing the resistance by such a large percentage, you can use the 25-pound dumbbells and put 1.25-pound ankle weights around your wrists. In effect, you would be using 26.25 pounds — a more reasonable progression in resistance of 5%.

Most selectorized machines have self-contained weight stacks with plates that usually weigh 10, 12.5, 15, 20 or 25 pounds. When using selectorized machines, you can make smaller progressions in the resistance by using saddle plates (or "add-on weights") that can be 1.25, 2.5 or 5 pounds. (Some selectorized machines enable you to make progressions in as little as one-pound increments without having to use or search for saddle plates.) If saddle plates are not available to make progressions, you can take an Olympic plate and secure it to the weight stack of the machine by first inserting a selector pin through the hole in the Olympic plate and then into one of the selectorized plates. This is often referred to as "pinning" an Olympic plate to the weight stack. You can also place any object that weighs about one or two pounds on top of a weight stack — as long as it will not fall off while you are using the equipment.

But again, the resistance you use must always be challenging. If you recently began a strength-training program or changed the exercises in your routine, it may take several workouts before you find a challenging weight. That is acceptable — simply continue to make progressions in the resistance as needed.

For those who want to achieve their physical potential, progressive overload has always been — and will always be — of utmost importance. To summarize: You must place a demand on your muscles that is beyond what they are accustomed. If you lifted 200 pounds today for 12 repetitions, then in a subsequent workout you either must attempt to do more repetitions or increase the resistance.

3. Perform the minimal number of sets necessary to produce an adequate level of muscular fatigue.

For many years, most people have done multiple-set training simply because that is what they have read or been told to do. The roots of this advice can be traced back to the time when virtually every authority in strength training came from the ranks of the professional strongmen, competitive weightlifters and, to a lesser degree, bodybuilders. In the early 1970s, the notion was advanced that people could improve their strength (and size) with far fewer sets — and, thus, less volume of training — than had been traditionally thought. The debate concerning the ideal number of sets has been raging ever since.

Know this: Science has been unable to determine how many sets of each exercise are necessary to produce optimal increases in muscular strength (and size). But the overwhelming majority of scientific evidence indicates that single-set training is at least as effective as multiple-set training. An exhaustive literature review in 1998 by Drs. Ralph Carpinelli and Robert Otto of Adelphi University (New York) and later reviews by Dr. Carpinelli examined all studies that compared different numbers of sets (dating back to 1956). Collectively, their research found five studies that showed multiple-set training was superior to single-set training *and 57 that did not.* Two of the studies that concluded multiple-set training was superior to single-set training involved only one exercise. One of these studies was done in 1962 and used only the bench press; the other study only reported data from the barbell squat. (Curiously, there were five other exercises used in the latter study, but no data were reported for them.)

So, the basis for performing single-set training — or a relatively low number of sets — has powerful and compelling support in the scientific literature. But is single-set training actually done in the "real world"? More importantly, can experienced or "trained" individuals obtain the same results from single-set training as they can from multiple-set training? The answer to both questions is "yes." The fact of the matter is that single-set training has been popular since the early 1970s. And to quote Drs. Carpinelli and Otto: "There is no evidence to suggest that the response to single or multiple sets in trained athletes would differ from that in untrained individuals." Indeed, numerous authorities advocate single-set training including the strength coaches for many collegiate and professional teams. Dan Riley — a veteran strength coach with more than 20 years of experience in the National Football League and another 8 years at the collegiate level (Penn State and Army) — notes, "Your goal must be to perform as few sets as possible while stimulating maximum gains. If performed properly, only one set is needed to generate maximum gains. In our standard routines, one set of each exercise is performed."

Recall that in order for your muscles to increase in strength (and size), they must experience an adequate level of fatigue. It is just that simple. Whether your muscles are fatigued in one set or several sets really does not matter — as long as you produce a sufficient level of muscular fatigue.

If doing one set of an exercise produces virtually the same results as several sets, then single-set training represents a more efficient means of strength training. After all, why perform several sets when you can obtain similar results from one set in a fraction of the time?

This is not to say that multiple-set training cannot be done. If performed properly, multiple-set training can certainly be effective in overloading your muscles. Multiple-set training has been used successfully by an enormous number of individuals for decades.

If you have a preference for multiple-set training, you should be aware of several things. First of all, simply doing multiple sets does not guarantee that you have overloaded your muscles. If the weights you use are not demanding enough then you will not produce sufficient muscular fatigue and your workout will not be as effective as possible. Remember, a large amount of low-intensity work does not necessarily produce an overload. So if you would rather do multiple sets, make sure that you are challenging your muscles with a progressive overload. In addition, keep in mind that performing too many sets (or too many exercises) can create a situation in which the demands on your muscles have surpassed your ability to recover. If this happens, your muscle tissue will be broken down in such an extreme manner that your body is unable to regenerate muscle tissue (essentially the resynthesis of myofibrillar proteins). Also, doing too many sets (or too many exercises) can significantly increase your risk of incurring an overuse injury such as tendinitis and bursitis. And as was indicated earlier, multiple-set training is relatively inefficient in terms of time so it is undesirable for time-conscious individuals. If you are like most people, time is a precious commodity — most people simply do not have much free time. The point is this: Keep your sets to the minimal amount that is needed to produce an adequate level of muscular fatigue.

To recap: Single-set training can be just as effective as multiple-set training. But again, if a single set of an exercise is to be productive, the set must be done with an appropriate level of intensity — that is, to the point of muscular fatigue. Your muscles should be thoroughly exhausted at the end of each exercise.

You should emphasize the *quality* of work done in the weight room rather than the *quantity* of work. Do not perform meaningless sets in the weight room — make every set count. The most efficient program is one that produces the *maximal* possible results in the *minimal* amount of time.

4. Reach concentric muscular fatigue within a prescribed number of repetitions or designated amount of time.

Determining an appropriate repetition range depends upon a number of factors and, even then, has some degree of variability. Understand first that strength training is not an aerobic activity that is comprised of long-term, low-intensity efforts. Rather, it is an anaerobic activity that is characterized by short-term, high-intensity efforts. Therefore, the duration of a series of repetitions — that is, a set — should be in the anaerobic domain. Efforts that last from a split second to several minutes are considered to be anaerobic (assuming, of course, that the level of effort is great enough to justify an anaerobic response). Since intense efforts at the lower end of this time frame carry a higher risk of injury and those at the upper end have a greater reliance on the aerobic pathways as the primary source of energy, narrowing the window of time to roughly 40 - 120 seconds represents a safe and effective range for strength training with higher durations assigned to larger muscles and lower durations to smaller ones. (Larger muscles — such as those in your hips and legs — should be trained for a slightly longer duration because of their greater size and work capacity.) Thus, time frames might be 90 - 120 seconds for a hip exercise, 60 - 90 seconds for a leg exercise, and 40 - 70 for an upper-body exercise.

Be that as it may, performing sets for a specified amount of time can be tricky and tedious. But you can use the aforementioned time frames to formulate repetition ranges. Suppose that you prefer to use a speed of movement that is six seconds per repetition. Dividing six seconds into the time frames that have been noted yields the following repetition ranges: 15 - 20 for your hips, 10 - 15 for your legs, and about 6 - 12 for your torso. (A repetition range of 8 - 12 is recommended for some upper-body exercises because of a rather abbreviated range of motion). Remember, these ranges are based upon six-second repetitions. Different repetition speeds require different repetition ranges. Suppose that you prefer to use a speed of movement that is 10 seconds per repetition. Dividing 10 seconds into the time frames that were mentioned earlier results in the following repetition ranges: 9 - 12 for your hips, 6 - 9 for your legs, and about 4 - 7 for your torso. Again, these ranges are based upon 10-second repetitions. (You are encouraged to experiment with different repetition speeds and vary them based upon your personal preferences and performance objectives.)

SPECIAL CONSIDERATIONS

The ranges that are based upon a six-second repetition will be effective for most SWAT officers. However, slightly higher repetition ranges are suggested for SWAT officers who are older or have orthopedic problems. In this case, repetition ranges might be 20 - 25 for exercises involving the hips, 15 - 20 for the legs, and 10 - 15 for the torso. These higher repetition ranges necessitate using somewhat lighter weights which reduces the orthopedic stress placed upon the bones, connective tissues, and joints. Slightly higher repetition ranges would also be recommended if you are doing rehabilitative training or have hypertension.

GENETIC CONSIDERATIONS

Because of their genetic make-up, some SWAT officers may require repetition ranges that are either a bit higher or lower than that prescribed for the general population. For example, some individuals have inherited a high percentage of slow-twitch (ST) fibers and would probably benefit more from strength training by doing slightly higher repetitions — such as those suggested in the previous paragraph — because their predominant muscle-fiber type is more suited for muscular endurance; conversely, some individuals have inherited a high percentage of fast-twitch (FT) fibers and would probably benefit more from strength training by doing slightly lower repetitions because their predominant muscle-fiber type is less suited for muscular endurance. Slightly lower repetition ranges of perhaps 12 - 15 for the hips, 9 - 12 for the legs, and 5 - 8 for the torso would likely produce a better response for someone who has inherited a high percentage of FT fibers in those bodyparts. In one study, sprinters trained with low repetitions, middle-distance runners with medium repetitions, and long-distance runners with high repetitions. All three groups experienced excellent and equal gains in strength. (In all likelihood, successful sprinters have inherited a high percentage of FT fibers and successful long-distance runners have inherited a high percentage of ST fibers.)

In a laboratory, fiber types can be distinguished by doing a biopsy in which a small plug of muscle tissue is removed and later analyzed under a microscope. Muscle biopsies are not ideal for assessing fiber types because they result in the destruction of tissue. Moreover, their accuracy has also been questioned. For one thing, fiber "headcounts" are subject to different interpretations. And since the distribution of fibers varies throughout a muscle, the site from which the biopsy is taken may not be indicative of the overall fiber-type mixture.

One way to guesstimate your fiber types is to assess their fatigue characteristics during a test of muscular endurance. To do this, you would determine the most weight that you can lift for one repetition — your one-repetition maximum (1-RM) — using good technique. Then, you would take 75% of your 1-RM and perform as many repetitions as possible using good technique. For instance, if you determine that your 1-RM is 80 pounds on the bicep curl, you would use 60 pounds for the endurance test [80 lbs x 0.75 = 60 lbs]. It would be expected that 10 repetitions could be done with 75% of a 1-RM. So if you can do a relatively high number of repetitions with 60 pounds (more than about 12), your biceps having a high percentage of ST fibers is likely; or if you can do a relatively low number of repetitions with 60 pounds (less than about 8), your biceps having a high percentage of FT fibers is likely. But remember: Since the composition and distribution of fibers can vary from muscle to muscle, the results of an endurance test are not necessarily reflective of your entire muscular system.

How much do individuals really vary in terms of their muscular endurance? Dr. Wayne Westcott reported data on 141 subjects who did an endurance test with 75% of their 1-RMs. Again, it would be expected that 10 repetitions could be done with this workload. And according to the data, the subjects completed an average of 10.5 repetitions. Yet only 16 of the 141 subjects (11.35%) did exactly 10 repetitions with 75% of their 1-RMs. Many of the subjects were in the neighborhood of 10 repetitions. In fact, 66 of the 141 subjects (46.81%) were able to do between 8 - 13 repetitions. But 75 of the 141 subjects (53.19%) did either less than 8 repetitions or more than 13. At the extremes, two subjects only did 5 repetitions and one managed 24. Researchers at the University of North Dakota also found wide variations in muscular endurance among 98 football players. In this study, four of the athletes had the same 1-RM in the bench press (300 pounds). But when tested with 75% of this weight (225 pounds), they did 9, 10, 11, and 16 repetitions. When tested with about 85% of their 1-RMs, six athletes did between 4 - 8 repetitions (6 repetitions would be expected). And when tested with about 92% of their 1-RMs, eight athletes did between 2 - 7 repetitions (4 repetitions would be expected). So while other factors may have certainly come into play, the influence that fiber types have on muscular endurance cannot be underemphasized or overlooked.

You can also make a logical guesstimate of your fiber types based upon performance. If you are successful in efforts that require muscular endurance, you probably have a high percentage of ST fibers and should perform slightly higher repetitions; similarly, if you are successful in efforts that require muscular strength (and/or power), you probably have a high percentage of FT fibers and should perform slightly lower repetitions.

Another way of making a reasonable guesstimate of your fiber types is to consider your muscular development. FT fibers have a much greater potential to increase in size (or hypertrophy) than ST fibers. Therefore, if you have a significant amount of muscular development, you probably have a high percentage of FT fibers; conversely, if you have an insignificant amount of muscular development, you probably have a high percentage of ST fibers (assuming, of course, that the low degree of muscular development is not the result of inactivity.)

One final point about FT and ST fibers: The use of lower repetitions is not suggested as a way to convert ST fibers to FT fibers. Nor is the use of higher repetitions suggested as a way to convert FT fibers to ST fibers. There is no scientific evidence that consistently supports the notion that ST fibers can be converted into FT fibers or vice versa. It appears as if one type of muscle fiber may take on certain metabolic characteristics of another type, but actual conversion does not occur. In other words, you cannot convert one fiber type into another any more than you can convert a pack mule into a racehorse. So if you were to take a pack mule and train it like a racehorse, you might get a slightly faster pack mule . . . but you will never get a racehorse. Performing different repetition ranges is done to maximize your response to training based upon your already-established predominant muscle-fiber type.

5. Perform each repetition with proper technique.

Most people have no understanding of — or pay little attention to — how they perform their repetitions. Regardless of the type of strength-training program that you utilize, a pro-

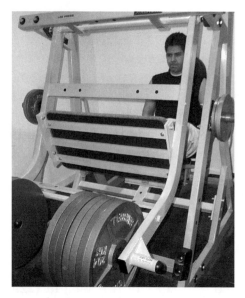

You should raise the weight in a deliberate, controlled manner without any explosive or jerking movements.

ductive program begins with a productive repetition. Remember, the repetition is the most basic and integral aspect of your strength-training program. If your repetitions are not productive, your sets will not be productive. If your sets are not productive, your workouts will not be productive. And if your workouts are not productive, your program will not be productive.

A repetition has four checkpoints: the positive (or raising) phase, the mid-range position, the negative (or lowering) phase, and the range of motion.

THE POSITIVE PHASE

A repetition starts with the raising of the weight. You should raise the weight in a deliberate, controlled manner without any explosive or jerking movements.

Raising a weight in a rapid, explosive fashion is not recommended for two main reasons. First of all, high-velocity repetitions that are performed in a ballistic manner are actually less productive than low-velocity repetitions that are performed in a controlled manner. Here is why: When weights are lifted explosively, the muscles produce tension during the initial part of the movement . . . but not for the last part. In simple terms, the weight is practically moving by itself. In effect, the load on the muscles is decreased — or eliminated — and so are the potential gains in muscular strength (and size).

Unfortunately, the reduced muscular loading that occurs as a result of excessive momentum is demonstrated in weight rooms across the world on a daily basis — albeit, in most cases, unknowingly. Have you ever seen others raise the weight so quickly on a leg-extension machine that the pad left their lower legs partway through the repetition? Well, think about it: The pad is attached to the movement arm of the machine that, in turn, is connected to the resistance by some means (such as a chain, cable, or strap). If the pad is no longer in contact with the lower legs, there is no load on the muscles. If there is no load on the muscles, there is no stimulus — or reason — for them to adapt. Sure, the lifter will obtain some benefit when the muscles were loaded during the first part of the repetition (when the pad was against the shins). However, the lifter will not obtain any benefit when the muscles were unloaded during the last part of the repetition (when the pad left the shins). There is no question that the more momentum is used to raise a weight, the less productive will be the repetitions.

Secondly — and more importantly — high-velocity repetitions also carry a greater risk of injury than low-velocity repetitions. Using an excessive amount of momentum to raise a weight increases the shearing forces encountered by a given joint; the faster a weight is raised, the higher these forces are amplified — especially at the point of explosion. In one study, a subject squatting with 80% of his four-repetition maximum incurred a 225-pound peak shearing force during a repetition that took 4.5 seconds to complete and a 270-pound peak shearing force during a repetition that took 2.1 seconds to complete. This is clear evidence that a slower speed of movement reduces the shearing forces on joints. When the forces exceed the structural limits of a joint, an injury occurs to the muscles, connective tissues, or bones. Also consider this statement made by Dr. Fred Allman, a past president of the American College of Sports Medicine: "It is even possible that many injuries . . . may be the result of weakened connective tissue caused by explosive training in the weight room." In other words, explosive lifting that is done *inside* the weight room can predispose you to a future injury *outside* the weight room. To ensure that your repetitions are safe and productive, it should take at least 1 - 2 seconds to raise the weight.

THE MID-RANGE POSITION

After raising the weight, you should pause briefly in the position of full muscular contraction or the mid-range position. Where is the mid-range position of a repetition? These two examples should help make it clear: When performing a leg extension, the mid-range position is where your legs are completely extended (or as straight as possible); when performing a bicep curl, the mid-range position is where your arms are completely flexed (or as bent as possible).

Most people are very weak in the mid-range position of a repetition because they rarely, if ever, emphasize it. Pausing momentarily in the mid-range position allows you to focus your attention on your muscles when they are fully contracted. Furthermore, a brief pause in the mid-range position permits a smooth transition between the raising and lowering of the weight, and helps reduce the influence of momentum. If you cannot pause momentarily in the mid-range position, it is likely that you are raising the weight too quickly and literally throwing it into position.

THE NEGATIVE PHASE

A repetition ends with the lowering of the weight. The importance of emphasizing the negative phase of a repetition cannot be overstated. Numerous studies have reported that repetitions involving both concentric and eccentric contractions produce greater increases in strength (and size) than those involving just concentric contractions.

Why? Because the same muscles that you use to raise a weight are also used to lower it. In a bicep curl, for example, your biceps are used in raising and lowering the weight. The only difference is that when you raise the weight, your biceps are shortening against the load and when you lower the weight, your biceps are lengthening against the load. So by emphasizing the lowering of the weight, each repetition becomes more productive. Because a "loaded" muscle lengthens as you lower the weight, emphasizing the negative phase of a repetition also ensures that the exercised muscle is being stretched properly and safely.

Recall that in a given exercise, your eccentric strength is greater than your concentric strength. This means that you can lower more weight than you can raise (again, in a given exercise). It stands to reason, that the lowering of the weight should take more time to complete than the raising of the weight. To ensure that your repetitions are safe and productive, it should take at least 3 - 4 seconds to lower the weight back to the starting position.

Effectively, it should take at least 4 - 6 seconds to perform a productive repetition. To a degree, the appropriate speed of movement for a repetition depends upon the range of motion (ROM) of the exercise. Keep in mind that all exercises do not have the same ROM. For instance, the elbow joint normally has a ROM that exceeds 135 degrees during the bicep curl and tricep extension; in comparison, the wrist joint normally has a ROM that is less than 90 degrees during wrist flexion and wrist extension. Hence, any exercise that has a relatively large ROM might take about six seconds per repetition; any exercise that has a relatively small ROM might take about four or five seconds per repetition.

Most authorities who are opposed to explosive, ballistic movements in the weight room consider a four- to six-second repetition to be an acceptable guideline for lifting a weight "under control" or "without an excessive amount of momentum." A 16-week study demonstrated a 50% increase in upper-body strength and a 33% increase in lower-body strength in a group that performed each repetition by raising the weight in two seconds and lowering it in four seconds. Furthermore, two different eight-week studies reported average increases in muscular strength of 55% in 17 subjects and 58.2% in 31 subjects. In both of these studies, the subjects used the same six-second guideline for raising and lowering the weight.

RANGE OF MOTION

A productive repetition is done throughout the greatest possible ROM that safety allows — from a full stretch to a full muscular contraction and back to a full stretch. Performing your repetitions throughout a full ROM will allow you to maintain (or perhaps increase) your flexibility. Moreover, it ensures that you are stimulating your entire muscle — not just a portion of it — thereby making the repetitions more productive. This point is underscored by many studies in which performing full-range repetitions were found to be a requirement for obtaining full-range effects. This does not imply that you should avoid limited-range repetitions altogether. During rehabilitative training, for example, you can exercise throughout a pain-free ROM and still manage to stimulate some gains in muscular strength (and size). Full-range repetitions are more productive, however, and should be performed whenever possible.

PRODUCTIVE REPETITIONS

Raising and lowering the weight in a deliberate, controlled manner without any jerking or explosive movements is much safer and more productive. To ensure that momentum did not play a significant role in the performance of the repetition, raise the weight in at least 1 - 2 seconds and lower it in at least 3 - 4 seconds. Remember, *how well* you lift a weight is more important than *how much* weight you lift. Your strength-training program will be safer and more productive when you perform each repetition with proper technique.

6. Strength train for no more than about one hour per workout.

When it comes to strength training, more is not necessarily better. Be aware that an inverse relationship exists between time and intensity: As the time of an activity increases, the level of intensity decreases. Stated otherwise, you cannot possibly train with a high level of intensity for a long period of time. Consider this analogy: With respect to anaerobic training, compare a workout that consists of eight 440-yard sprints to a workout that consists of twelve 440-yard sprints. In the workout with eight sprints, the time of your activity would be relatively low, but your level of intensity would be relatively high; in the workout with the twelve sprints, the time of your activity would be relatively high, but your intensity would be relatively low. So as the time of your activity goes up, your level of intensity goes down.

The fact is that you can train for a short period of time with a high level of intensity or a long period of time with a low level of intensity. But you cannot possibly train with a high level of intensity for a long period of time. In order to train with a fairly high level of intensity, you must train for a relatively brief period of time. If you lengthen the duration of your workout — by increasing either the number of exercises or sets that you normally perform — you must reduce your level of intensity. And, of course, using a lower level of intensity is not desirable.

Carbohydrates are your preferred fuel during intense activity. They circulate in your bloodstream as glucose, and are stored in your liver and muscles as glycogen. Most people exhaust their carbohydrate stores after about one hour of intense activity. For this reason, your strength training should be completed in approximately one hour or less. Under normal circumstances, if you are in the weight room for much more than about one hour then you are probably not training with an appropriate level of intensity. (Note that this one-hour window of time will dictate the number of exercises and sets that you can perform in your workout.)

The exact duration of your workout depends upon several factors such as the size of the facility, the amount of accessible equipment, the preparation for each exercise/set (such as adjusting seats, changing plates, moving pins, and so on), the number of people using the facility, the transition time between each exercise/set, and the availability of a training partner. Generally speaking, however, you should be able to complete your workout in no more than about one hour.

You can make your workouts more efficient — and more intense — by taking as little recovery as possible between exercises/sets. The length of your recovery interval depends upon your current level of fitness. Initially, you may require several minutes of recovery between exercises/sets to "catch your breath" or feel that you can produce a maximal level of effort. With improved fitness, your pace can be quickened to the point where you are moving as quickly as possible between exercises/sets. (The speed with which you do your repetitions should not be quickened — just the pace between exercises/sets.) Performing strength training with a minimal amount of recovery time between exercises and sets will elicit improvements in your metabolic fitness that cannot be approached by traditional multiple-set training. (Metabolic training is detailed in Chapter 12.)

7. Perform no more than about 15 exercises per workout.

Most SWAT officers can perform a comprehensive, total-body workout in the weight room using 15 exercises or less. The focal point for most of these exercises should be your major muscles (that is, your hips, legs, and torso). Include one exercise for your hips, hamstrings, quadriceps, calves/dorsi flexors, biceps, triceps, forearms, abdominals, and lower back. Because your shoulder joint allows movement at many different angles, you should perform two exercises for your chest, upper back (your "lats"), and shoulders. You can choose any exercises that you prefer to address those bodyparts.

Some SWAT officers may need to do slightly more than 15 exercises. For instance, if you also participate in a combat sport — such as football, rugby, boxing, judo, or wrestling — a comprehensive, total-body workout should include an additional 2 - 4 exercises for your neck to strengthen and protect your cervical area against possible catastrophic injury. (A general summary of the recommended volume of exercises and repetition ranges for SWAT officers is given in Figure 7.1.)

Once again, more is not necessarily better when it comes to strength training. Performing too many exercises can produce too much stress which will impede compensatory adaptation. A total-body workout that contains 20 exercises could be metabolically devastating for someone who has a low level of tolerance for strength training. And the more exercises that you perform, the more difficult it will be for you to maintain a desirable level of intensity.

This is not to say that you cannot do an extra exercise or two in order to emphasize a particular bodypart. As long as you continue to make improvements in your strength, you are not performing too many exercises. So if your workout consists of 20 exercises and you are making progress, then you are not overtraining. But if you start to level off or "plateau" in one or more exercises, it is probably because you are overtraining — the volume of your training has exceeded your ability to recover.

8. Train your muscles from largest to smallest.

The order in which you perform your exercises is essential in producing optimal improvements in your muscular strength (and size). The order of your exercises also determines which muscle(s) you emphasize or target.

As a rule of thumb, the idea is to train your most important muscles as early as possible in your workout. It stands to reason that you would want to address those muscles while you are fresh, both mentally as well as physically. In effect, your workout should begin with exercises that influence your largest muscles and proceed to those that involve your smallest ones.

THE LOWER BODY

Your largest and most powerful muscles are found in your lower body, specifically your hips and legs. What is the best order of exercise for training your lower body? Consider this: Multiple-joint movements that are done for your lower body — such as the leg press and deadlift — require the use of your upper legs for assistance. Your upper legs — your hamstrings and quadriceps — are the "weak link" in those exercises because they have a smaller amount of muscle mass. So if you fatigue your upper legs first, you will weaken an already

BODYPART	EXERCISES	REPETITION RANGE
Hips	1	15 - 20
Hamstrings	1	10 - 15
Quadriceps	1	10 - 15
Calves or Dorsi Flexors	1	10 - 15
Chest	2	6 - 12
Upper Back (or "lats")	2	6 - 12
Shoulders	2	6 - 12 or 8 - 12
Biceps	1	6 - 12
Triceps	1	6 - 12
Forearms	1	8 - 12
Abdominals	1	8 - 12
Lower Back	1	10 - 15
Neck (optional)	2 - 4	8 - 12

FIGURE 7.1: SUMMARY OF THE RECOMMENDED VOLUME OF EXERCISES AND REPETITION RANGES

Your workout should begin with exercises that influence your largest muscles and proceed to those that involve your smallest ones.

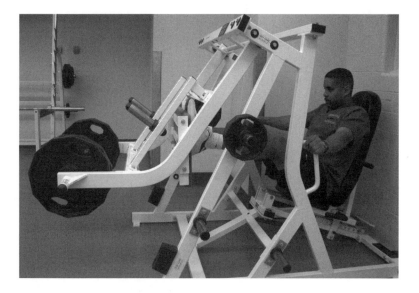

weak link, thereby limiting the workload placed on the muscles of your hips. Consequently, training your hips before your upper legs is usually best.

What would happen if you trained your upper legs immediately prior to your hips? In other words, what if you did the leg extension (for your quadriceps) and then the leg press (for your hips)? That order of exercise would be effective in really fatiguing your quadriceps, but you would not get much out of it for your hips.

That being said, do you follow your hips with an exercise for your hamstrings or one for your quadriceps? If you did an exercise for your hips that also provided a significant amount of work for your hamstrings — such as the hip extension or a hip-and-back movement — then you might want to train your quadriceps next, so that your hamstrings get a little breather and allow them to momentarily recover; on the other hand, if you did an exercise for your hips that also provided a great deal of work for your quadriceps — such as the leg press or deadlift — then you might want to train your hamstrings next so that your quadriceps receive a slight respite and allow them to momentarily recover.

But there is another reason why you might opt to exercise your hamstrings before your quadriceps. After performing the leg extension — and assuming that you did the exercise with a high level of effort — you should notice that your quadriceps are "pumped." This is because they became engorged with blood that was redirected from other areas of your body in order to deliver oxygen to your working muscles. With such a large amount of blood pooled in your quadriceps, it might be uncomfortable for you to do the prone leg curl since your "pumped" front thighs would be compressed against the back pad of the machine. This would not be an issue, however, if you elected to do the seated leg curl where there is no compression of the quadriceps.

After training your upper legs, you should proceed to your lower legs. If you train your calves (on the back part of your lower leg) and your dorsi flexors (on the front part of your lower leg) in the same workout, the order in which you do so really does not matter.

So in general, you should start with your hips and literally work down your legs. In other words, the best sequence would be hips, upper legs (hamstrings and quadriceps) and lower legs (calves or dorsi flexors).

THE UPPER BODY

Once you have exercised your lower body, attention can now be directed to your upper body. What is the best order of exercise for training your upper body? Not to be redundant, but from a conceptual standpoint, it sounds quite similar to what was discussed previously for your lower body. Multiple-joint movements that are performed for your upper body — such as the bench press, seated row, and seated press — require the use of your arms to assist the movement. Your arms — your biceps, triceps, and forearms — are the "weak link" in those exercises because they are smaller. So if you fatigue your arms first, you will weaken an already weak link thereby limiting the workload placed on the muscles of your torso. As a result, training your upper back before your biceps and your biceps before your forearms; and your chest and/or shoulders before your triceps is usually best.

What would happen if you trained your triceps immediately prior to your chest and/or shoulders or your biceps immediately prior to your upper back? In other words, what if you did the tricep extension and then the bench press or the bicep curl and then the seated row? Those orders of exercise would be effective in really fatiguing your arms, but you would not get much out of it for your chest or upper back.

Having said that, do you follow your torso with an exercise for your biceps or one for your triceps? If your last exercise before training your arms involved your chest and/or shoulders with assistance from your triceps — such as the bench press or seated press — then you might want to train your biceps next so that your triceps get some relief and allow them to momentarily recover; conversely, if your last exercise before training your arms involved your upper back with assistance from your biceps (and forearms) — such as the pull-up or seated row — then you might want to train your triceps next so that your biceps (and forearms) receive a slight respite and allow them to momentarily recover.

Here is another reason why you might want to train your biceps before your triceps: After doing a movement for your triceps — and assuming that you did it with a high level of effort — you should notice that the muscle is "pumped" (for the same reasons expressed earlier when discussing the quadriceps). With such a large amount of blood pooled in your triceps, it might not be comfortable for you to perform a bicep curl in which the backs of your arms are placed on a pad and your triceps are compressed. But this would not be a concern if you chose to perform the bicep curl in a position where there is no compression of the triceps.

You have at least two options for the order in which you train your chest, upper back, and shoulders. One way is to do all of the exercises for a given muscle — your chest, for example — and then move to the next muscle. Another way is to alternate "pushing" movements with "pulling" movements. (To avoid confusion, noting that all muscles "pull" when they contract is important; however, muscle contractions cause joints to extend and flex which produce movements that can be described as either "pushing" or "pulling.") Your chest, anterior portion of your shoulders, and triceps are involved during pushing movements while your upper back, posterior portion of your shoulders, and biceps are used during pulling movements.) In a "push-pull" application, you might do the following sequence for your torso: bench press (push), seated row (pull), incline press (push), underhand lat pulldown (pull), front raise (push), bent-over raise (pull), tricep extension (push), and bicep curl (pull). Performing all of the exercises for a given muscle before moving to another muscle will produce a large amount of fatigue since the muscle being exercised gets little relief (assuming, of course, that the time taken between exercises/sets is minimal); alternating exercises in a push-pull fashion allows one muscle to recover while another muscle is being trained. (You are encouraged to experiment with these two applications and vary them based upon your personal preferences and performance objectives.)

So in general, you should start with your chest, upper back, and shoulders and literally work down your arms. In other words, the best order of exercise would be torso (chest, upper back, and shoulders), upper arms (biceps and triceps), and lower arms (forearms).

THE MID-SECTION

Not fatiguing your mid-section early in your workout is important. Your abdominals stabilize your rib cage and serve as respiratory muscles during intense activity to facilitate forced expiration. Therefore, early fatigue of your abdominals would detract from your performance in other exercises that involve your larger, more powerful muscles.

Your lower back should be the very last muscle that you exercise. Fatiguing your lower back earlier in your workout will also hinder your performance in other exercises. So, the last area that you should train in your workout is your mid-section. And the best order of exercise would be to train your abdominals followed by your lower back.

THE NECK

SWAT officers who also participate in combat sports should train their neck muscles. If you include exercises for your neck in your workout, you can do them at the beginning, in the middle (following your lower-body movements), or at the end of your routine. However, training your neck at the beginning of your workout or just after you complete your lower-body exercises (that is, prior to beginning your upper-body exercises) makes most sense. This violates the "largest-to-smallest" rule, but at the end of your workout, you will be — and should be — physically and mentally drained. If you wait until this point to train your neck, you will be less likely to address this all-important area with a desirable level of effort or enthusiasm. Training your neck earlier in your workout when you are less fatigued will yield a more favorable response.

SUMMARY

In summary, the best order of exercise in a total-body workout would usually look like this: hips, upper legs (hamstrings and quadriceps), lower legs (calves or dorsi flexors), torso (chest, upper back, and shoulders), upper arms (biceps and triceps), lower arms (forearms), abdominals, and finally your lower back. If included, your neck should be trained at the beginning of your workout or just after you complete your lower-body exercises.

If you prefer to do a "split routine" — in which you "split" your bodyparts into several workouts instead of one total-body workout — the aforementioned order of exercise would still apply. In a workout that only targeted your chest, shoulders, and triceps, for example, you should still address those bodyparts from largest to smallest.

9. Strength train 2 - 3 times per week on nonconsecutive days.

Intense strength training places great demands on your muscles. In order to adapt to those demands, your muscles must receive an adequate amount of recovery between workouts.

Compensatory adaptation to the demands occurs during the recovery process. Believe it or not, your muscles do not get stronger during your workout . . . your muscles get stronger *after* your workout. If the demands are of sufficient magnitude, a muscle is literally torn.

Although these tears are quite small — microscopic, in fact — the recovery process is essential to allow the damaged muscle enough time to repair itself. Think of this as allowing a wound to heal. If you had a scab and picked at it every day, you would delay the healing process. But if you left it alone, you would permit the damaged tissue time to heal. So in a sense, the recovery following a workout is a process in which damaged tissue — in this case, muscle tissue — is healed.

There are individual variations in recovery ability — everyone has different levels of tolerance for exercise. However, a period of at least 48 hours is usually necessary for muscle tissue to recover sufficiently from an intense workout in the weight room. Keep in mind, too, that intense strength training relies heavily upon carbohydrates as the primary source of energy. Adequate recovery is required to return the carbohydrate (or glycogen) stores to their pre-training levels. Approximately 48 hours are also needed to replenish carbohydrate stores that are depleted as a result of intense physical exertion. As such, performing your strength training 2 - 3 times per week on nonconsecutive days (such as on Monday, Wednesday, and Friday) is suggested. This advice is consistent with the recommendation of the American College of Sports Medicine. (Note that this assumes total-body workouts.) Can you achieve significant improvements in strength by doing just two weekly workouts? Absolutely. In one study that involved 117 subjects, a group that trained two times per week experienced approximately 80 percent of the gains in strength of the group that trained three times per week.

An appropriate frequency (and volume) of strength training can be likened to doses of medication. In order for medicine to improve a condition, it must be taken at specific intervals and in certain amounts. Taking medicine at a greater frequency or in a larger quantity beyond what is needed can have harmful effects. Similarly, an "overdose" of strength training — in which workouts are done too often or have too much volume — can also be detrimental.

Most individuals respond well from three total-body workouts per week. But because of a low tolerance for strength training, others respond more favorably from two total-body workouts per week. (In rare circumstances, an individual may respond better from one total-body workout per week.) Performing any more than three "doses" of total-body workouts per week will gradually become counterproductive if the demands placed upon your muscles exceed your recovery ability.

Most authorities have suggested that a muscle begins to lose strength (and size) if it is not adequately stimulated within 48 - 96 hours of a previous workout. Some anecdotal reports suggest that it may be more than this time frame — at least for some individuals. Clearly, however, a loss of muscular strength (and size) will occur after some period of extended inactivity. If you are an athlete, continuing strength training even while in-season or while competing is important. However, the workouts should be reduced to twice a week, due to the increased activity level of practices and competitions. One workout should be done as soon as possible following a competition and another not within 48 hours of the next competition. So, an athlete who competes on Saturdays and Tuesdays should do strength training on Sundays and Wednesdays (or Thursdays — providing that it is not within 48 hours of the next competition). From time to time, an athlete may only be able to do strength training once per week because of a particularly heavy schedule such as competing three times in one week or several days in a row.

How do you know if your muscles have had an adequate amount of recovery? You should see a gradual improvement in the amount of resistance and/or number of repetitions that you are able to do over the course of several weeks. If not, then you are probably not getting enough recovery between your workouts — which, again, could be the result of performing too many sets, too many repetitions, or too many exercises. Remember, strength training will be effective if it provides an *overload* not an *overdose*.

THE SPLIT ROUTINE

A method that has been popularized by bodybuilders and competitive weightlifters is known as the "split routine." When using a split routine, the body is divided — or "split" — into different parts that are trained on different days. There are many possibilities for a split routine. One example would be to split the muscles such that the hips, legs, and mid-section are trained on Monday and Thursday; the chest, shoulders, and triceps on Tuesday and Friday; and the upper back, biceps, and forearms on Wednesday and Saturday. So in this split routine, each muscle would be trained twice per week during six workouts.

Despite the popularity of split routines, they are no more effective than total-body workouts. In a study involving 30 women, one group did a split routine consisting of four workouts per week (two for the upper body and two for the lower body) and another group did two total-body workouts per week. (A third group served as the control and did not train.) After 20 weeks of training, the researchers concluded that both protocols were equally effective in improving maximum strength, increasing lean-body mass, and decreasing body fat.

Split routines can be productive as long as they encourage progressive overload and provide adequate recovery. However, split routines often fall short in the latter area. If a split routine is designed correctly, a person will not train the same muscles two days in a row. Recall that it takes about 48 hours for your body to replenish its stockpiles of carbohydrates following an intense workout. (Again, carbohydrates are the principal fuel during intense exercise.) So if you trained your lower body on Monday with a desirable level of intensity, you exhausted much of your carbohydrate stores. Even if you train different muscles on Tuesday, your body may not have had enough time to fully recover those carbohydrate stores. Keep in mind, too, that even though you may train part of your body in a workout, you still stress your entire anaerobic energy pathways (which provide metabolic support for your efforts). Your energy systems do not recover in parts — they recover as a whole. The researchers in the aforementioned study that compared split routines to total-body workouts noted that doing fewer workouts per week in the weight room "would free more days for recovery or other types of training." This is an important consideration for competitive athletes who must invest significant amounts of time in aerobic, anaerobic, and skill training; it is an equally important consideration for SWAT officers who must invest significant amounts of time in various forms of physical and tactical training.

If you prefer to use a split routine, make sure that you group your muscles based upon their functions and relations with other muscles. For instance, your triceps and shoulders are used to train your chest, and your biceps and forearms are used to train your upper back. As such, muscles with common functions should be trained together.

One final point: From a performance perspective, split routines do not make sense because they are not specific to the muscular involvement in most physical activities. When you use a split routine, you train different muscles on different days. However, a selective use of muscles almost never happens during a physical activity. Rather, you are required to integrate all of your muscles at once. Therefore, it makes little sense for you to prepare for physical activities by training your muscles separately on different days.

10. Keep accurate records of your performance.

Many people believe that they do not need to use a workout card because they can remember their resistance and repetitions. In all likelihood, they have probably been lifting the same resistance and doing the same repetitions for so long that the numbers have become firmly entrenched in their long-term memories. The fact of the matter is that keeping written records that are accurate and detailed is absolutely critical, if strength training is to be as productive as possible.

Why? For one thing, records document the history of what you accomplished during every exercise of every strength session. Moreover, maintaining records is an extremely valuable tool to monitor your progress and make your workouts more meaningful. Records can also be used to identify exercises in which you have reached a plateau. In the unfortunate event of an injury, you can also gauge the effectiveness of your rehabilitative training if you have a record of your pre-injury levels of strength.

A workout card can have an infinite number of appearances and need not be elaborate. However, you should be able to record your bodyweight, the date of each workout, the resistance used for each exercise, the number of repetitions performed for each exercise, the order in which the exercises were completed, and any necessary seat adjustments.

Some of the more common exercises can be listed on the workout card (such as the leg extension, bench press, and bicep curl). Or, the workout card can contain blank spaces so that you can fill in your own menu of exercises. The recommended repetition ranges should also be given for each exercise. (Appendices C and D contain workout cards for single-set training and multiple-set training, respectively.)

RECORDING DATA

Perhaps the best way to illustrate the correct way for you to record your data on a workout card — as well as to understand the application of the double-progressive technique — is to detail several imaginary workouts. In the upcoming discussion, please refer to Figure 7.2 where data from four workouts (using single-set training) have been recorded for the period of January 3 - 10. Due to space constraints, the data for our fictional SWAT officer — Officer Tom DeLorme — have been limited to details of the first eight exercises in his total-body workout. (It must be stressed that a total-body workout normally includes more exercises than are about to be discussed in the following illustration.)

January 3: Officer DeLorme started his workout by performing neck lateral flexion (to the right and left). He was able to do 11 repetitions with 105 pounds in both exercises. After training his neck, he performed the leg press as his hip exercise. Note that he used 275 pounds and managed 18 repetitions. He then did 15 repetitions on the prone leg curl with 100 pounds. Using 160 pounds on the leg extension, he performed 10 repetitions. Officer DeLorme's third and final leg exercise (his sixth overall) was the seated calf raise. In this movement, he did 17 repetitions with 120 pounds. In the bench press, he managed 8 repetitions with 180 pounds. As a second chest exercise (his eighth overall), the officer chose the bent-arm fly. Here, he performed 8 repetitions with a pair of 40-pound dumbbells.

January 5: Two days later during his second workout of the week, Officer DeLorme again began with his neck exercises. This time, however, he elected to perform two different exercises: neck flexion and neck extension (using manual resistance or "MR"). After completing these two exercises, the officer moved to the leg press. Because he was not able to do the maximal number of repetitions during his previous workout, note that he used the same resistance. On this date, however, he performed 20 repetitions with 275 pounds — an improvement of 2 repetitions. In his previous workout, he was able to do the maximal number of repetitions on the prone leg curl, so he increased the resistance by 2.5 pounds — from 100 to 102.5. The officer managed 14 repetitions with the new resistance. During the leg extension, he again used 160 pounds, but was able to do 11 repetitions — one more than the last time. Since Officer DeLorme exceeded the maximal number of repetitions on the seated calf raise in his previous workout, he increased the resistance from 120 to 122.5 pounds and did 16 repetitions with it. In the bench press, he repeated 180 pounds and managed 9 repetitions — an improvement of one repetition compared to his preceding workout. During the bent-arm fly, the officer again used 40-pound dumbbells and improved his repetitions from 8 to 9.

January 7: Officer DeLorme started off his third and final workout of the week by doing neck lateral flexion (again to the right and left). Since he did not do the maximal number of repetitions the last time that he performed those two exercises, he used the same resistance, but was able to do 12 repetitions. His next exercise was the leg press in which he increased the resistance by 5 pounds — from 275 to 280 — and did 19 repetitions. For the second consecutive workout, the officer managed 14 repetitions with 102.5 pounds on the prone leg curl. On the leg extension, he used the same resistance as the previous workout — 160 pounds — but was able to do one more repetition. He increased the resistance on the seated calf raise from 122.5 to 125 pounds and performed 15 repetitions. The officer again used 180 pounds on the bench press and was able to perform 10 repetitions — one more than his previous workout. In the bent-arm fly, he used 40-pound dumbbells again and did the same number of repetitions as the last time.

January 10: During his first workout of the second week, Officer DeLorme began his workout with neck flexion and neck extension (using manual resistance). On this date, he decided to change his hip exercise from the leg press to the deadlift (with a trap bar) and was able to do 20 repetitions with 205 pounds. Next, he moved to the prone leg curl and performed 15 repetitions with 102.5 pounds — an improvement of one repetition compared to his previous workout. Using 160 pounds on the leg extension, he again did 12 repetitions. Officer DeLorme completed his lower-body exercises by doing 14 repetitions on the seated calf raise with an increased resistance of 127.5 pounds. In the bench press, he again did 10 repetitions with 180 pounds. And in the bent-arm fly, he performed 10 repetitions — one more than in his last workout — with the 40-pound dumbbells.

January 12: The resistance for each exercise has been recorded for this workout based upon Officer DeLorme's performance in his prior workout. Note that the resistance was increased on neck lateral flexion (right and left) as well as the deadlift and prone leg curl because he performed the maximal number of repetitions during his previous workout. The resistance remained the same on the leg extension, bench press, and bent-arm fly. Finally, the officer chose to perform dorsi flexion (with manual resistance) as his lower-leg exercise instead of the seated calf raise.

The bottom line: Do not underestimate the importance of using a workout card in making your strength training more productive and more meaningful.

Name: Tom DeLorme			Date	Mon. 01/03	Wed. 01/05	Fri. 01/07	Mon. 01/10	Wed. 01/12
			BW					
	Exercise	Reps	Seat	wt / reps	wt / reps	wt / reps	wt / reps	wt / reps
Neck (2-4)	Neck Lateral Flexion/R	8-12	5	105 / 11		105 / 12		107.5
	Neck Lateral Flexion/L	8-12	5	105 / 11		105 / 12		107.5
	Neck Flexion	8-12	5		MR / 12		MR / 12	
	Neck Extension	8-12	5		MR / 12		MR / 12	
Hips (1)	Leg Press	15-20	7½	275 / 18	275 / 20	280 / 19		
	Deadlift	15-20					205 / 20	207.5
Upper Legs (2)	Prone Leg Curl	10-15		100 / 15	102.5 / 14	102.5 / 14	102.5 / 15	102.5
	Leg Extension	10-15	3½	160 / 10	160 / 11	160 / 12	160 / 12	160
Lower Legs (1)	Seated Calf Raise	10-15		120 / 17	122.5 / 16	125 / 15	127.5 / 14	
	Dorsi Flexion	10-15						MR
Chest (2)	Bench Press	6-12		180 / 8	180 / 9	180 / 10	180 / 10	180
	Bent-Arm Fly	6-12	5	40 / 8	40 / 9	40 / 9	40 / 10	40

FIGURE 7.2: RECORDING WORKOUT DATA (SINGLE-SET TRAINING)

Chapter 8
Free-Weight Exercises

In 1902, the Milo Barbell Company — founded by Alvin Calvert — manufactured and sold the first adjustable, plate-loading barbell in the United States. The plate-loading barbell — patterned after the Berg-Hantel barbell from Germany — was a tremendous break-through in weight training. For the first time, a barbell could be loaded in a relatively short period of time with any amount of weight that was desired. Previously, a different barbell was necessary for a different weight.

Today, free weights are extremely popular pieces of equipment that are inexpensive and can last for years with little or no maintenance. Most commercial fitness centers outfit their strength-training areas with at least some free-weight equipment.

ADVANTAGES OF FREE WEIGHTS

Free weights have the following advantages over machines:

1. If you are trying to outfit a weight room with a limited or tight budget, the most important consideration in your choice of equipment may very well be the cost. Machines are generally much more expensive than free weights. You could easily pay more than $40,000 for a complete "line" of state-of-the-art selectorized equipment (10 - 12 machines). That same number of plate-loaded machines would be much less expensive, but remember a possible "hidden" cost: A few thousand pounds of plates may need to be purchased to serve as the resistance for the machines. A considerable amount of free-weight equipment could be purchased for much less of an investment.

2. Most machines that are geared toward commercial use are designed to perform only one or two functions. A bicep-curl machine, for example, can only be used to exercise the biceps. In comparison, a bar and several hundred pounds of plates can allow you to perform movements for just about every major muscle in your body. So, free weights offer more variety per dollar.

3. When it comes to free weights, "one size fits all" can be applied. Indeed, free weights can accommodate just about everyone regardless of their size from the tallest SWAT officer to the shortest. On the other hand, those who are at an extreme in terms of skeletal height and/or limb length may not be able to fit properly on some machines. For this reason, machines present a major drawback for some individuals who wish to strengthen their muscles.

4. Having to balance free weights requires a greater involvement of synergistic muscles. (A muscle is said to act as a "synergist" if it is used to prevent an undesired movement of a joint.) Keep in mind, though, that the significance of this remains unclear. Ken Mannie, a strength and conditioning coach with more than 15 years of experience at the collegiate level (including stints at the University of Toledo and Michigan State University), points out that "the rate and level at which [the synergistic muscles] act merit additional study."

THE USE OF DUMBBELLS

A dumbbell is essentially a shorter version of a barbell that is intended for use with one hand. There are several advantages of using dumbbells in a workout. First of all, dumbbells can provide variety to your routine. Variety can be furnished in at least two ways. For one thing, every exercise that can be performed with a barbell can also be performed with dumbbells. This means that every barbell exercise has a dumbbell counterpart that can be used as an alternative movement. Secondly, you have the added option of being able to use a different grip with dumbbells. For example, you can perform a dumbbell bench press with a "parallel grip" (that is, your palms facing each other) as well as the traditional bench-press grip.

Perhaps the biggest advantage in using dumbbells, however, is that each of your limbs must work independently of the other. Most people are often stronger (and more flexible) on one side of their body than the other. Usually, this is not a significant difference. But when there is a gross difference in the strength between limbs, the use of dumbbells is highly recommended. This is also an important consideration for rehabilitative strength training. (Chapter 13 discusses rehabilitative strength training in great detail.) In this case, an individual may even have to work one limb at a time while using a lighter weight for the weaker limb. In short, the advantages of dumbbells are pure and simple: variety and an independent workload.

THE EXERCISES

This chapter will describe and illustrate the safest and most productive exercises that can be performed with free weights. Included in the discussions of each exercise are the muscle(s) involved (if more than one muscle is involved, the first muscle listed is the prime mover), suggested repetitions (the time that the targeted muscles should be loaded is shown in parentheses), type of movement, starting position, performance description, and training tips for making the exercise safer and more productive. The exercises described in this chapter are the deadlift, standing calf raise, bench press, incline press, decline press, dip, bent-arm fly, bent-over row, chin, pull-up, pullover, seated press, lateral raise, front raise, bent-over raise, internal rotation, external rotation, upright row, shoulder shrug, bicep curl, tricep extension, wrist flexion, wrist extension, finger flexion, sit-up, knee-up, side bend, and back extension.

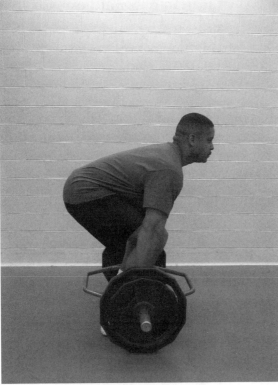

Start/Finish Position

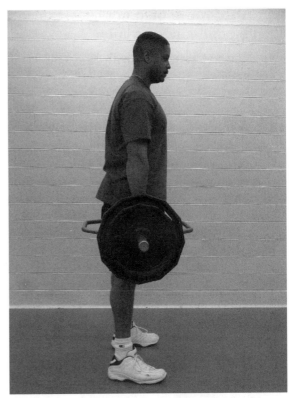

Mid-Range Position

DEADLIFT

Muscles Involved: gluteus maximus (buttocks), hamstrings, quadriceps, and erector spinae (lower back)

Suggested Repetitions: 15 - 20 (or 90 - 120 seconds)

Type of Movement: multiple joint

Starting Position: Step inside the opening of the trap bar and spread your feet slightly wider than shoulder-width apart. Reach down and grasp the bar on the outside of your legs with a "parallel grip" (your palms facing each other). Lower your hips until your upper legs are almost parallel to the floor. Flatten your back and look up slightly. Place most of your bodyweight on your heels, not on the balls of your feet.

Performance Description: Stand upright by straightening your legs and torso. Pause briefly in this mid-range position (your hips, legs, and lower back extended), and then lower the weight under control to the starting position (your hips, legs, and lower back flexed) to ensure an adequate stretch.

Training Tips:

- Do not lift your hips too early as you perform this exercise. Raising your hips too soon negates their effectiveness and causes you to perform the exercise almost entirely with your lower back. Ideally, your hips, legs, and lower back should work together. However, your hips and legs should do most of the work.

- You should not "lock" or "snap" your knees in the mid-range position of a repetition. This removes the load from the target muscles and may hyperextend your knees.

Also, you should not hyperextend your torso (that is, lean backward excessively) in the mid-range position.

- Keep your arms straight, head up, and back relatively flat as you perform this exercise.

- Do not bounce the weight off the floor between repetitions.

- You can also perform this exercise with an Olympic bar and dumbbells. When doing this exercise with an Olympic bar, you should use an "alternating grip" (your dominant palm forward and nondominant palm backward); when doing this exercise with dumbbells, you should use a "parallel grip" and keep the weights at your sides.

- You can use wrist straps if you have difficulty in maintaining your grip on the bar (or the dumbbells).

- This exercise may be contraindicated if you have low-back pain, hyperextended elbows, or an exceptionally long torso and/or legs.

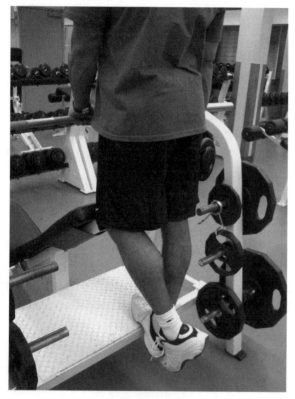

Start/Finish Position

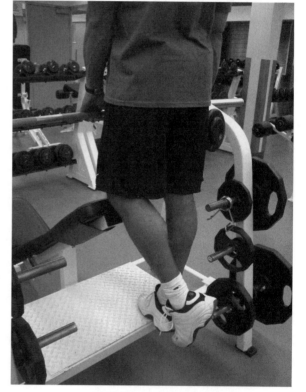

Mid-Range Position

STANDING CALF RAISE

Muscles Involved: gastrocnemius (calves)

Suggested Repetitions: 10 - 15 (or 60 - 90 seconds)

Type of Movement: single joint

Starting Position: Hold a dumbbell in your right hand and stand on something that is solid and at least several inches high. Hold onto a piece of equipment with your left hand to maintain your balance and position your leg so that the ball of your right foot is on the edge. Lower your right heel and cross your left foot behind your right ankle.

Performance Description: Keep your right leg straight and rise up onto your toes as high as possible. Pause briefly in this mid-range position (your ankle extended), and then lower the weight under control to the starting position (your heel near the floor) to ensure a proper stretch. After performing a set with your right leg, repeat the exercise for the other side of your body (with the dumbbell in your left hand).

Training Tips:

- You will need to stand on something at least several inches high in order to obtain a better stretch.

- Using your hip and leg as you perform this exercise is natural. However, movement of your hip and leg should not be excessive or used to raise the weight — movement should only occur around your ankle joint.

- Traditionally, this exercise is done with a weight placed on the shoulders — either a barbell or the movement arm of a machine. This should be avoided whenever possible, however, because it compresses the spinal column.

- You can use wrist straps if you have difficulty in maintaining your grip on the dumbbell.

- This exercise may be contraindicated if you have shin splints.

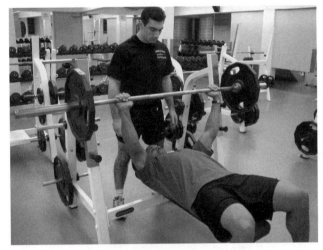

Start/Finish Position

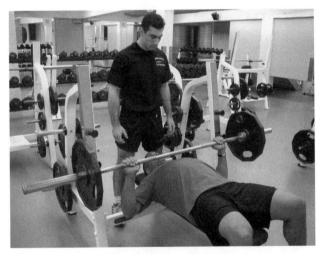

Mid-Range Position

BENCH PRESS

Muscles Involved: chest, anterior deltoid, and triceps

Suggested Repetitions: 6 - 12 (or 40 - 70 seconds)

Type of Movement: multiple joint

Starting Position: Lie down on the back pad of the bench and place your feet flat on the floor. Grasp the bar and spread your hands slightly wider than shoulder-width apart. Lift the bar out of the uprights or have a spotter give you assistance. Keep your arms almost fully extended (that is, without "locking" your elbows).

Performance Description: Lower the bar under control until it touches the middle part of your chest. Without bouncing the weight off your chest, push the bar up to the starting position (your arms almost fully extended).

Training Tips:

- For reasons of safety, you should not perform this exercise without a spotter.

- You should not use an excessively wide grip since this will reduce your range of motion.

- Keep your hips flat on the back pad and your feet flat on the floor as you perform this exercise. If you have low-back pain, you can place your feet on the end of the back pad or a stool. This will flatten your lumbar area against the back pad and reduce the stress in your low-back region.

- You should not "lock" or "snap" your elbows in the mid-range position of a repetition. This removes the load from the target muscles and may hyperextend your elbows.

- Do not bounce the weight off your chest between repetitions.

- You should move the bar upward and backward as you press the weight.

- You can also perform this exercise with dumbbells which can offer a different range of motion, alleviating stress on the shoulder joints and tendons.

- This exercise may be contraindicated if you have shoulder-impingement syndrome or a rotator cuff injury.

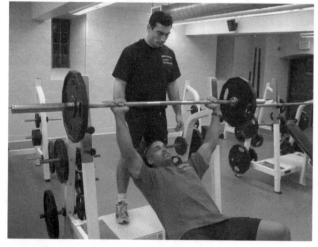
Start/Finish Position

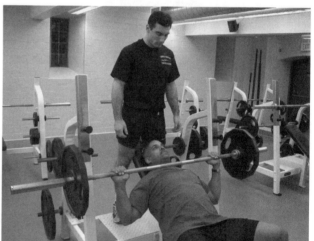
Mid-Range Position

INCLINE PRESS

Muscles Involved: chest (upper portion), anterior deltoid, and triceps

Suggested Repetitions: 6 - 12 (or 40 - 70 seconds)

Type of Movement: multiple joint

Starting Position: Sit down on the seat pad of the bench, lie back against the back pad, and place your feet flat on the floor (or against a footrest if one is provided). Grasp the bar and space your hands slightly wider than shoulder-width apart. Lift the bar out of the uprights or have a spotter give you assistance. Keep your arms almost fully extended (that is, without "locking" your elbows).

Performance Description: Lower the bar under control until it touches the upper part of your chest (near your collarbones). Without bouncing the weight off your chest, push the bar up to the starting position (your arms almost fully extended).

Training Tips:

- For reasons of safety, you should not perform this exercise without a spotter.

- You should not use an excessively wide grip since this reduces your range of motion.

- Keep your hips flat on the seat pad and your feet flat on the floor (or a footrest if one is provided) as you perform this exercise. If you have low-back pain, you can place your feet on a stool (if a footrest is not provided). This will flatten your lumbar area against the back pad and reduce the stress in your low-back region.

- You should not "lock" or "snap" your elbows in the mid-range position of a repetition. This removes the load from the target muscles and may hyperextend your elbows.

- Do not bounce the weight off your chest between repetitions.

- You should move the bar upward and backward as you press the weight.

- You can also perform this exercise with dumbbells which can offer a different range of motion, alleviating stress on the shoulder joints and tendons.

- This exercise may be contraindicated if you have shoulder-impingement syndrome or a rotator cuff injury.

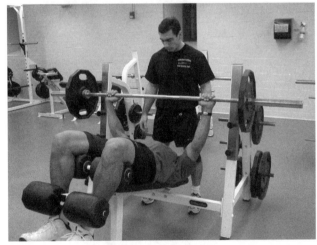

Start/Finish Position

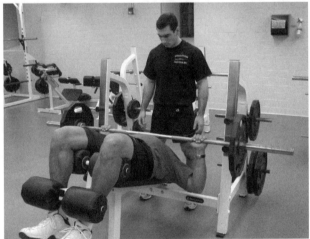

Mid-Range Position

DECLINE PRESS

Muscles Involved: chest (lower portion), anterior deltoid, and triceps

Suggested Repetitions: 6 - 12 (or 40 - 70 seconds)

Type of Movement: multiple joint

Starting Position: Lie down on the back pad of the bench and place your lower legs behind the roller pads. Grasp the bar and space your hands slightly wider than shoulder-width apart. Lift the bar out of the uprights or have a spotter give you assistance. Keep your arms almost fully extended (that is, without "locking" your elbows).

Performance Description: Lower the bar under control until it touches the lower part of your chest (near the tip of your breastbone). Without bouncing the weight off your chest, push the bar up to the starting position (your arms almost fully extended).

Training Tips:

- For reasons of safety, you should not perform this exercise without a spotter.

- You should not use an excessively wide grip since this will reduce your range of motion.

- Keep your hips flat on the back pad as you perform this exercise.

- You should not "lock" or "snap" your elbows in the mid-range position of a repetition. This removes the load from the target muscles and may hyperextend your elbows.

- Do not bounce the weight off your chest between repetitions.

- You should move the bar upward and backward as you press the weight.

- You can also perform this exercise with dumbbells which can offer a different range of motion, alleviating stress on the shoulder joints and tendons.

- This exercise may be contraindicated if you have shoulder-impingement syndrome or a rotator cuff injury.

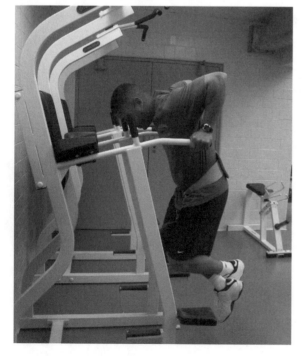 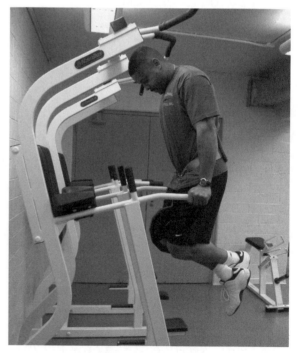

Start/Finish Position   *Mid-Range Position*

DIP

Muscles Involved: chest (lower portion), anterior deltoid, and triceps

Suggested Repetitions: 6 - 12 (or 40 - 70 seconds)

Type of Movement: multiple joint

Starting Position: Grasp the handles with a "parallel grip" (your palms facing each other). Bend your arms such that your upper arms are roughly parallel to the floor. Lift your feet off the floor, bend your knees, and cross your ankles.

Performance Description: Push yourself up until your arms are almost fully extended (that is, without "locking" your elbows). Pause briefly in this mid-range position (your arms almost fully extended), and then lower your body under control to the starting position (your arms flexed) to obtain a sufficient stretch.

Training Tips:

- Avoid swinging your body back and forth as you perform this exercise — movement should only occur around your shoulder and elbow joints.

- You should not "lock" or "snap" your elbows in the mid-range position of a repetition. This removes the load from the target muscles and may hyperextend your elbows.

- If you can do 12 repetitions or more in strict form using your bodyweight, you can increase the workload on your muscles by attaching extra weight to your waist, performing the exercise with a slower speed of movement or having a spotter apply manual resistance to your waist.

- After reaching concentric muscular fatigue, you can overload your muscles further by stepping up to the mid-range position and lowering your body under control to the starting position for 3 - 5 negative repetitions.

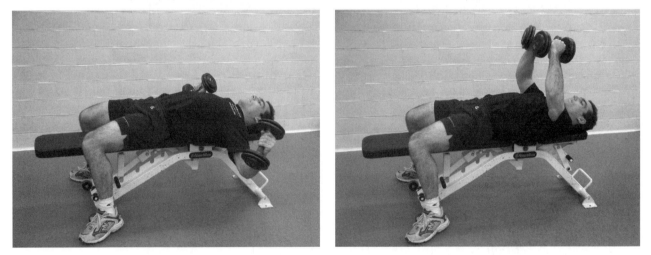

Start/Finish Position   *Mid-Range Position*

BENT-ARM FLY

Muscles Involved: chest and anterior deltoid

Suggested Repetitions: 6 - 12 (or 40 - 70 seconds)

Type of Movement: single joint

Starting Position: Sit down near the end of the back pad of the bench, reach down, and grasp two dumbbells. Lift the dumbbells, lie down on the back pad, and place your feet flat on the floor. Position the dumbbells on both sides of your torso so that they are even with your chest. (One or two spotters can assist you in positioning heavy dumbbells.) Point your palms toward your knees and move the dumbbells up and away from your chest until the angle between your upper and lower arms is about 90 degrees.

Performance Description: Without significantly changing the angle between your upper and lower arms, bring the dumbbells together above your chest. Pause briefly in this mid-range position (the dumbbells directly over your chest), and then return the weights under control to the starting position (the dumbbells away from each other) to obtain a sufficient stretch.

Training Tips:

• Maintain about a 90-degree angle between your upper and lower arms as you raise and lower the dumbbells. (Imagine that you are hugging a tree.) If you straighten your arms as you raise the dumbbells, you will change the exercise from a bent-arm fly into a bench press.

• Keep your hips flat on the back pad and your feet flat on the floor as you perform this exercise. If you have low-back pain, you can place your feet on the end of the back pad or a stool. This will flatten your lumbar area against the back pad and reduce the stress in your low-back region.

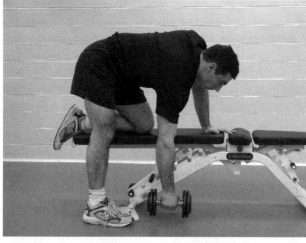

Start/Finish Position

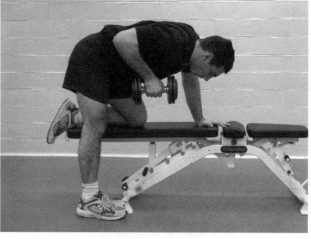

Mid-Range Position

BENT-OVER ROW

Muscles Involved: upper back ("lats"), biceps, and forearms

Suggested Repetitions: 6 - 12 (or 40 - 70 seconds)

Type of Movement: multiple joint

Starting Position: Place your left hand and left knee on the back pad of the bench, and position your right foot on the floor at a comfortable distance from the bench. Reach down with your right hand and grasp a dumbbell. Lift the dumbbell slightly off the floor and keep your right arm straight. Your right palm should be facing the bench.

102

Performance Description: Keep your upper arm close to your torso and pull the dumbbell up to your right shoulder. Pause briefly in this mid-range position (your arm flexed), and then return the dumbbell under control to the starting position (your arm fully extended) to ensure an adequate stretch. After performing a set with your right arm, repeat the exercise for the other side of your body (with your right hand and right knee on the back pad for support).

Training Tips:

- Changing the position of your shoulder as you perform this exercise is natural. However, movement of your shoulder should not be excessive or used to throw the dumbbell — movement should only occur around your shoulder and elbow joints.

- You can also do this exercise with your upper arm positioned farther away from your torso. Keep in mind, however, that this will produce a greater involvement of your posterior deltoid and trapezius. In this case, your upper arm would be almost perpendicular to your torso in the mid-range position and your palm would be facing backward slightly.

- You can use wrist straps if you have difficulty in maintaining your grip on the dumbbell.

- This exercise may be contraindicated if you have a hyperextended elbow.

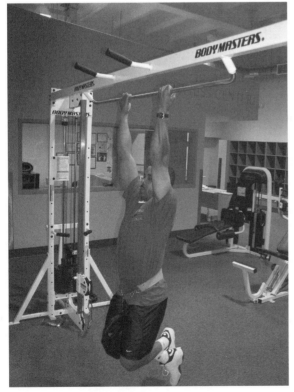

Start/Finish Position

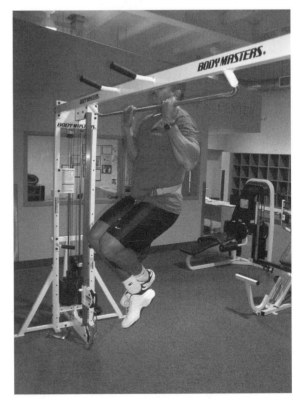

Mid-Range Position

CHIN

Muscles Involved: upper back ("lats"), biceps, and forearms

Suggested Repetitions: 6 - 12 (or 40 - 70 seconds)

Type of Movement: multiple joint

Starting Position: Reach up, grasp the bar with your palms facing you, and space your hands approximately shoulder-width apart. Bring your body to a "dead hang" and cross your ankles.

Performance Description: Pull yourself up so that your upper chest touches the bar and draw your elbows backward. Pause briefly in this mid-range position (your arms flexed), and then lower your body under control back to the starting position (your arms fully extended) to obtain a proper stretch.

Training Tips:

- Avoid swinging your body back and forth as you perform this exercise — movement should only occur around your shoulder and elbow joints.

- Touching your upper chest to the bar rather than your chin will increase your range of motion. Drawing your elbows backward in the mid-range position will increase the workload performed by your upper back.

- If you cannot do 6 repetitions in strict form using your bodyweight, you can exercise the same muscles in a similar fashion by performing the underhand lat pulldown (as described in Chapter 9).

- If you can do 12 repetitions or more in strict form using your bodyweight, you can increase the workload on your muscles by attaching extra weight to your waist, performing the exercise with a slower speed of movement, or having a spotter apply manual resistance to your waist.

- After reaching concentric muscular fatigue, you can overload your muscles further by stepping up to the mid-range position, and lowering your body under control to the starting position for 3 - 5 negative repetitions.

- You can use wrist straps if you have difficulty in maintaining your grip on the bar.

- This exercise may be contraindicated if you have hyperextended elbows.

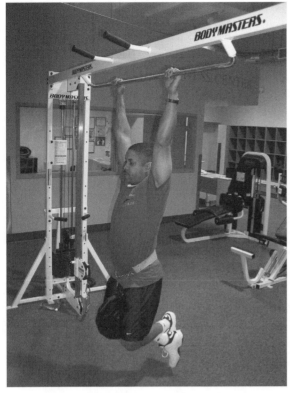

Start/Finish Position

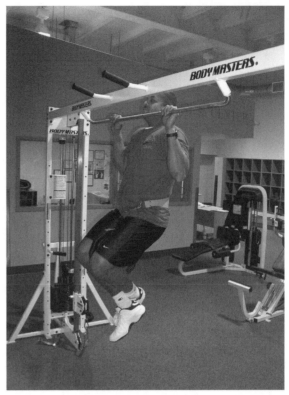

Mid-Range Position

PULL-UP

Muscles Involved: upper back ("lats"), biceps, and forearms

Suggested Repetitions: 6 - 12 (or 40 - 70 seconds)

Type of Movement: multiple joint

Starting Position: Reach up, grasp the bar with your palms facing away from you, and space your hands several inches wider than shoulder-width apart. Bring your body to a "dead hang" and cross your ankles.

Performance Description: Pull yourself up so that your upper chest touches the bar and draw your elbows backward. Pause briefly in this mid-range position (your arms flexed), and then lower your body under control to the starting position (your arms fully extended) to obtain an adequate stretch.

Training Tips:

• Avoid swinging your body back and forth as you perform this exercise — movement should only occur around your shoulder and elbow joints.

• You should not use an excessively wide grip since this will reduce your range of motion.

• Touching your upper chest to the bar rather than your chin will increase your range of motion. Drawing your elbows backward in the mid-range position will increase the workload performed by your upper back.

• If you cannot do 6 repetitions in strict form using your bodyweight, you can exercise the same muscles in a similar fashion by performing the overhand lat pulldown (as described in Chapter 9).

- If you can do 12 repetitions or more in strict form using your bodyweight, you can increase the workload on your muscles by attaching extra weight to your waist, performing the exercise with a slower speed of movement, or having a spotter apply manual resistance to your waist.

- After reaching concentric muscular fatigue, you can overload your muscles further by stepping up to the mid-range position, and lowering your body under control to the starting position for 3 - 5 negative repetitions.

- Performing pull-ups with an overhand grip (your palms facing away from you) is not as biomechanically efficient as doing chins with an underhand grip (your palms facing toward you). But this exercise is still quite productive when performed in the manner described above.

- You can use wrist straps if you have difficulty in maintaining your grip on the bar.

- You can also perform this exercise by pulling yourself up so that the upper part of your trapezius touches the bar behind your head. However, this may be contraindicated if you have shoulder-impingement syndrome. This exercise may also be contraindicated if you have hyperextended elbows.

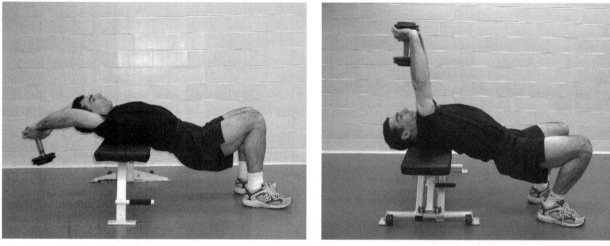

Start/Finish Position   *Mid-Range Position*

PULLOVER

Muscles Involved: upper back ("lats")

Suggested Repetitions: 6 - 12 (or 40 - 70 seconds)

Type of Movement: single joint

Starting Position: Sit down near the middle of the back pad of the bench, reach down and grasp a dumbbell. Lift the dumbbell and lie down across the back pad of the bench. Position your shoulder blades such that your torso is perpendicular to the length of the pad and place your feet flat on the floor. Hold the dumbbell by placing your palms against the innermost plate (not the handle). Position your elbows near or slightly past your head, and keep your arms relatively straight. (A spotter can assist you in positioning a heavy weight.)

Performance Description: Without bending your arms, pull the dumbbell directly over your head. Pause briefly in this mid-range position (the dumbbell directly over your head), and then lower the dumbbell under control to the starting position (your elbows near or slightly past your head) to ensure an adequate stretch.

Training Tips:

- You can also perform this exercise with a barbell (spacing your hands about 4 - 6 inches apart).

- This exercise may be contraindicated if you have low-back pain or shoulder-impingement syndrome.

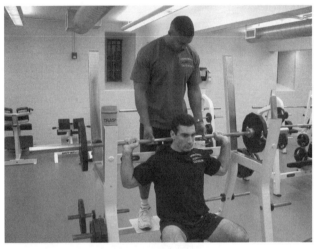

Start/Finish Position

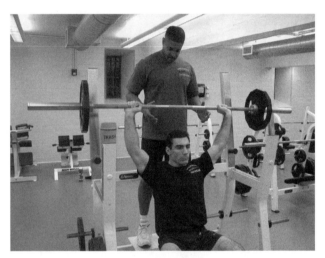

Mid-Range Position

SEATED PRESS

Muscles Involved: anterior deltoid and triceps

Suggested Repetitions: 6 - 12 (or 40 - 70 seconds)

Type of Movement: multiple joint

Starting Position: Sit down on the seat pad of the bench, lean back against the back pad, and place your feet flat on the floor (or against a footrest if one is provided). Grasp the bar and spread your hands slightly wider than shoulder-width apart. Lift the bar out of the uprights or have a spotter give you assistance. Place the bar behind your head on the upper part of your trapezius. (If the bench does not have uprights, two spotters can place the bar in the same position.)

Performance Description: Push the bar up until your arms are almost fully extended (that is, without "locking" your elbows). Pause briefly in this mid-range position (your arms almost fully extended), and then return the weight under control to the starting position (your arms flexed) to provide a proper stretch.

Training Tips:

- For reasons of safety, you should not perform this exercise without a spotter.

- You should not use an excessively wide grip since this will reduce your range of motion.

- Keep your hips flat on the seat pad, your torso against the back pad, and your feet flat on the floor (or a footrest if one is provided) as you perform this exercise. If you have low-back pain, you can place your feet on a stool/footrest. This will flatten your lumbar area against the back pad and reduce the stress in your low-back region.

- You should not "lock" or "snap" your elbows in the mid-range position of a repetition. This removes the load from the target muscles and may hyperextend your elbows.

- You can also perform this exercise with dumbbells.

- This exercise may be contraindicated if you have shoulder-impingement syndrome. In this case, however, raising and lowering the bar in front of your head rather than behind it will reduce the stress on an impinged shoulder. This exercise may also be contraindicated if you have low-back pain.

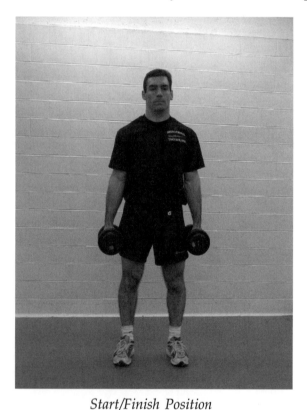
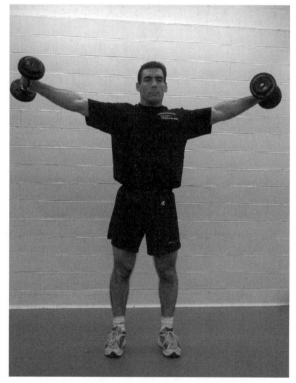

Start/Finish Position   *Mid-Range Position*

LATERAL RAISE

Muscles Involved: middle deltoid and trapezius (upper portion)

Suggested Repetitions: 6 - 12 (or 40 - 70 seconds)

Type of Movement: single joint

Starting Position: Reach down and grasp a dumbbell in each hand. Stand upright by straightening your legs and torso (as if performing a deadlift). Hold the dumbbells at the sides of your body with your palms facing your legs and spread your feet about shoulder-width apart.

Performance Description: Keep your arms fairly straight and raise the dumbbells away from the sides of your body until your arms are parallel to the floor. Pause briefly in this mid-range position (your arms parallel to the floor), and then lower the dumbbells under control to the starting position (your arms at your sides) to ensure an adequate stretch.

Training Tips:

- Avoid throwing the dumbbells by using your legs or by swinging your torso back and forth — movement should only occur around your shoulder joints.

- You should not raise your arms beyond a point that is parallel to the floor.

- Your palms should be facing the floor in the mid-range position.

- You can do this exercise unilaterally (one limb at a time) in the event that you have a shoulder or arm injury, or a gross difference in the strength between your limbs. You can also do it in this fashion if you desire a training variation.

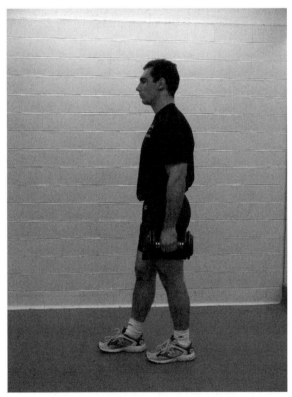

Start/Finish Position

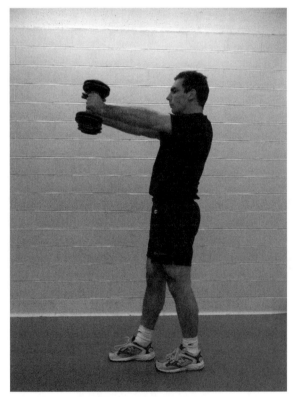

Mid-Range Position

FRONT RAISE

Muscle Involved: anterior deltoid

Suggested Repetitions: 6 - 12 (or 40 - 70 seconds)

Type of Movement: single joint

Starting Position: Reach down and grasp a dumbbell in each hand. Stand upright by straightening your legs and torso (as if performing a deadlift). Hold the dumbbells at the sides of your body with your palms facing your legs and spread your feet a comfortable distance apart with one foot slightly in front of the other.

Performance Description: Keep your arms fairly straight and raise the dumbbells in front of your body until your arms are parallel to the floor. Pause briefly in this mid-range position (your arms parallel to the floor), and then return the dumbbells under control to the starting position (your arms at your sides) to obtain a proper stretch.

Training Tips:

• Avoid throwing the dumbbells by using your legs or by swinging your torso back and forth — movement should only occur around your shoulder joints.

• You should not raise your arms beyond a point that is parallel to the floor.

• Your palms should be facing each other in the mid-range position.

• You can do this exercise unilaterally (one limb at a time) in the event that you have a shoulder or arm injury, or a gross difference in the strength between your limbs. You can also do it in this fashion if you desire a training variation.

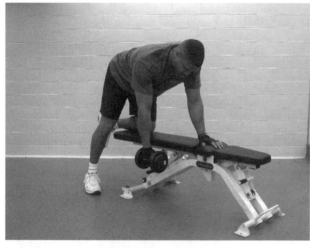 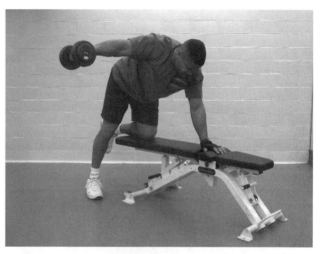

Start/Finish Position   *Mid-Range Position*

BENT-OVER RAISE

Muscle Involved: posterior deltoid and trapezius (middle portion)

Suggested Repetitions: 6 - 12 (or 40 - 70 seconds)

Type of Movement: single joint

Starting Position: Place your left hand and left knee on the back pad of the bench, and position your right foot on the floor at a comfortable distance from the bench. Reach down with your right hand and grasp a dumbbell. Lift the dumbbell slightly off the floor and keep your right arm straight. Your right palm should be facing the bench.

Performance Description: Keep your right arm fairly straight, and raise the dumbbell away from your body until your arm is parallel to the floor. Pause briefly in this mid-range position (your arm parallel to the floor), and then return the dumbbell under control to the starting position (your arm near the bench) to obtain a proper stretch. After performing a set with your right arm, repeat the exercise for the other side of your body (with your right hand and right knee on the back pad for support).

Training Tips:

- Changing the position of your shoulder as you perform this exercise is natural. However, movement of your shoulder should not be excessive or used to throw the dumbbell — movement should only occur around your shoulder joint.

- You should not raise your arm beyond a point that is parallel to the floor.

- Your palm should be facing the floor and your upper arm perpendicular to your torso in the mid-range position.

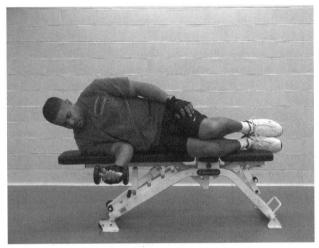
Start/Finish Position

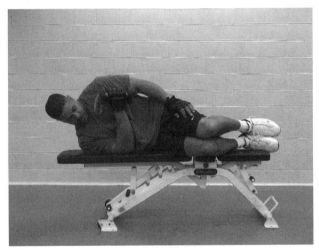
Mid-Range Position

INTERNAL ROTATION

Muscles Involved: internal rotators

Suggested Repetitions: 8 - 12 (or 50 - 70 seconds)

Type of Movement: single joint

Starting Position: Grasp a dumbbell with your right hand, lie down on the back pad of the bench on your right side, and draw your knees toward your torso. Position your right elbow just in front of your torso, and bend your right arm so that the angle between your upper and lower arms is about 90 degrees. Point your right palm upward.

Performance Description: Without moving your right elbow or changing the angle of your right arm, pull the dumbbell to your left upper arm. Pause briefly in this mid-range position (dumbbell near your left side), and then lower the weight under control to the starting position (dumbbell away from your left side) to ensure a sufficient stretch.

111

After performing a set with your right arm, repeat the exercise for the other side of your body (by lying on your left side).

Training Tips:

- You should not lie directly on your upper arm as you perform this exercise.

- Doing this exercise on a bench (instead of the floor) will increase your range of motion and permit a greater stretch.

- You can also perform this exercise using surgical tubing or elastic cord as the resistance. The tubing should be secured to an object that will not move such as a machine. Simply grasp the free end of the tubing and pull it horizontally toward your body in the fashion described above. In this case, you would do the exercise while standing. (Refer to the pictures of internal rotation in Chapter 9.)

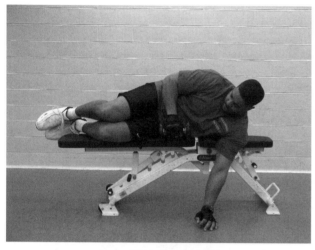

Start/Finish Position   *Mid-Range Position*

EXTERNAL ROTATION

Muscles Involved: external rotators

Suggested Repetitions: 8 - 12 (or 50 - 70 seconds)

Type of Movement: single joint

Starting Position: Grasp a dumbbell with your right hand, lie down on the back pad of the bench on your left side, and draw your knees toward your torso. Position your left arm just in front of your torso and lean back slightly. Keep your right elbow against your side, and bend your right arm so that the angle between your upper and lower arms is about 90 degrees. Point your right palm downward.

Performance Description: Without moving your right elbow or changing the angle of your right arm, raise the dumbbell as high as possible. Pause briefly in this mid-range position (dumbbell away from your left side), and then lower the weight under control to the starting position (dumbbell near your left side) to obtain a proper stretch. After performing a set with your right arm, repeat the exercise for the other side of your body (by lying on your right side).

Training Tips:

- Doing this exercise on a bench (instead of the floor) will increase your range of motion and permit a greater stretch.

- You can also perform this exercise with surgical tubing or elastic cord as the resistance. The tubing should be secured to an object that will not move such as a machine. Simply grasp the free end of the tubing and pull it horizontally away from your body in the fashion described above. In this case, you would do the exercise while standing.

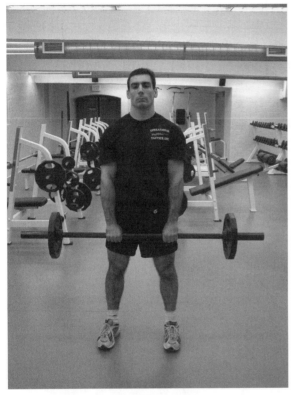

Start/Finish Position

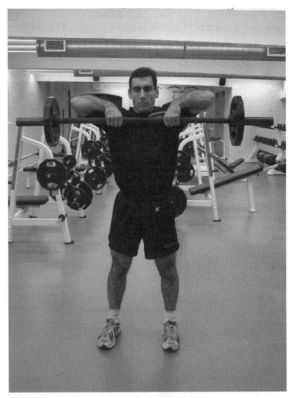

Mid-Range Position

UPRIGHT ROW

Muscles Involved: trapezius (upper portion), biceps, and forearms

Suggested Repetitions: 6 - 12 (or 40 - 70 seconds)

Type of Movement: multiple joint

Starting Position: Reach down and grasp the bar with your hands spaced about 8 - 10 inches apart and your palms facing you. Stand upright by straightening your legs and torso (as if performing a deadlift). Spread your feet approximately shoulder-width apart.

Performance Description: Pull the bar up until it is just below your chin. (Your elbows should be slightly higher than your hands in this position.) Pause briefly in this mid-range position (your arms flexed), and then return the bar under control to the starting position (your arms fully extended) to ensure a proper stretch.

Training Tips:

- Avoid throwing the weight by using your legs or by swinging your torso back and forth — movement should only occur around your shoulder and elbow joints.

- You can also perform this exercise with dumbbells. In this case, you should grasp the dumbbells with your palms facing you and hold them in front of your body about 8 - 10 inches apart.

- For better biomechanical leverage, you should keep the bar (or the dumbbells) close to your body as you perform this exercise.

- You can use wrist straps if you have difficulty in maintaining your grip on the bar (or the dumbbells).

- This exercise may be contraindicated if you have shoulder-impingement syndrome. In this case, however, raising and lowering the bar to the lower part of your chest (near the tip of your breastbone) rather than to the upper part of it will reduce the stress on an impinged shoulder. This exercise may also be contraindicated if you have low-back pain or hyperextended elbows.

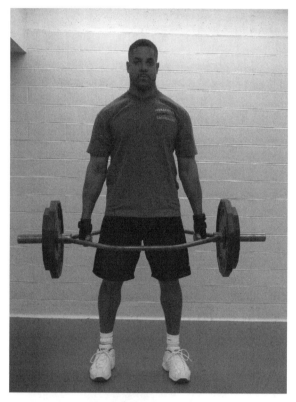

Start/Finish Position

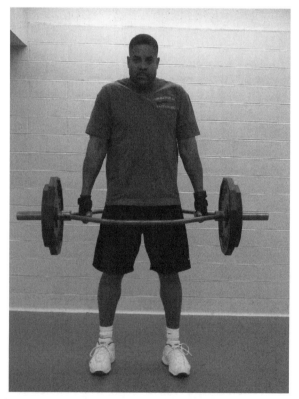

Mid-Range Position

SHOULDER SHRUG

Muscle Involved: trapezius (upper portion)

Suggested Repetitions: 8 - 12 (or 50 - 70 seconds)

Type of Movement: single joint

Starting Position: Step inside the opening of the trap bar and spread your feet approximately shoulder-width apart. Reach down and grasp the bar on the outside of your legs with a "parallel grip" (your palms facing each other). Stand upright by straightening your legs and torso (as if performing a deadlift). (Two spotters can assist you in positioning a heavy weight.)

Performance Description: Keep your arms and legs fairly straight, and pull the bar up as high as possible trying to touch your shoulders to your ears (as if to say, "I do not know"). Pause briefly in this mid-range position (your shoulders near your ears), and then lower the weight under control to the starting position (your shoulders away from your ears) to obtain an adequate stretch.

Training Tips:

- "Rolling" your shoulders as you perform this exercise is not necessary or advisable.

- Avoid throwing the weight by using your legs or by swinging your torso back and forth — movement should only occur around your shoulder joints.

- You can also perform this exercise with an Olympic bar and dumbbells. When doing this exercise with an Olympic bar, you should grasp the bar with both hands approximately shoulder-width apart with your palms facing you. When doing this exercise with dumbbells, you should use a "parallel grip" and keep the weights at your sides. For better biomechanical leverage, you should also keep the Olympic bar and dumbbells close to your body as you perform this exercise.

- You can use wrist straps if you have difficulty in maintaining your grip on the bar (or the dumbbells).

- This exercise may be contraindicated if you have low-back pain or hyperextended elbows.

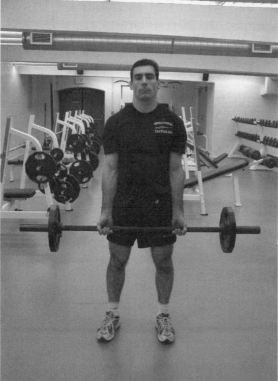
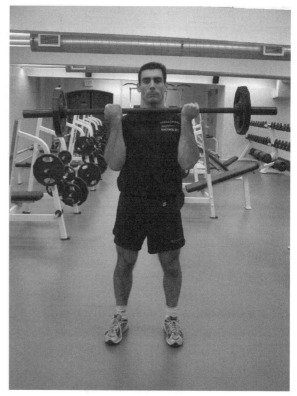

Start/Finish Position   *Mid-Range Position*

BICEP CURL

Muscles Involved: biceps and forearms

Suggested Repetitions: 6 - 12 (or 40 - 70 seconds)

Type of Movement: single joint

Starting Position: Reach down and grasp the bar with your hands spaced slightly wider than shoulder-width apart and your palms facing away from you. Stand upright by straightening your legs and torso (as if performing a deadlift). Spread your feet approximately shoulder-width apart.

Performance Description: Keep your elbows against the sides of your torso and pull the bar below your chin by bending your arms. Pause briefly in this mid-range position (your arms flexed), and then lower the weight under control to the starting position (your arms fully extended) to provide a sufficient stretch.

Training Tips:

• Avoid throwing the weight by using your legs or by swinging your torso back and forth — movement should only occur around your elbow joints.

• Changing the position of your elbows as you perform this exercise is natural. However, movement of your elbows should not be excessive.

• You can also perform this exercise with dumbbells or the "E-Z curl bar." When doing this exercise with dumbbells, you should start the movement using a "parallel grip" (your palms facing each other) with the weights at your sides. As you pull the dumbbells up to your shoulders, you should gradually supinate (turn) your hands so that they are facing you in the mid-range position. You would reverse this action when you return the dumbbells to the starting position.

- This exercise may be contraindicated if you have hyperextended elbows.

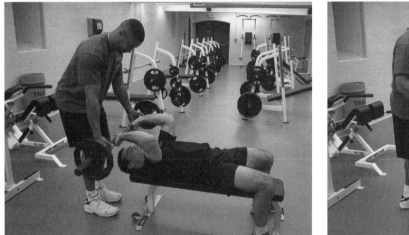 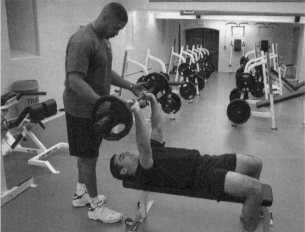

Start/Finish Position   *Mid-Range Position*

TRICEP EXTENSION

Muscle Involved: triceps

Suggested Repetitions: 6 - 12 (or 40 - 70 seconds)

Type of Movement: single joint

Starting Position: Sit down near the end of the back pad of the bench, reach down, and grasp the bar with your palms facing you. Lift the bar, lie down on the back pad, and place your feet flat on the floor. Position your upper arms so that they are roughly perpendicular to the floor, point your elbows toward your knees, and spread your hands about 4 - 6 inches apart. (A spotter can assist you in positioning a heavy weight.) Lower the bar until it is near your forehead. (How near the bar is to your forehead depends on the length of your lower arms).

Performance Description: Keep your upper arms perpendicular to the floor and your elbows pointing toward your knees, and push the bar up by straightening your arms. Pause briefly in this mid-range position (your arms extended), and then return the weight under control to the starting position (your arms flexed) to obtain a proper stretch.

Training Tips:

- Your upper arms should remain perpendicular to the floor and your elbows should be pointed toward your knees as you perform this exercise.

- Keep your hips flat on the back pad and your feet flat on the floor as you perform this exercise. If you have low-back pain, you can place your feet on the end of the back pad or a stool. This will flatten your lumbar area against the back pad and reduce the stress in your low-back region.

- You can also perform this exercise while sitting or standing. In both cases, you would keep your upper arms perpendicular to the floor and raise and lower the weight behind your head.

- You can also perform this exercise with dumbbells or the "E-Z curl bar."

- This exercise may be contraindicated if you have shoulder-impingement syndrome.

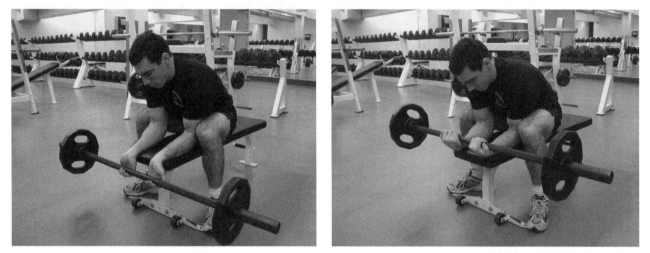

Start/Finish Position   *Mid-Range Position*

WRIST FLEXION

Muscles Involved: wrist flexors

Suggested Repetitions: 8 - 12 (or 50 - 70 seconds)

Type of Movement: single joint

Starting Position: Reach down and grasp the bar with your palms facing away from you. Lift the bar, sit down near the end of the back pad of the bench, and place the backs of your forearms directly over your upper legs. (You can also place your forearms flat on the back pad between your legs.) Place your thumbs underneath the bar alongside your fingers and spread your hands about 4 - 6 inches apart. Lean forward slightly so that the angle between your upper and lower arms is about 90 degrees or less. Your wrists should be over your kneecaps (or over the edge of the back pad if you placed your forearms on it).

Performance Description: Pull the bar up as high as possible by bending your wrists. Pause briefly in this mid-range position (your wrists flexed), and then lower the weight under control to the starting position (your wrists extended) to provide a sufficient stretch.

Training Tips:

- Your forearms should remain directly over your upper legs throughout the performance of this exercise.

- Placing your thumbs underneath the bar alongside your fingers will give you a greater range of motion.

- Avoid throwing the weight by using your legs or by swinging your torso back and forth — movement should only occur around your wrist joints.

- You can also perform this exercise with dumbbells.

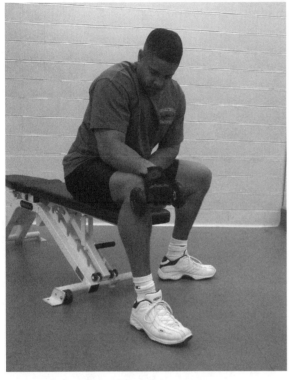

Start/Finish Position

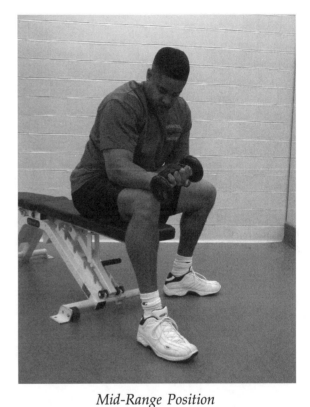

Mid-Range Position

WRIST EXTENSION

Muscles Involved: wrist extensors

Suggested Repetitions: 8 - 12 (or 50 - 70 seconds)

Type of Movement: single joint

Starting Position: Reach down and grasp a dumbbell with your right hand. Lift the dumbbell, sit down near the end of the back pad of the bench, and place the front of your right forearm directly over your right upper leg so that your palm is facing down. (You can also place your forearms flat on the back pad between your legs.) Lean forward slightly so that the angle between your upper and lower arms is about 90 degrees or less. Your right wrist should be over your right kneecap (or over the edge of the back pad if you placed your forearm on it).

Performance Description: Pull the dumbbell up as high as possible by bending your wrist. Pause briefly in this mid-range position (your wrist extended), and then lower the weight under control to the starting position (your wrist flexed) to obtain an adequate stretch. After performing a set with your right arm, repeat the exercise for the other side of your body.

Training Tips:

- Your forearm should remain directly over your upper leg throughout the performance of this exercise.

- Avoid throwing the weight by using your leg or by swinging your torso back and forth — movement should only occur around your wrist joint.

- This exercise is more comfortable on your wrist when it is performed one limb at a time with a dumbbell rather than both limbs at a time with a barbell.

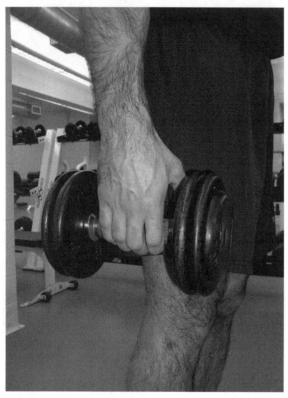

Start/Finish Position

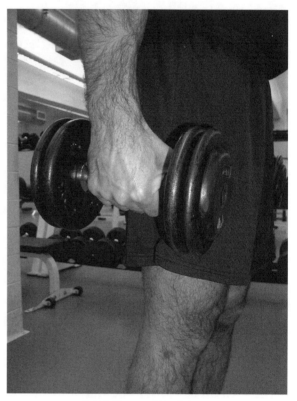

Mid-Range Position

FINGER FLEXION

Muscles Involved: finger flexors

Suggested Repetitions: 8 - 12 (or 50 - 70 seconds)

Type of Movement: single joint

Starting Position: Reach down and grasp a dumbbell in each hand. Stand upright by straightening your legs and torso (as if performing a deadlift). Hold the dumbbells at the sides of your body with your palms facing your legs and spread your feet about shoulder-width apart. Allow the dumbbells to roll down your hands to your fingertips.

Performance Description: Keep your arms fairly straight and pull the dumbbells up to your thumbs. Pause briefly in this mid-range position (your fingers flexed), and then lower the dumbbells under control to the starting position (your fingers extended) to ensure an adequate stretch.

Training Tips:

- Avoid throwing the dumbbells by using your legs or arms — movement should only occur around your finger joints.

- Squeeze the dumbbells as hard as possible in the mid-range position.

- Attempt to lower the dumbbells all the way down to your fingertips — to the point where the dumbbells almost drop from your fingers.

- You can also perform this exercise with a barbell (keeping the bar in front of your legs, and grasping it with either your palms facing or away from you).

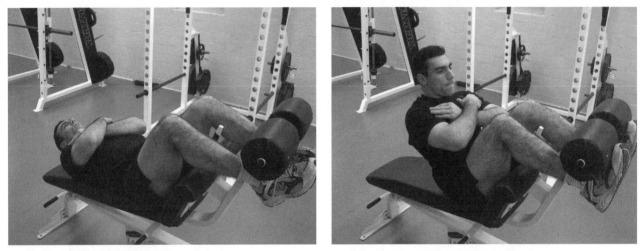

Start/Finish Position   *Mid-Range Position*

SIT-UP

Muscles Involved: rectus abdominis and iliopsoas

Suggested Repetitions: 8 - 12 (or 50 - 70 seconds)

Type of Movement: single joint

Starting Position: Lie down on the back pad of the abdominal bench and place the backs of your lower legs on top of the thigh pads, and your feet under the roller pads. Position yourself so that the angle between your upper and lower legs is about 90 degrees. Fold your arms across your chest and lift your head off the back pad. (The upper portion of your shoulder blades should not be touching the back pad.)

Performance Description: Pull your torso forward until it is just short of being perpendicular to the floor. Pause briefly in this mid-range position (your torso flexed), and then lower your torso under control to the starting position (your torso extended) to obtain a proper stretch.

Training Tips:

- Your abdominals are used primarily during the first 30 degrees or so of this exercise. (Thereafter, your hip flexors accept most of the workload.) So, bringing your torso all the way to your upper legs is not necessary. You should stop, however, before you reach a point where your torso is perpendicular to the floor.

121

- You should not contact the back pad with the upper portion of your shoulder blades between repetitions. This removes the load from the target muscles.

- You should always bend your knees when performing this exercise to reduce the stress on your lower back.

- Avoid throwing your torso forward or snapping your head forward as you perform this exercise — movement should only occur around your hip joint and mid-section.

- If you can do 12 repetitions or more in strict form using your bodyweight, you can increase the workload on your muscles by holding a weight across your chest, increasing the angle of the back pad, performing the exercise with a slower speed of movement, or having a spotter apply manual resistance to your shoulders.

- After reaching concentric muscular fatigue, you can overload your muscles further by grasping the backs of your upper legs, pulling your torso to the mid-range position, and lowering your torso under control to the starting position for 3 - 5 negative repetitions.

- This exercise may be contraindicated if you have low-back pain.

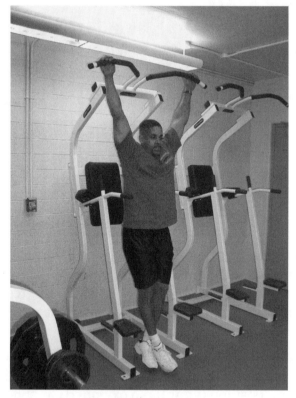
Start/Finish Position

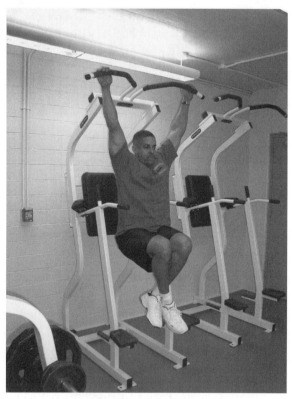
Mid-Range Position

KNEE-UP

Muscles Involved: iliopsoas and rectus abdominis (lower portion)

Suggested Repetitions: 8 - 12 (or 50 - 70 seconds)

Type of Movement: single joint

Starting Position: Reach up, grasp the bar with your palms facing away from you, and space your hands several inches wider than shoulder-width apart. Bring your body to a "dead hang" and cross your ankles.

Performance Description: Pull your knees up as close to your chest as possible. Pause briefly in this mid-range position (your knees near your chest), and then lower your legs under control to the starting position (your legs hanging down) to ensure a proper stretch.

Training Tips:

- Avoid swinging your body back and forth as you perform this exercise — movement should only occur around your hip and knee joints.

- If you can do 12 repetitions or more in strict form using your bodyweight, you can increase the workload on your muscles by performing the exercise with a slower speed of movement or having a spotter apply manual resistance to your upper legs.

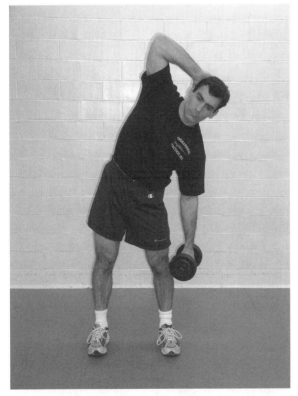

Start/Finish Position

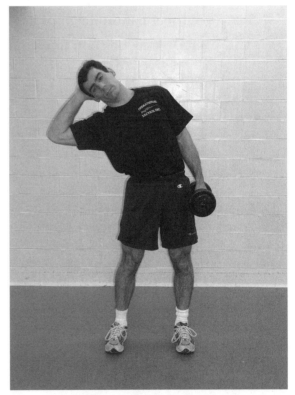

Mid-Range Position

SIDE BEND

Muscles Involved: obliques and erector spinae (lower back)

Suggested Repetitions: 8 - 12 (or 50 - 70 seconds)

Type of Movement: single joint

Starting Position: Reach down and grasp a dumbbell in your left hand. Stand upright by straightening your legs and torso. Hold the dumbbell at the side of your body with your palm facing your leg and spread your feet about shoulder-width apart. Place your right palm against the right side of your head. Without moving your hips, bend your torso to the left as far as possible.

Performance Description: Without moving your hips, bend your torso to the right as far as possible. Pause briefly in this mid-range position (your torso bent to the right), and then lower the dumbbell under control to the starting position (your torso bent to the left) to ensure a sufficient stretch. After performing a set for the right side of your body, repeat the exercise for the other side of your body (holding the dumbbell in your right hand).

Training Tips:

- Changing the position of your hips as you perform this exercise is natural. However, movement of your hips should not be excessive or used to throw the dumbbell — movement should only occur around your mid-section.

- Do not bend forward at the waist as you perform this exercise.

- Keep your feet flat on the floor as you perform this exercise.

- This exercise may be contraindicated if you have low-back pain.

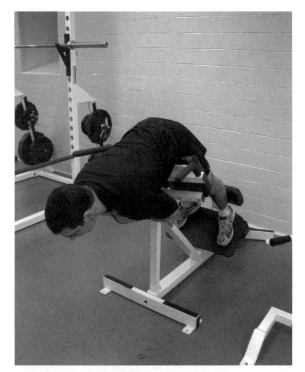
Start/Finish Position

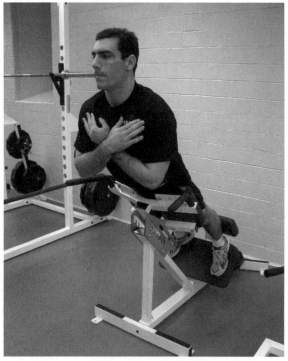
Mid-Range Position

BACK EXTENSION

Muscles Involved: erector spinae (lower back)

Suggested Repetitions: 10 - 15 (or 60 - 90 seconds)

Type of Movement: single joint

Starting Position: Place your feet flat on the foot platform and the backs of your lower legs against the leg pads. Position your pelvis against the hip pads so that your navel (or "belly button") is above the edges. Allow your torso to hang straight down over the edges of the hip pads and fold your arms across your chest.

Performance Description: Raise your torso until it is approximately aligned with your upper legs. Pause briefly in this mid-range position (your torso extended), and then lower your torso under control to the starting position (your torso flexed) to obtain a sufficient stretch.

Training Tips:

- You should not raise your torso beyond a point where it is approximately aligned with your upper legs.

- Avoid throwing your torso backward or snapping your head backward as you perform this exercise — movement should only occur around your hip joint and mid-section.

- If you can do 15 repetitions or more in strict form using your bodyweight, you can increase the workload on your muscles by holding a weight across your chest, performing the exercise with a slower speed of movement, or having a spotter apply manual resistance to your upper back.

- This exercise may be contraindicated if you have low-back pain.

Chapter 9
Machine Exercises

The two most popular types of machines are selectorized and plate-loaded. With a selectorized machine, adjustments in resistance are made by inserting a selector pin or key into a stack of flat weight plates that travel up and down metal guide rods; with a plate-loaded machine, adjustments in resistance are made by adding or removing standard plates from horns that are located on the movement arms.

There is some debate as to who introduced selectorized machines to the fitness community. Legend has it that the first Nautilus™ machine — a prototype pullover model — was built by Arthur Jones in 1948 on a front porch in Tulsa, Oklahoma. But it was not until late 1970 — after 27 different prototypes of the pullover machine were built and tested — that the first Nautilus™ machine was actually sold and delivered to a customer.

In 1957, the original Universal Gym Company developed the first multi-station selectorized machine. Invented by Harold Zinkin, this revolutionary machine featured several different exercises or "stations" with separate stacks of weight plates that could accommodate many individuals at one time.

In the early 1980s, Nautilus™ began to manufacture and sell plate-loaded machines — which were referred to as "leverage machines." These machines were actually the forerunners of the Hammer Strength™ machines that were introduced in 1988.

So, selectorized and plate-loaded machines have a relatively short history. But since their introduction, their use and popularity have grown considerably. Besides Nautilus™ and Hammer Strength™ there are currently several other major manufacturers of selectorized and plate-loaded machines including Body Masters™, Cybex™, and MedX™.

ADVANTAGES OF MACHINES

Machines have the following advantages over free weights:

1. Some exercises cannot be easily performed or performed at all with free weights including hip abduction, hip adduction, leg curl, leg extension, and lat pulldown as

well as those for the neck. These machine exercises and others have a valuable role in a comprehensive strength-training program.

2. Most machines can provide variable resistance. As an exercise is performed, the bio-mechanical leverage of your skeletal system changes — which makes the movement feel easier in some positions and harder in others. A properly designed machine auto-matically varies the resistance to match the changes in your biomechanical leverage. In positions of inferior leverage (and inferior strength), the machine creates a mechanical advantage and a lower level of resistance; as your skeletal system moves into a position of superior leverage (and superior strength), the machine creates a mechanical disadvantage and a higher level of resistance. The end result is greater muscular effort throughout the range of motion (ROM). During a typical free-weight exercise, there is adequate resistance for your muscles in their weakest positions, but not enough in their strongest positions. Because of this, the amount of resistance that you can use is limited to that which you can handle in your position of least leverage. There are, however, a few free-weight exercises that provide somewhat adequate resistance throughout most of the ROM including wrist flexion/extension, shoulder shrug, and calf raise. Incidentally, the idea of variable resistance dates back to 1898.

3. Most machines do not require you to balance the weight like you would when using free weights. Having to do this can be viewed as a drawback. Some individuals — particularly those who have very little experience in strength training — might worry more about balancing the weight effectively than about performing the exercise prop-erly. Furthermore, you are likely to spend excessive energy in balancing the weight. With most machines, the weight is already balanced for you, so that you will be able to concentrate on the proper performance of the exercise. Because synergistic muscles are not involved when the weight is balanced, machines can also work the target muscles to a greater degree.

4. Workouts are generally more time-efficient when machines are used. Some individu-als do not have an abundance of extra time to spend in the weight room. The resis-tance on selectorized machines can be set by simply moving a pin rather than by con-stantly changing plates.

5. In general, machines provide direct resistance over a greater ROM compared to a similar free-weight exercise. A machine pullover, for example, can provide direct re-sistance over as much as 270 degrees ROM around your shoulder joint. By compari-son, a barbell or dumbbell pullover provides only about 100 degrees of direct resis-tance for the same musculature — that is, your upper back (or "lats"). Therefore, a pullover done with a machine is much more efficient than a pullover done with free weights because the targeted muscles are exercised over a greater ROM. This holds true for just about all machine exercises compared to their free-weight counterparts.

6. Many free-weight exercises do not provide the target muscles with an adequate stretch. For instance, a barbell bench press restricts the stretching of your chest muscles — you could stretch them farther, but are unable to do so because the bar must stop at your chest. A machine bench press utilizes movement arms that do not interfere with your ROM. This enables you to obtain a greater stretch, so that you do not compromise

your flexibility. Note that performing free-weight exercises with dumbbells can allow you to obtain a better stretch than with a barbell.

7. Machines are more practical than free weights during rehabilitation. Suppose that you injured your left knee. Many free-weight exercises would be quite difficult or uncomfortable (if not impossible) to perform. However, you could still train your entire torso, your right leg, and possibly even both hips if you have access to machines. You could even continue to exercise on most machines with very little discomfort even if your arm or leg was immobilized in a cast. For instance, if your wrist was casted such that you were unable to grasp a barbell or dumbbell, you could still perform many upper-body exercises on machines including the pec fly, pullover, and lateral raise.

8. A spotter is rarely needed for safety purposes when using machines. Any barbell exercise that involves lifting a weight over your head — such as a bench press or incline press — should only be done with a spotter. With machines, getting pinned underneath a bar or stuck with a weight in a compromising position is virtually impossible.

THE EXERCISES

This chapter will describe and illustrate the safest and most productive exercises that can be performed with machines. (Generic descriptions are given in this chapter that can be applied to equipment from different manufacturers.) Included in the discussions of each exercise are the muscle(s) involved (if more than one muscle is involved, the first muscle listed is the prime mover), suggested repetitions (the time that the targeted muscles should be loaded is shown in parentheses), type of movement, starting position, performance description, and training tips for making the exercise safer and more productive. The exercises described in this chapter are the leg press, hip abduction, hip adduction, prone leg curl, seated leg curl, leg extension, standing calf raise, seated calf raise, dorsi flexion, chest press, pec fly, seated row, underhand lat pulldown, overhand lat pulldown, pullover, shoulder press, lateral raise, internal rotation, external rotation, upright row, scapulae retraction, bicep curl, tricep extension, wrist flexion, wrist extension, abdominal, side bend, rotary torso, back extension, neck flexion, neck extension, and neck lateral flexion.

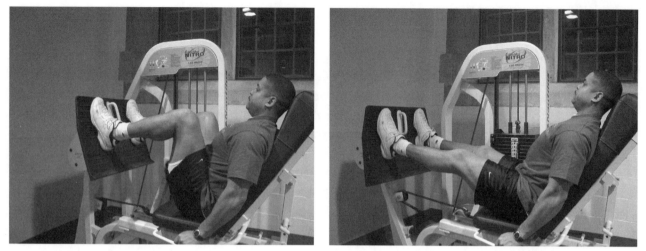

Start/Finish Position   *Mid-Range Position*

LEG PRESS

Muscles Involved: gluteus maximus (buttocks), hamstrings, and quadriceps

Suggested Repetitions: 15 - 20 (or 90 - 120 seconds)

Type of Movement: multiple joint

Starting Position: Adjust the position of the seat pad (as described below in the training tips). Sit down on the seat pad, lean back against the back pad, and place your feet on the foot pedal so that they are slightly wider than shoulder-width apart. Position your lower legs so that they are roughly perpendicular to the floor. Lightly grasp the handles located on the sides of the seat pad.

Performance Description: Push the foot pedal forward until your legs are almost fully extended (that is, without "locking" your knees). Pause briefly in this mid-range position (your hips and legs extended), and then return the weight under control to the starting position (your hips and legs flexed) to provide a proper stretch.

Training Tips:

- Adjust the position of the seat pad so that the angle between your upper and lower legs is about 90 degrees in the starting position.

- On some machines, you can adjust the angle of the back pad. As the back pad is positioned less upright, there is more emphasis on the gluteus maximus (your buttocks). Note that in the positions that are less upright, you must move the seat closer to the foot pedal to maintain the same range of motion as the more upright positions.

- You should exert force through your heels, not the balls of your feet.

- You should not "lock" or "snap" your knees in the mid-range position of a repetition. This removes the load from the target muscles and may hyperextend your knees.

- When performing this exercise with a selectorized machine, do not slam the weights together between repetitions; when performing this exercise with a plate-loaded machine, do not bounce the movement arms off the rubber stoppers.

- You can do this exercise unilaterally (one limb at a time) in the event that you have a leg or knee injury, or a gross difference in the strength between your limbs. You can also do it in this fashion if you desire a training variation.

- This exercise may be contraindicated if you have hyperextended knees.

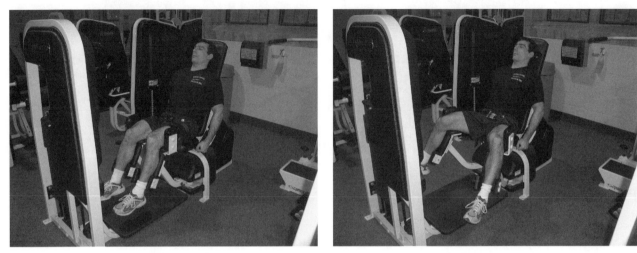

Start/Finish Position   *Mid-Range Position*

HIP ABDUCTION

Muscle Involved: gluteus medius

Suggested Repetitions: 10 - 15 (or 60 - 90 seconds)

Type of Movement: single joint

Starting Position: Adjust the position of the back pad so that the angle is as upright as possible (if it is adjustable). Sit down on the seat pad, place your legs on top of the leg pads, and lie against the back pad. Secure the waist belt (if one is provided) and lightly grasp the handles located on the sides of the seat pad.

Performance Description: Spread your legs apart as far as possible by pulling against the thigh pads. Pause briefly in this mid-range position (your legs apart), and then lower the weight under control to the starting position (your legs together) to obtain a proper stretch.

Training Tips:

- If your legs are relatively short, you may have to use an additional back pad.

- Keep your torso against the back pad as you perform this exercise — movement should only occur around your hip joint.

- Attempt to raise the weight as high as possible in the mid-range position of every repetition to ensure that you are obtaining a maximal contraction of the target muscles throughout the duration of the exercise.

- When performing this exercise with a selectorized machine, do not slam the weights together between repetitions.

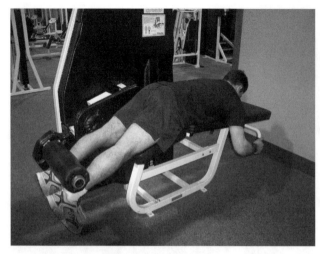

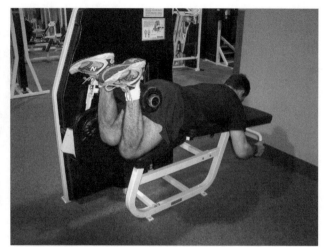

Start/Finish Position *Mid-Range Position*

PRONE LEG CURL

Muscles Involved: hamstrings

Suggested Repetitions: 10 - 15 (or 60 - 90 seconds)

Type of Movement: single joint

Starting Position: Adjust the position of the roller pads (as described below in the training tips). Lie face down on the back pad and place your lower legs underneath the roller pads. Position the tops of your kneecaps so that they are just over the edge of the back pad, not on the pad. (By doing this, your knees will be approximately even with the axis of rotation of the machine.) Lightly grasp the handles located on the sides of the back pad.

Performance Description: Pull your heels as close to your hips as possible by pulling against the roller pads. Pause briefly in this mid-range position (your heels near your hips), and then lower the weight under control to the starting position (your legs fully extended) to ensure a sufficient stretch.

Training Tips:

• Adjust the position of the roller pads so that they are near the bottom part of your calves (just above your ankles) in the starting position. On some machines, a single leg pad is used rather than two roller pads.

• Keep your torso against the back pad as you perform this exercise. However, you can raise your hips as you perform this exercise since this actually increases your range of motion. Otherwise, movement should only occur around your knee joints.

• The angle between your upper and lower legs should be about 90 degrees or less in the mid-range position. This could be deceiving if the pad is humped or angled rather than parallel to the floor.

• When performing this exercise with a selectorized machine, do not slam the weights together between repetitions; when performing this exercise with a plate-loaded machine, do not bounce the movement arms off the rubber stoppers.

- You can do this exercise unilaterally (one limb at a time) in the event that you have a leg or knee injury, or a gross difference in the strength between your limbs. You can also do it in this fashion if you desire a training variation.

- This exercise may be contraindicated if you have low-back pain or hyperextended knees.

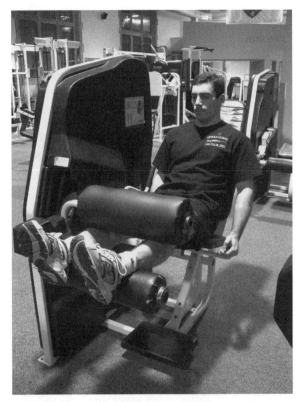
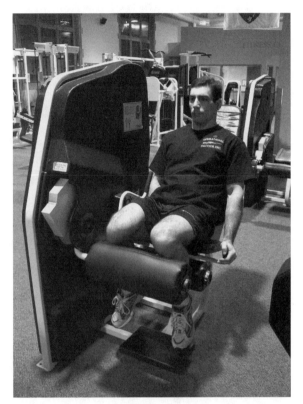

Start/Finish Position　　　　　　　　*Mid-Range Position*

SEATED LEG CURL

Muscles Involved: hamstrings

Suggested Repetitions: 10 - 15 (or 60 - 90 seconds)

Type of Movement: single joint

Starting Position: Adjust the position of the bottom roller pad and back pad (as described below in the training tips). Sit down on the seat pad and place your lower legs between the roller pads. Position your knees so that they are approximately even with the axis of rotation of the machine. Lightly grasp the handles located on the sides of the seat pad.

Performance Description: Pull your heels as close to your hips as possible by pulling against the bottom roller pad. Pause briefly in this mid-range position (your heels near your hips), and then lower the weight under control to the starting position (your legs fully extended) to ensure a sufficient stretch.

Training Tips:

- Adjust the position of the bottom roller pad so that it is near the bottom part of your calves (just above your ankles) in the starting position. On some machines, a single leg pad is used rather than two roller pads.

- Adjust the position of the back pad so that your knees are approximately even with the axis of rotation of the machine.

- Keep your torso against the back pad as you perform this exercise — movement should only occur around your knee joints.

- The angle between your upper and lower legs should be about 90 degrees or less in the mid-range position. This could be deceiving if the pad is angled rather than parallel to the floor.

- When performing this exercise with a selectorized machine, do not slam the weights together between repetitions; when performing this exercise with a plate-loaded machine, do not bounce the movement arms off the rubber stoppers.

- You can do this exercise unilaterally (one limb at a time) in the event that you have a leg or knee injury, or a gross difference in the strength between your limbs. You can also do it in this fashion if you desire a training variation.

- Performing this exercise in the seated position produces less stress in the low-back region than performing it in the prone position.

- This exercise may be contraindicated if you have hyperextended knees.

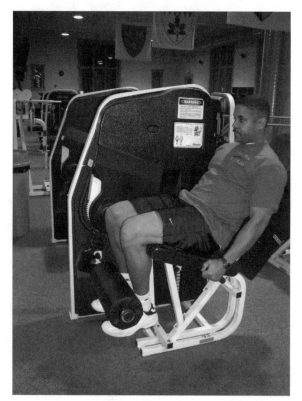 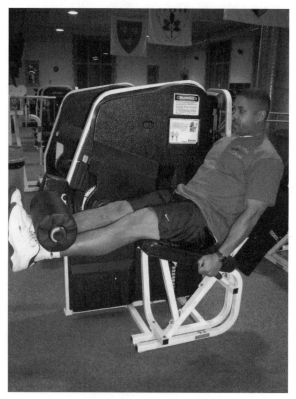

Start/Finish Position   *Mid-Range Position*

LEG EXTENSION

Muscles Involved: quadriceps

Suggested Repetitions: 10 - 15 (or 60 - 90 seconds)

Type of Movement: single joint

Starting Position: Adjust the position of the roller pad and back pad (as described below in the training tips). Sit down on the seat pad and place the backs of your knees against the end of it. Position your feet behind the roller pad and secure the waist belt (if one is provided). Lightly grasp the handles located on the sides of the seat pad.

Performance Description: Extend your lower legs as high as possible by pushing against the roller pad. Pause briefly in this mid-range position (your legs fully extended), and then return the weight under control to the starting position (your legs flexed) to obtain a proper stretch.

Training Tips:

- Adjust the position of the roller pad so that it is near the bottom part of your shins (just above your ankles) in the starting position. On some machines, a single leg pad is used rather a roller pad.

- Adjust the position of the back pad so that your knees are approximately even with the axis of rotation of the machine. There should be little or no space between your hips and the back pad.

- If your upper legs are relatively short, you may have to use an additional back pad (if the back pad of the machine does not adjust).

- Keep your torso against the back pad as you perform this exercise — movement should only occur around your knee joints.

- Attempt to raise the weight as high as possible in the mid-range position of every repetition to ensure that you are obtaining a maximal contraction of the target muscles throughout the duration of the exercise.

- When performing this exercise with a selectorized machine, do not slam the weights together between repetitions; when performing this exercise with a plate-loaded machine, do not bounce the movement arms off the rubber stoppers.

- You can do this exercise unilaterally (one limb at a time) in the event that you have a leg or knee injury, or a gross difference in the strength between your limbs. You can also do it in this fashion if you desire a training variation.

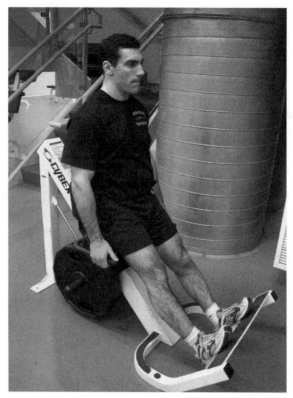

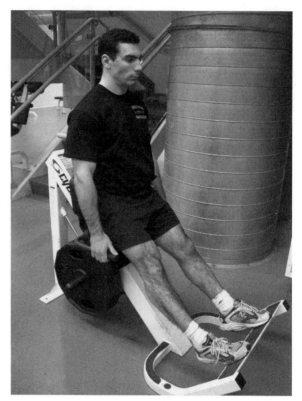

Start/Finish Position *Mid-Range Position*

STANDING CALF RAISE

Muscles Involved: gastrocnemius (calves)

Suggested Repetitions: 10 - 15 (or 60 - 90 seconds)

Type of Movement: single joint

Starting Position: Place your hips on the seat pad and your lower back against the back pad. Position your feet on the foot plate, grasp the handles located on the sides of the seat pad (if ones are provided), and straighten your legs. Position your legs so that the balls of your feet are on the edge of the foot plate and lower your heels.

Performance Description: Keep your legs straight and rise up onto your toes as high as possible. Pause briefly in this mid-range position (your ankles extended), and then lower the weight under control to the starting position (your heels near the floor) to provide a proper stretch.

Training Tips:

• Using your hips and legs as you perform this exercise is natural. However, movement of your hips and legs should not be excessive or used to raise the weight — movement should only occur around your ankle joints.

• Traditionally, this exercise is done with a weight placed on the shoulders — either a barbell or the movement arm of a machine. This should be avoided whenever possible, however, because it compresses the spinal column.

- Attempt to raise the weight as high as possible in the mid-range position of every repetition to ensure that you are obtaining a maximal contraction of the target muscles throughout the duration of the exercise.

- You can do this exercise unilaterally (one limb at a time) in the event that you have a leg or ankle injury, or a gross difference in the strength between your limbs. You can also do it in this fashion if you desire a training variation.

- This exercise may be contraindicated if you have shin splints.

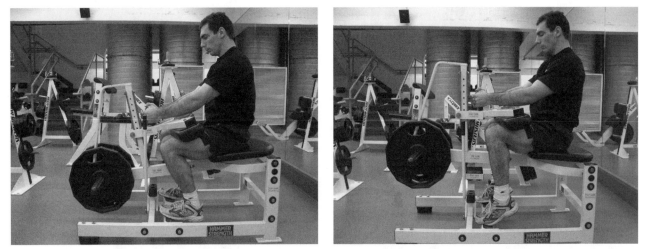

Start/Finish Position   *Mid-Range Position*

SEATED CALF RAISE

Muscles Involved: gastrocnemius and soleus (calves)

Suggested Repetitions: 10 - 15 (or 60 - 90 seconds)

Type of Movement: single joint

Starting Position: Sit down on the seat pad, place the balls of your feet on the edge of the foot plate, and lower your heels. Lower the leg pads until they are against your upper legs. Rise up onto your toes slightly and release the lever arm located on the side of the machine. (This will free the movement arm so that you have a full range of motion.) Grasp the handle (if one is provided) and lower your heels.

Performance Description: Rise up onto your toes as high as possible. Pause briefly in this mid-range position (your ankles extended), and then lower the weight under control to the starting position (your heels near the floor) to provide a proper stretch. When you have finished performing the exercise, rise up onto your toes slightly and return the lever arm located on the side of the machine. (This will hold the movement arm in place.)

Training Tips:

- Avoid throwing the weight by using your arms or by swinging your torso back and forth — movement should only occur around your ankle joints.

- Traditionally, this exercise is done with a weight placed on the shoulders — either a barbell or the movement arm of a machine. This should be avoided whenever possible, however, because it compresses the spinal column.

- Attempt to raise the weight as high as possible in the mid-range position of every repetition to ensure that you are obtaining a maximal contraction of the target muscles throughout the duration of the exercise.

- You can do this exercise unilaterally (one limb at a time) in the event that you have a leg or ankle injury, or a gross difference in the strength between your limbs. You can also do it in this fashion if you desire a training variation.

- This exercise may be contraindicated if you have shin splints.

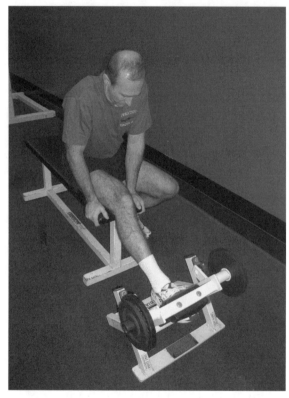

Start/Finish Position   *Mid-Range Position*

DORSI FLEXION

Muscles Involved: dorsi flexors

Suggested Repetitions: 10 - 15 (or 60 - 90 seconds)

Type of Movement: single joint

Starting Position: Sit down near the end of the back pad of a bench and place the back of your right knee against the end of it. Position your right foot between the foot pads.

Performance Description: Without moving your torso, pull your right foot up as high as possible. Pause briefly in this mid-range position (your ankles flexed), and then lower the weight under control to the starting position (your ankles fully extended) to provide a proper stretch. After performing a set with your right ankle, repeat the exercise for the other side of your body.

Training Tips:

- Avoid throwing the weight by swinging your torso back and forth — movement should only occur around your ankle joint.

- Attempt to raise the weight as high as possible in the mid-range position of every repetition to ensure that you are obtaining a maximal contraction of the target muscles throughout the duration of the exercise.

- This exercise may be contraindicated if you have shin splints.

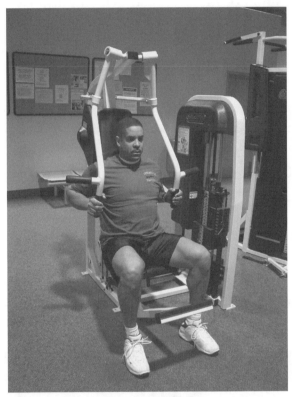
Start/Finish Position

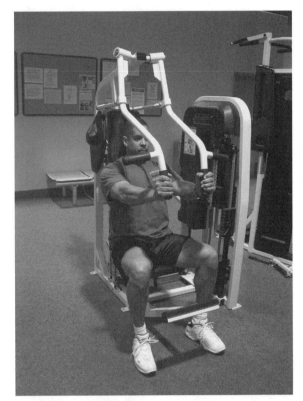
Mid-Range Position

CHEST PRESS

Muscles Involved: chest, anterior deltoid, and triceps

Suggested Repetitions: 6 - 12 (or 40 - 70 seconds)

Type of Movement: multiple joint

Starting Position: Adjust the position of the seat pad (as described below in the training tips). Sit down on the seat pad, secure the waist belt (if one is provided), and lean back against the back pad. Place your feet on the foot lever and push it forward with your legs. Grasp the handles of the movement arms with a "parallel grip" (your palms facing each other). Remove your feet from the foot lever and place them flat on the floor. (If your feet do not reach the floor, bring your legs together and cross your ankles.) Position your hands just below your shoulders.

Performance Description: Push the movement arms forward until your arms are almost fully extended (that is, without "locking" your elbows). Pause briefly in this mid-range position (your arms almost fully extended), and then lower the weight under control to the starting position (your hands near your shoulders) to obtain a sufficient stretch. After completing the exercise, place your feet on the foot lever, remove your hands from the handles of the movement arms, and use your legs to return the weight to the rest of the stack.

Training Tips:

- Adjust the position of the seat pad so that your hands are just below your shoulders in the starting position.

- On some machines, you can adjust the position of the back pad. Moving it forward will increase your range of motion.

- On some machines, you can perform this exercise with a traditional barbell grip in which your palms face the floor. However, using a "parallel grip" reduces the stress in your shoulder joints.

- Keep your hips flat on the seat pad and your torso against the back pad as you perform this exercise — movement should only occur around your shoulder and elbow joints.

- You should not "lock" or "snap" your elbows in the mid-range position of a repetition. This removes the load from the target muscles and may hyperextend your elbows.

- When performing this exercise with a selectorized machine, do not slam the weights together between repetitions.

- You can do this exercise unilaterally (one limb at a time) in the event that you have a shoulder or arm injury, or a gross difference in the strength between your limbs. You can also do it in this fashion if you desire a training variation.

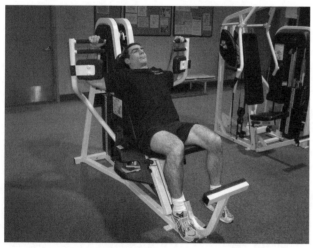

Start/Finish Position

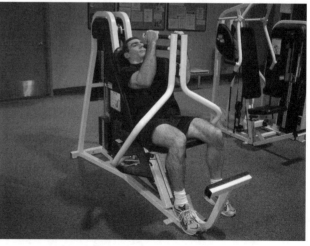

Mid-Range Position

PEC FLY

Muscles Involved: chest and anterior deltoid

Suggested Repetitions: 6 - 12 (or 40 - 70 seconds)

Type of Movement: single joint

Starting Position: Adjust the position of the seat pad (as described below in the training tips). Sit down on the seat pad, secure the seat belt (if one is provided), and lie back against the back pad. Place your feet on the foot lever and push it forward with your legs. Position your lower arms against the arm pads and lightly grasp the handles. Remove your feet from the foot lever, bring your legs together, and cross your ankles.

Performance Description: Keep your torso and head against the back pad, and bring your elbows as close together as possible by pushing against the arm pads. Pause briefly in this mid-range position (your arms together), and then lower the weight under control to the starting position (your arms apart) to provide an adequate stretch. After completing the exercise, place your feet on the foot lever, remove your lower arms from the arm pads, and use your legs to return the weight to the rest of the stack.

Training Tips:

- Adjust the position of the seat pad so that the top part of your shoulder is approximately even with the axis of rotation of the machine, and your elbows are slightly higher than your shoulders in the starting position. On some machines, this can also be accomplished by adjusting the position of the back pad.

- If your torso is relatively short, you may have to use an additional seat pad and/or back pad (if the seat pad and back pad of the machine do not adjust).

- Keep your hips flat on the seat pad, and your torso and head against the back pad as you perform this exercise — movement should only occur around your shoulder joints.

- Keep your lower arms against the arm pads as you perform this exercise. You should exert force against the arm pads, not the handles.

- When performing this exercise with a selectorized machine, do not slam the weights together between repetitions; when performing this exercise with a plate-loaded machine, do not bounce the movement arms off the rubber stoppers.

- You can do this exercise unilaterally (one limb at a time) in the event that you have a shoulder or arm injury, or a gross difference in the strength between your limbs. You can also do it in this fashion if you desire a training variation.

- The pec fly — which is often referred to as the "pec dec" — is the free-weight equivalent of the bent-arm fly performed with dumbbells.

- This exercise may be contraindicated if you have shoulder-impingement syndrome.

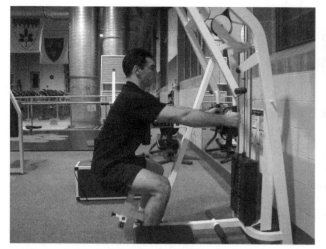
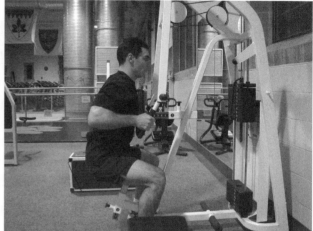

Start/Finish Position   *Mid-Range Position*

SEATED ROW

Muscles Involved: upper back ("lats"), biceps, and forearms

Suggested Repetitions: 6 - 12 (or 40 - 70 seconds)

Type of Movement: multiple joint

Starting Position: Adjust the position of the seat pad (as described below in the training tips). Sit down on the seat pad, slide your hips backward slightly, and lean forward against the chest pad. Place your feet flat on the floor or on the footrest (if one is provided). Grasp the handles of the movement arms with a "parallel grip" (your palms facing each other).

Performance Description: Keep your upper arms close to your torso and pull the handles just below your shoulders. Pause briefly in this mid-range position (your arms flexed), and then lower the weight under control to the starting position (your arms fully extended) to ensure a sufficient stretch.

Training Tips:

• Adjust the position of the seat pad so that your hands are just below your shoulders in the mid-range position.

• On some machines, you can adjust the position of the chest pad. If the chest pad is adjustable, position it so that when you grasp the handles in the starting position, the weight you intend to lift is separated slightly from the rest of the weight stack. In other words, your arms are fully extended. (This produces a greater stretch of your upper back and biceps).

• Changing the position of your torso as you perform this exercise is natural. However, movement of your torso should not be excessive or used to throw the weight -- movement should only occur around your shoulder and elbow joints.

• When performing this exercise with a selectorized machine, do not slam the weights together between repetitions; when performing this exercise with a plate-loaded machine, do not bounce the movement arms off the rubber stoppers.

- You can do this exercise unilaterally (one limb at a time) in the event that you have a shoulder or arm injury, or a gross difference in the strength between your limbs. You can also do it in this fashion if you desire a training variation.

- Performing this exercise with a "parallel grip" (your palms facing each other) is more biomechanically efficient than doing it with an overhand grip (your palms facing downward). However, this exercise is still productive when performed with an overhand grip in the manner described above.

- You can use wrist straps if you have difficulty in maintaining your grip on the handles.

- This exercise may be contraindicated if you have hyperextended elbows.

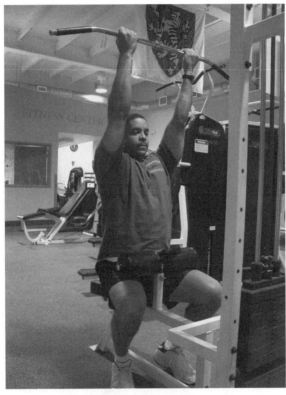

Start/Finish Position

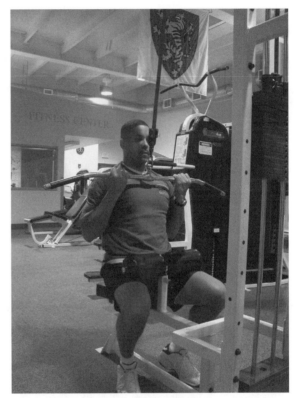

Mid-Range Position

UNDERHAND LAT PULLDOWN

Muscles Involved: upper back ("lats"), biceps, and forearms

Suggested Repetitions: 6 - 12 (or 40 - 70 seconds)

Type of Movement: multiple joint

Starting Position: Reach up, grasp the bar (or handles) with your palms facing you, and space your hands approximately shoulder-width apart. Sit down on the seat pad, place your upper legs under the roller pads, and lean back slightly.

Performance Description: Pull the bar (or handles) down to your upper chest and draw your elbows backward. Pause briefly in this mid-range position (your arms flexed), and then return the weight under control to the starting position (your arms fully extended) to obtain a proper stretch.

Training Tips:

- Avoid swinging your torso back and forth as you perform this exercise — movement should only occur around your shoulder and elbow joints.

- Touching the bar to your upper chest rather than your chin will increase your range of motion. Drawing your elbows backward in the mid-range position will increase the workload performed by your upper back.

- On some machines, you can do this exercise unilaterally (one limb at a time) in the event that you have a shoulder or arm injury, or a gross difference in the strength between your limbs. You can also do it in this fashion if you desire a training variation.

- You can use wrist straps if you have difficulty in maintaining your grip on the bar.

- This exercise may be contraindicated if you have hyperextended elbows.

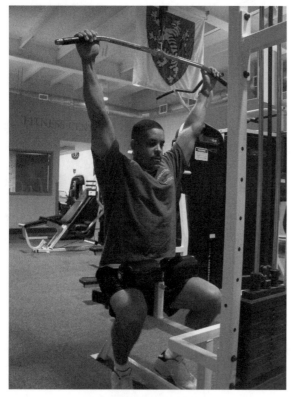
Start/Finish Position

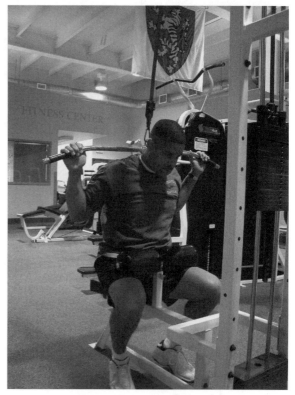
Mid-Range Position

OVERHAND LAT PULLDOWN

Muscles Involved: upper back ("lats"), biceps, and forearms

Suggested Repetitions: 6 - 12 (or 40 - 70 seconds)

Type of Movement: multiple joint

Starting Position: Reach up, grasp the bar (or handles) with your palms facing away from you, and space your hands several inches wider than shoulder-width apart. Sit down on the seat pad and place your upper legs under the roller pads.

Performance Description: Pull the bar (or handles) behind your head to the base of your neck and draw your elbows downward. Pause briefly in this mid-range position (your arms flexed), and then lower the weight under control to the starting position (your arms fully extended) to obtain an adequate stretch.

Training Tips:

- Avoid swinging your torso back and forth as you perform this exercise — movement should only occur around your shoulder and elbow joints.

- You should not use an excessively wide grip since this will reduce your range of motion.

- On some machines, you can do this exercise unilaterally (one limb at a time) in the event that you have a shoulder or arm injury, or a gross difference in the strength between your limbs. You can also do it in this fashion if you desire a training variation.

- Performing a lat pulldown with an overhand grip (your palms facing away from you) is not as biomechanically efficient as doing it with an underhand grip (your palms facing toward you). But this exercise is still quite productive when performed with an overhand grip in the manner described above.

- You can use wrist straps if you have difficulty in maintaining your grip on the bar.

- This exercise may be contraindicated if you have shoulder-impingement syndrome. In this case, however, raising and lowering the bar (or handles) in front of your head rather than behind it will reduce the stress on an impinged shoulder. This exercise may also be contraindicated if you have hyperextended elbows.

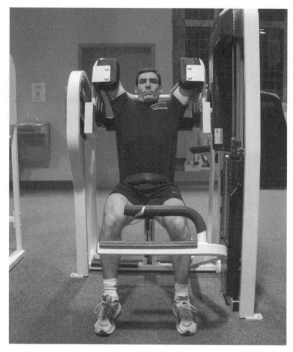

Start/Finish Position

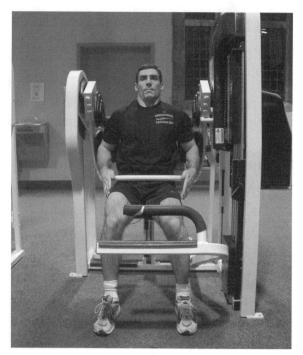

Mid-Range Position

PULLOVER

Muscles Involved: upper back ("lats")

Suggested Repetitions: 6 - 12 (or 40 - 70 seconds)

Type of Movement: single joint

Starting Position: Adjust the position of the seat pad (as described below in the training tips). Sit down on the seat pad, secure the waist belt, and lean back against the back pad. Place your feet on the foot lever and push it forward with your legs. Position the backs of your upper arms against the elbow pads, place your hands on the movement arm so that your palms are facing the bar, and open your hands (that is, extend your fingers). Remove your feet from the foot lever and place them flat on the floor. (If your feet do not reach the floor, bring your legs together and cross your ankles.) Position your elbows near or slightly past your head.

Performance Description: Pull the movement arm down to your mid-section by exerting force against the elbow pads. Pause briefly in this mid-range position (the movement arm against your mid-section), and then lower the weight under control to the starting position (your elbows near or slightly past your head) to ensure a sufficient stretch. After completing the exercise, place your feet on the foot lever, remove your upper arms from the elbow pads, and use your legs to return the weight to the rest of the stack.

Training Tips:

• Adjust the position of the seat pad so that the top parts of your shoulders are slightly below the axis of rotation of the machine when sitting upright with your arms hanging straight down.

- If your arms are relatively short, you may have to use an additional back pad (if the back pad of the machine does not adjust). If performing this exercise while keeping your upper arms against the elbow pads is still difficult, you can grasp the movement arm with an underhand grip and pull with your hands instead of your upper arms. This will not allow you to isolate the muscles of your upper back, but it will make the exercise more comfortable for you to perform.

- Keep your torso against the back pad as you perform this exercise — movement should only occur around your shoulder joints.

- Keep your hands open and fingers extended so that you exert force against the elbow pads with your upper arms, not your hands. This is critical in order for you to isolate your upper back.

- When performing this exercise with a selectorized machine, do not slam the weights together between repetitions; when performing this exercise with a plate-loaded machine, do not bounce the movement arms off the rubber stoppers.

- You can do this exercise unilaterally (one limb at a time) in the event that you have a shoulder or arm injury, or a gross difference in the strength between your limbs. You can also do it in this fashion if you desire a training variation.

- This exercise may be contraindicated if you have low-back pain or shoulder-impingement syndrome.

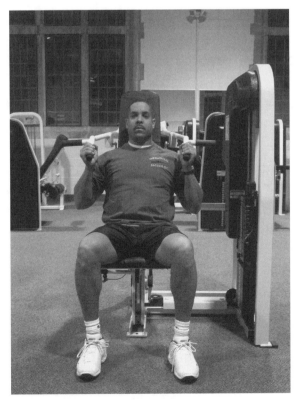

Start/Finish Position

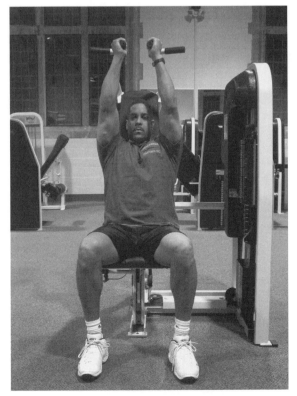

Mid-Range Position

SHOULDER PRESS

Muscles Involved: anterior deltoid and triceps

Suggested Repetitions: 6 - 12 (or 40 - 70 seconds)

Type of Movement: multiple joint

Starting Position: Adjust the position of the seat pad (as described below in the training tips). Sit down on the seat pad, secure the waist belt (if one is provided), and lean back against the back pad. Reach up and grasp the handles of the movement arms with a "parallel grip" (your palms facing each other). Place your feet flat on the floor. (If your feet do not reach the floor, bring your legs together and cross your ankles.)

Performance Description: Push the movement arms up until your arms are almost fully extended (that is, without "locking" your elbows). Pause briefly in this mid-range position (your arms almost fully extended), and then lower the weight under control to the starting position (your hands near your shoulders) to ensure a proper stretch.

Training Tips:

- Adjust the position of the seat pad so that your hands are just below your shoulders in the starting position.

- On some machines, you can adjust the position of the back pad. Moving it forward will increase the range of motion.

- On some machines, you can perform this exercise with a traditional barbell grip in which your palms face away from you. However, using a "parallel grip" reduces the stress in your shoulder joints.

- Keep your hips flat on the seat pad and your torso against the back pad as you perform this exercise. If you have low-back pain, you can place your feet on a stool. This will flatten your lumbar area against the back pad and reduce the stress in your low-back region.

- You should not "lock" or "snap" your elbows in the mid-range position of a repetition. This removes the load from the target muscles and may hyperextend your elbows.

- When performing this exercise with a selectorized machine, do not slam the weights together between repetitions; when performing this exercise with a plate-loaded machine, do not bounce the movement arms off the rubber stoppers.

- You can do this exercise unilaterally (one limb at a time) in the event that you have a shoulder or arm injury, or a gross difference in the strength between your limbs. You can also do it in this fashion if you desire a training variation.

- This exercise may be contraindicated if you have low-back pain or shoulder-impingement syndrome.

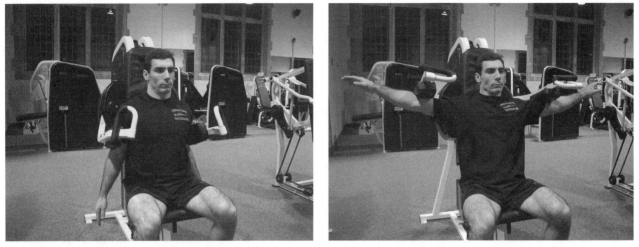

Start/Finish Position   *Mid-Range Position*

LATERAL RAISE

Muscles Involved: middle deltoid and trapezius (upper portion)

Suggested Repetitions: 6 - 12 (or 40 - 70 seconds)

Type of Movement: single joint

Starting Position: Adjust the position of the seat pad (as described below in the training tips). Sit down on the seat pad, secure the waist belt (if one is provided), and lean back against the back pad. Position your upper arms against the arm pads. Straighten your arms and position your palms such that they are facing each other. Place your feet flat on the floor. (If your feet do not reach the floor, bring your legs together and cross your ankles.)

Performance Description: Keep your arms fairly straight and raise them away from the sides of your body until they are parallel to the floor. Pause briefly in this mid-range position (your arms parallel to the floor), and then lower the weight under control to the starting position (your arms at your sides) to provide a proper stretch.

Training Tips:

- Adjust the position of the seat pad so that the back part of your shoulder is approximately even with the axis of rotation of the machine.

- Keep your hips flat on the seat pad and your torso against the back pad as you perform this exercise — movement should only occur around your shoulder joints.

- You should not raise your arms beyond a point that is parallel to the floor.

- Your palms should be facing the floor in the mid-range position.

- When performing this exercise with a selectorized machine, do not slam the weights together between repetitions; when performing this exercise with a plate-loaded machine, do not bounce the movement arms off the rubber stoppers.

- You can do this exercise unilaterally (one limb at a time) in the event that you have a shoulder injury or a gross difference in the strength between your limbs. You can also do it in this fashion if you desire a training variation.

149

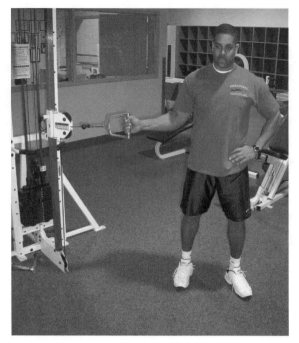

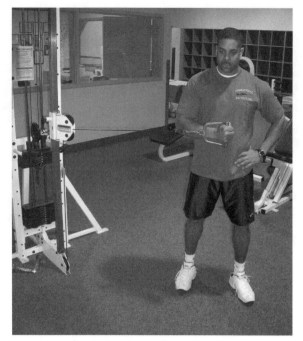

Start/Finish Position   *Mid-Range Position*

INTERNAL ROTATION

Muscles Involved: internal rotators

Suggested Repetitions: 8 - 12 (or 50 - 70 seconds)

Type of Movement: single joint

Starting Position: Adjust the position of the pulley so that it is approximately even with your right elbow. Grasp the handle with your right hand and turn your feet to the left so that the right side of your body is facing the pulley. Slide your feet away from the machine so that the weight you intend to lift is separated slightly from the rest of the weight stack. Position your left hand on your left hip and spread your feet about shoulder-width apart. Place your right elbow against the right side of your torso, and bend your right arm so that the angle between your upper and lower arms is about 90 degrees. (By doing this, your right lower arm will be approximately parallel to the floor.) Position the handle away from your mid-section.

Performance Description: Without moving your right elbow away from the side of your torso or changing the angle of your right arm, pull the handle to your mid-section. Pause briefly in this mid-range position (handle against your mid-section), and then return the weight under control to the starting position (handle away from your mid-section) to ensure a sufficient stretch. After performing a set with your right arm, repeat the exercise for the other side of your body.

Training Tips:

- Keep your elbow against the side of your torso and your lower arm parallel to the floor as you perform this exercise.

- Do not rotate your torso as you perform this exercise — movement should only occur around your shoulder joint.

- Your palm should be facing you in the mid-range position.

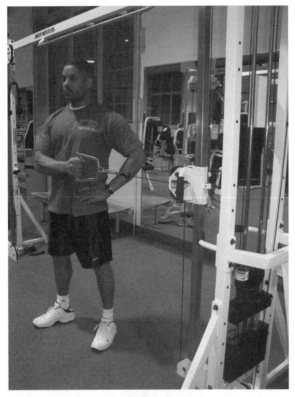

Start/Finish Position

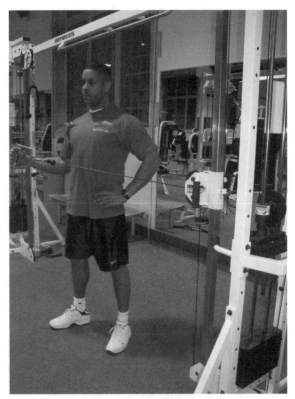

Mid-Range Position

EXTERNAL ROTATION

Muscles Involved: external rotators

Suggested Repetitions: 8 - 12 (or 50 - 70 seconds)

Type of Movement: single joint

Starting Position: Adjust the position of the pulley so that it is approximately even with your right elbow. Grasp the handle with your right hand and turn your feet to the right so that the left side of your body is facing the pulley. Slide your feet away from the machine so that the weight you intend to lift is separated slightly from the rest of the weight stack. Position your left hand on your left hip and spread your feet about shoulder-width apart. Place your right elbow against the right side of your torso, and bend your right arm so that the angle between your upper and lower arms is about 90 degrees. (By doing this, your right lower arm will be approximately parallel to the floor.) Position the handle against your mid-section.

Performance Description: Without moving your right elbow away from the side of your torso or changing the angle of your right arm, pull the handle away from your mid-section. Pause briefly in this mid-range position (handle away from your mid-section), and then return the weight under control to the starting position (handle against your mid-section) to ensure a sufficient stretch. After performing a set with your right arm, repeat the exercise for the other side of your body.

Training Tips:

- Keep your elbow against the side of your torso and your lower arm parallel to the floor as you perform this exercise.

- Do not rotate your torso as you perform this exercise — movement should only occur around your shoulder joint.

- Your palm should be facing you in the starting position.

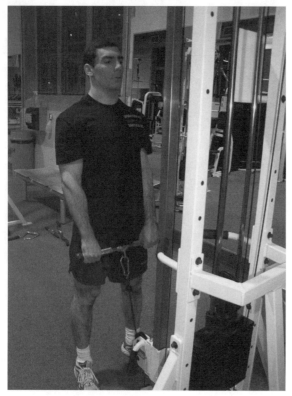

Start/Finish Position

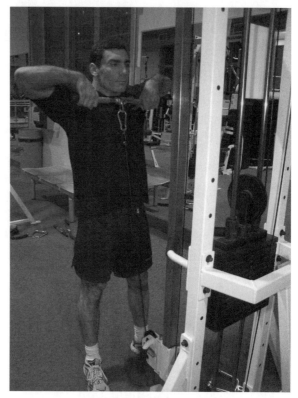

Mid-Range Position

UPRIGHT ROW

Muscles Involved: trapezius, biceps, and forearms

Suggested Repetitions: 6 - 12 (or 40 - 70 seconds)

Type of Movement: multiple joint

Starting Position: Adjust the position of the pulley so that it is near the floor. Reach down and grasp the bar with your hands spaced about 8 - 10 inches apart and your palms facing you. Stand upright by straightening your legs and torso (as if performing a deadlift). Take a slight step backwards and spread your feet approximately shoulder-width apart.

Performance Description: Pull the bar up until it is just below your chin. (Your elbows should be slightly higher than your hands in this position.) Pause briefly in this mid-range position (your arms flexed), and then return the bar under control to the starting position (your arms fully extended) to ensure a proper stretch.

Training Tips:

- Avoid throwing the weight by using your legs, or by swinging your torso back and forth — movement should only occur around your shoulder and elbow joints.

- For better biomechanical leverage, you should keep the bar close to your body as you perform this exercise.

- You can do this exercise unilaterally (one limb at a time) in the event that you have a shoulder or arm injury, or a gross difference in the strength between your limbs. You can also do it in this fashion if you desire a training variation.

- You can use wrist straps if you have difficulty in maintaining your grip on the bar.

- This exercise may be contraindicated if you have shoulder-impingement syndrome. In this case, however, raising and lowering the bar to the lower part of your chest (near the tip of your breastbone) rather than to the upper part of it will reduce the stress on an impinged shoulder. This exercise may also be contraindicated if you have low-back pain or hyperextended elbows.

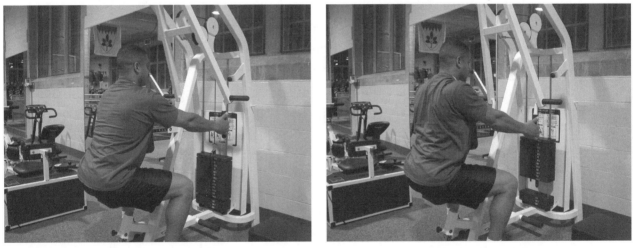

Start/Finish Position   *Mid-Range Position*

SCAPULAE RETRACTION

Muscles Involved: trapezius (middle portion)

Suggested Repetitions: 8 - 12 (or 50 - 70 seconds)

Type of Movement: single joint

Starting Position: Adjust the position of the seat pad (as described below in the training tips). Sit down on the seat pad, slide your hips backward slightly, and lean forward against the chest pad. Place your feet flat on the floor or on the footrest (if one is provided). Grasp the handles of the movement arms with a "parallel grip" (your palms facing each other).

Performance Description: Keep your arms fairly straight and pinch your shoulder blades together. Pause briefly in this mid-range position (your shoulder blades together), and then lower the weight under control to the starting position (your shoulder blades apart) to ensure a sufficient stretch.

Training Tips:

- Adjust the position of the seat pad so that your hands are slightly lower than your shoulders in the starting position.

- On some machines, you can adjust the position of the chest pad. If the chest pad is adjustable, position it so that when you grasp the handles in the starting position, the weight you intend to lift is separated slightly from the rest of the weight stack. In other words, your arms are fully extended. (This produces a greater stretch of your upper back and biceps).

- Changing the position of your torso as you perform this exercise is natural. However, movement of your torso should not be excessive or used to throw the weight — movement should only occur around your shoulder joints.

- When performing this exercise with a selectorized machine, do not slam the weights together between repetitions; when performing this exercise with a plate-loaded machine, do not bounce the movement arms off the rubber stoppers.

- You can do this exercise unilaterally (one limb at a time) in the event that you have a shoulder or arm injury, or a gross difference in the strength between your limbs. You can also do it in this fashion if you desire a training variation.

- You can use wrist straps if you have difficulty in maintaining your grip on the handles.

- This exercise may be contraindicated if you have hyperextended elbows.

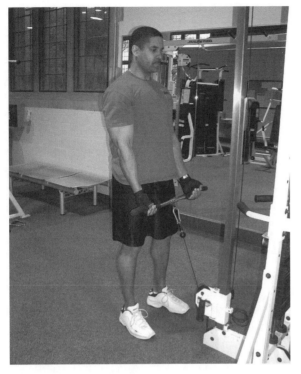

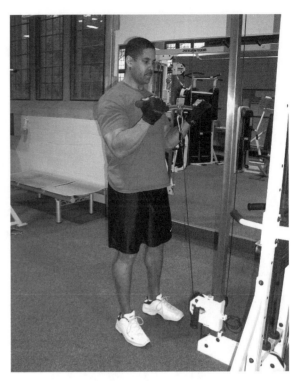

Start/Finish Position   *Mid-Range Position*

BICEP CURL

Muscles Involved: biceps and forearms

Suggested Repetitions: 6 - 12 (or 40 - 70 seconds)

Type of Movement: single joint

Starting Position: Adjust the position of the pulley so that it is near the floor. Reach down and grasp the bar with your hands spaced slightly wider than shoulder-width apart and your palms facing away from you. Stand upright by straightening your legs and torso (as if performing a deadlift). Take a slight step backwards and spread your feet approximately shoulder-width apart.

Performance Description: Keep your elbows against the sides of your torso and pull the bar below your chin by bending your arms. Pause briefly in this mid-range position (your arms flexed), and then lower the weight under control to the starting position (your arms fully extended) to provide a sufficient stretch.

Training Tips:

- Avoid throwing the weight by using your legs, or by swinging your torso back and forth — movement should only occur around your elbow joints.

- Changing the position of your elbows as you perform this exercise is natural. However, movement of your elbows should not be excessive.

- You can do this exercise unilaterally (one limb at a time) with a handle instead of a bar in the event that you have an arm injury or a gross difference in the strength between your limbs. You can also do it in this fashion if you desire a training variation.

- This exercise may be contraindicated if you have hyperextended elbows.

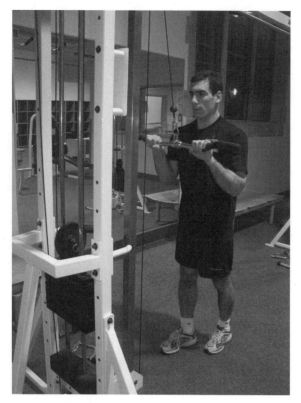

Start/Finish Position

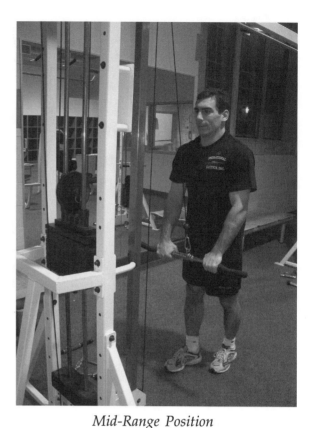

Mid-Range Position

TRICEP EXTENSION

Muscle Involved: triceps

Suggested Repetitions: 6 - 12 (or 40 - 70 seconds)

Type of Movement: single joint

Starting Position: Adjust the position of the pulley so that it is above your head. Reach up and grasp the bar with your hands spaced about 4 - 6 inches apart and your palms facing downward. Take a slight step backwards and place one foot slightly in front of the other. Pull the bar down until your elbows are against the sides of your torso.

Performance Description: Keep your elbows against the sides of your torso and push the bar down by straightening your arms. Pause briefly in this mid-range position (your arms fully extended), and then return the weight under control to the starting position (your arms flexed) to ensure a proper stretch.

Training Tips:

- Your elbows should remain in contact with the sides of your torso as you perform this exercise.

- Avoid swinging your torso back and forth as you perform this exercise — movement should only occur around your elbow joints.

- You can do this exercise unilaterally (one limb at a time) with a handle instead of a bar in the event that you have an arm injury or a gross difference in the strength between your limbs. You can also do it in this fashion if you desire a training variation.

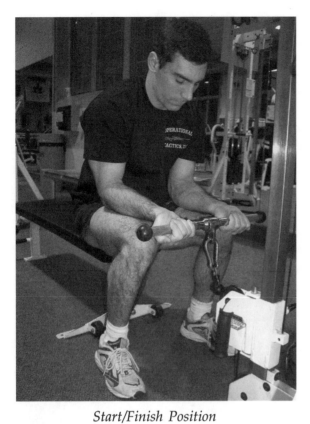

Start/Finish Position

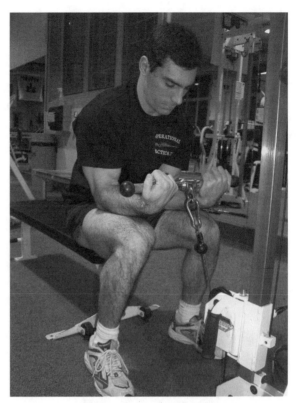

Mid-Range Position

WRIST FLEXION

Muscles Involved: wrist flexors

Suggested Repetitions: 8 - 12 (or 50 - 70 seconds)

Type of Movement: single joint

Starting Position: Adjust the position of the pulley so that it is near the floor. Place a bench several feet in front of the pulley. Reach down and grasp the bar with your palms facing away from you. Lift the bar, sit down near the end of the back pad of the bench, and place the backs of your forearms directly over your upper legs. (You can also place your forearms flat on the back pad between your legs.) Place your thumbs underneath the bar alongside your fingers and spread your hands about 4 - 6 inches apart. Lean forward slightly so that the angle between your upper and lower arms is about 90 degrees or less. Your wrists should be over your kneecaps (or over the edge of the back pad if you placed your forearms on it).

Performance Description: Pull the bar up as high as possible by bending your wrists. Pause briefly in this mid-range position (your wrists flexed), and then lower the weight under control to the starting position (your wrists extended) to provide a sufficient stretch.

Training Tips:

- Your forearms should remain directly over your upper legs throughout the performance of this exercise.

- Placing your thumbs underneath the bar alongside your fingers will give you a greater range of motion.

- Avoid throwing the weight by using your legs, or by swinging your torso back and forth — movement should only occur around your wrist joints.

- You can do this exercise unilaterally (one limb at a time) with a handle instead of a bar in the event that you have a wrist injury or a gross difference in the strength between your limbs. You can also do it in this fashion if you desire a training variation.

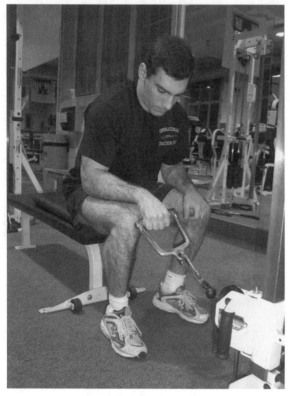

Start/Finish Position

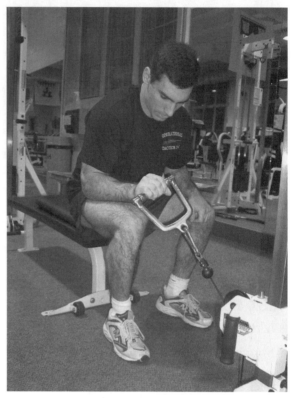

Mid-Range Position

WRIST EXTENSION

Muscles Involved: wrist extensors

Suggested Repetitions: 8 - 12 (or 50 - 70 seconds)

Type of Movement: single joint

Starting position: Adjust the position of the pulley so that it is near the floor. Place a bench several feet in front of the pulley. Reach down and grasp the handle with your right hand. Lift the handle, sit down near the end of the back pad of the bench, and place the front of your right forearm directly over your right upper leg so that your palm is facing down. (You can also place your forearms flat on the back pad between your legs.) Lean forward slightly so that the angle between your upper and lower arms is about 90 degrees or less. Your right wrist should be over your right kneecap (or over the edge of the back pad if you placed your forearm on it).

Performance Description: Pull the handle up as high as possible by bending your wrist. Pause briefly in this mid-range position (your wrist extended), and then lower the weight under control to the starting position (your wrist flexed) to obtain an adequate stretch. After performing a set with your right arm, repeat the exercise for the other side of your body.

Training Tips:

- Your forearm should remain directly over your upper leg throughout the performance of this exercise.

- Avoid throwing the weight by using your leg or by swinging your torso back and forth — movement should only occur around your wrist joint.

- This exercise is more comfortable on your wrist when it is performed one limb at a time with a handle rather than both limbs at a time with a bar.

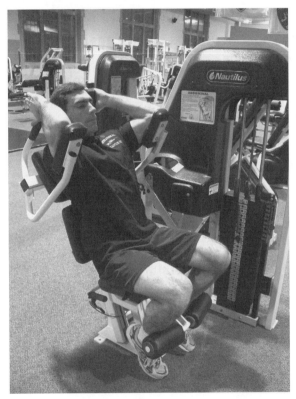

Start/Finish Position

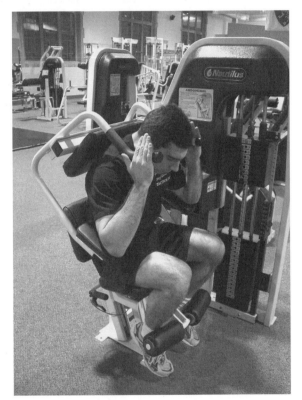

Mid-Range Position

ABDOMINAL

Muscles Involved: rectus abdominis and iliopsoas

Suggested Repetitions: 8 - 12 (or 50 - 70 seconds)

Type of Movement: single joint

Starting Position: Adjust the position of the seat pad (as described below in the training tips). Sit down on the seat pad, place your lower legs behind the roller pads, and lean back against the back pad. Position the backs of your upper arms against the elbow pads, place your hands on the handles so that your palms are facing each other, and open your hands (that is, extend your fingers).

Performance Description: Pull your torso down as far as possible by exerting force against the elbow pads. Pause briefly in this mid-range position (your torso flexed), and then lower the weight under control to the starting position (your torso extended) to obtain a proper stretch.

Training Tips:

- Adjust the position of the seat pad so that your navel (or "belly button") is approximately even with the axis of rotation of the machine.

- Your abdominals are used primarily during the first 30 degrees or so of this exercise. (Thereafter, your hip flexors accept most of the workload.) So, bringing your torso all the way to your upper legs is not necessary.

- Avoid throwing your torso forward or snapping your head forward as you perform this exercise — movement should only occur around your hip joint and mid-section.

- Keep your hands open and fingers extended so that you exert force against the elbow pads with your upper arms, not your hands. This is critical in order for you to isolate your abdominals.

- If performing this exercise while keeping your upper arms against the elbow pads is difficult, you can grasp the handles with a "parallel grip" (your palms facing each other) and pull with your hands instead of your upper arms. This will not allow you to isolate the muscles of your abdominals, but it will make the exercise more comfortable for you to perform.

- When performing this exercise with a selectorized machine, do not slam the weights together between repetitions; when performing this exercise with a plate-loaded machine, do not bounce the movement arm off the rubber stoppers.

- This exercise may be contraindicated if you have low-back pain or shoulder-impingement syndrome.

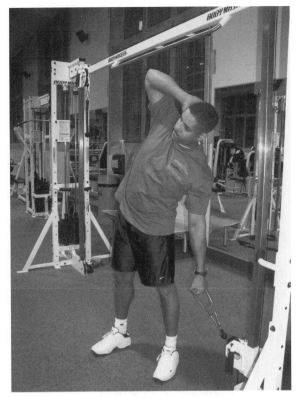

Start/Finish Position

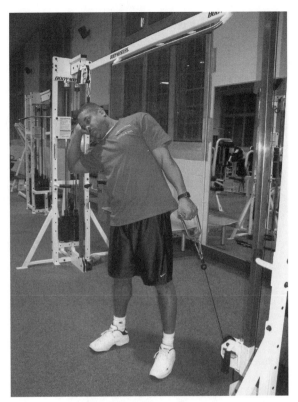

Mid-Range Position

SIDE BEND

Muscles Involved: obliques and erector spinae (lower back)

Suggested Repetitions: 8 - 12 (or 50 - 70 seconds)

Type of Movement: single joint

Starting Position: Adjust the position of the pulley so that it is near the floor. Reach down and grasp the handle with your left hand. Stand upright by straightening your legs and torso. Turn your feet to the right so that the left side of your body is facing the pulley. Slide your feet away from the machine so that the weight you intend to lift is separated slightly from the rest of the weight stack. Hold the handle at the side of your body with your palm facing your leg and spread your feet about shoulder-width apart. Place your right palm against the right side of your head. Without moving your hips, bend your torso to the left as far as possible.

Performance Description: Without moving your hips, bend your torso to the right as far as possible. Pause briefly in this mid-range position (your torso bent to the right), and then lower the weight under control to the starting position (your torso bent to the left) to ensure a sufficient stretch. After performing a set for the right side of your body, repeat the exercise for the other side of your body (holding the handle with your right hand).

Training Tips:

- Changing the position of your hips as you perform this exercise is natural. However,

161

movement of your hips should not be excessive or used to throw the weight — movement should only occur around your mid-section.

- Do not bend forward at the waist as you perform this exercise.

- Keep your feet flat on the floor as you perform this exercise.

- This exercise may be contraindicated if you have low-back pain.

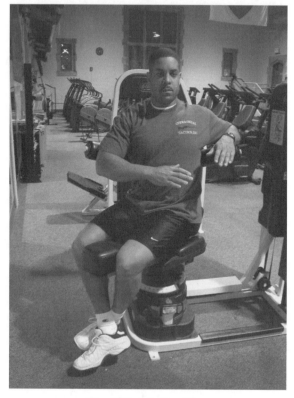

Start/Finish Position

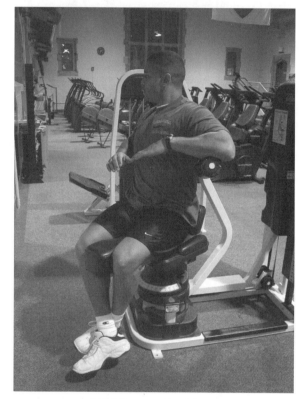

Mid-Range Position

ROTARY TORSO

Muscles Involved: obliques and erector spinae (lower back)

Suggested Repetitions: 8 - 12 (or 50 - 70 seconds)

Type of Movement: sing1le joint

Starting Position: Sit down on the seat pad so that the yoke is between your legs. Turn your torso to the left and lean back against the back pad. Bend your right arm and place the back of it against the right roller pad. Bend your left arm and place it over the left roller pad. Bring your legs together (with the yoke between them) and cross your ankles.

Performance Description: Rotate your torso to the right as far as possible by exerting force against the right roller pad. Pause briefly in this mid-range position (your torso rotated to the right), and then lower the weight under control to the starting position (your torso rotated to the left) to ensure a sufficient stretch. After performing a set for the right side of your body, repeat the exercise for the other side of your body.

Training Tips:

- On some machines, you can adjust the position of the seat pad. If the seat pad is adjustable, position it so that it offers the greatest degree of torso rotation in the starting position.

- When performing this exercise, one side of your body should be active and the other side should be passive.

- Changing the position of your hips as you perform this exercise is natural. However, movement of your hips should not be excessive or used to throw the weight — movement should only occur around your mid-section.

- Your torso should remain upright as you perform this exercise.

- Your head should rotate in union with your torso as you perform this exercise.

- When performing this exercise with a selectorized machine, do not slam the weights together between repetitions.

- This exercise may be contraindicated if you have low-back pain.

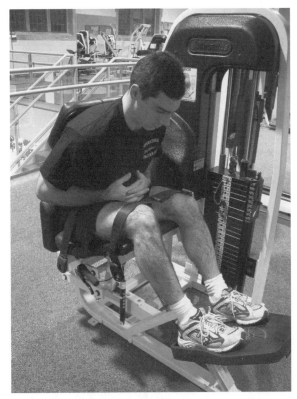

Start/Finish Position

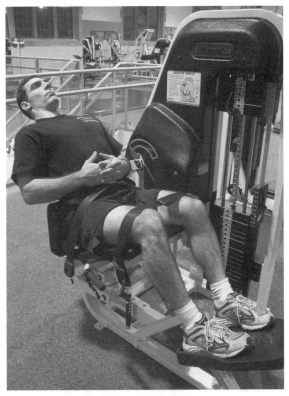

Mid-Range Position

BACK EXTENSION

Muscles Involved: erector spinae (lower back)

Suggested Repetitions: 10 - 15 (or 60 - 90 seconds)

Type of Movement: single joint

Starting Position: Adjust the position of the seat pad (as described below in the training tips). Sit down on the seat pad, place your feet flat on the foot platform, and position your back against the back pad. Secure the thigh belt (if one is provided) and the waist belt. Interlock your fingers and place your palms against your mid-section.

Performance Description: Extend your torso backward as far as possible by pushing against the back pad. Pause briefly in this mid-range position (your torso extended), and then lower the weight under control to the starting position (your torso flexed) to ensure a sufficient stretch.

Training Tips:

- Adjust the position of the seat pad so that your navel (or "belly button") is approximately even with the axis of rotation of the machine.

- On some machines, you can adjust the position of the foot platform. If the foot platform is adjustable, position it so that when your feet are flat on it there is no space between the back of your upper legs and the seat pad.

- Avoid throwing your head backward as you perform this exercise — movement should only occur around your hip joint and mid-section.

- Keep your hips flat on the seat pad and your feet flat on the foot platform as you perform this exercise.

- When performing this exercise with a selectorized machine, do not slam the weights together between repetitions.

- This exercise may be contraindicated if you have low-back pain.

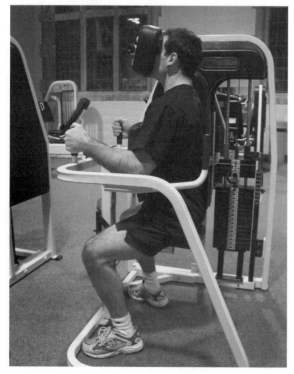 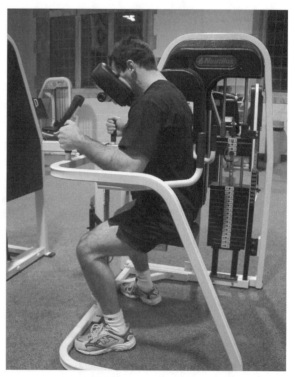

Start/Finish Position   *Mid-Range Position*

NECK FLEXION

Muscle Involved: sternocleidomastoideus (both sides acting together)

Suggested Repetitions: 8 - 12 (or 50 - 70 seconds)

Type of Movement: single joint

Starting Position: Adjust the position of the seat pad (as described below in the training tips). Sit down on the seat pad and position the front part of your head against the face pads. Place your feet flat on the floor, grasp the handles, and position your head so that it is perpendicular to the floor.

Performance Description: Without moving your torso, pull your head as close to your chest as possible by exerting force against the face pads. Pause briefly in this mid-range position (your chin near your chest), and then lower the weight under control to the starting position (your head perpendicular to the floor) to provide an adequate stretch.

Training Tips:

- Adjust the position of the seat pad so that the front part of your head is centered on the face pads when sitting upright.

- On some machines, there is an adjustable torso pad. If the machine has a torso pad, position it so that it will be directly below the face pads in the mid-range position.

- Do not move your head backward beyond a point that it is perpendicular to the floor as you perform this exercise.

- Changing the position of your torso as you perform this exercise is natural. However, movement of your torso should not be excessive or used to throw the weight — movement should only occur around your neck.

- Keep your hips on the seat pad and your feet flat on the floor as you perform this exercise.

- When performing this exercise with a selectorized machine, do not slam the weights together between repetitions; when performing this exercise with a plate-loaded machine, do not bounce the movement arm off the rubber stoppers.

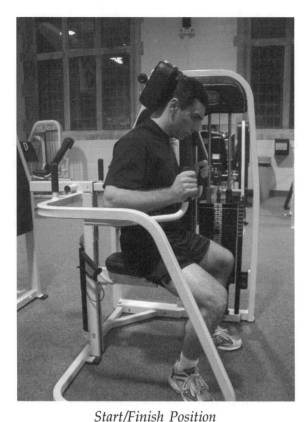

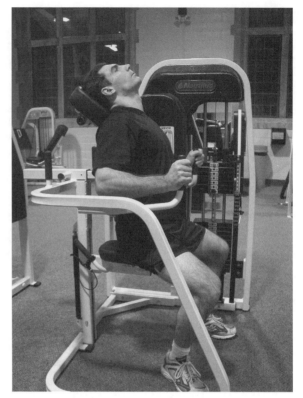

Start/Finish Position   *Mid-Range Position*

NECK EXTENSION

Muscles Involved: neck extensors and trapezius (upper portion)

Suggested Repetitions: 8 - 12 (or 50 - 70 seconds)

Type of Movement: single joint

Starting Position: Adjust the position of the seat pad (as described below in the training tips). Sit down on the seat pad and position the back part of your head against the face pads. Place your feet flat on the floor, grasp the handles, and position your chin near your chest.

Performance Description: Without moving your torso, extend your head backward as far as possible by exerting force against the face pads. Pause briefly in this mid-range position (your neck extended), and then return the weight under control to the starting position (your chin near your chest) to ensure an adequate stretch.

Training Tips:

- Adjust the position of the seat pad so that the back part of your head is centered on the face pads when sitting upright.

- On some machines, there is an adjustable torso pad. If the machine has a torso pad, position it so that it will be directly under the face pads in the mid-range position.

- Changing the position of your torso as you perform this exercise is natural. However, movement of your torso should not be excessive or used to throw the weight — movement should only occur around your neck.

- Keep your hips on the seat pad and your feet flat on the floor as you perform this exercise.
- When performing this exercise with a selectorized machine, do not slam the weights together between repetitions; when performing this exercise with a plate-loaded machine, do not bounce the movement arm off the rubber stoppers.

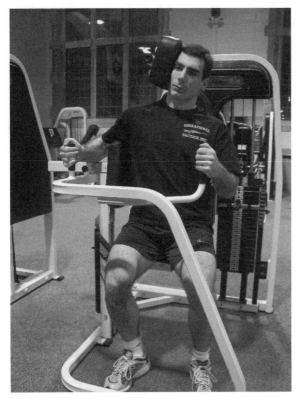

Start/Finish Position

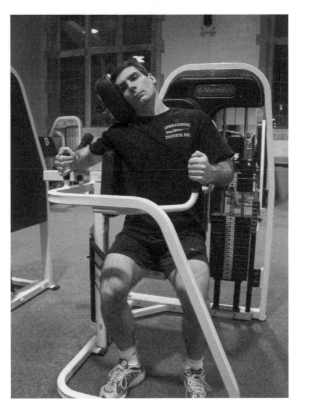

Mid-Range Position

NECK LATERAL FLEXION

Muscle Involved: sternocleidomastoideus (one side acting singly)

Suggested Repetitions: 8 - 12 (or 50 - 70 seconds)

Type of Movement: single joint

Starting Position: Adjust the position of the seat pad (as described below in the training tips). Sit down on the seat pad and position the right side of your head against the face pads. Place your feet flat on the floor, grasp the handles, and position your head near your left shoulder.

Performance Description: Without moving your torso, pull your head to your right shoulder by exerting force against the face pads. Pause briefly in this mid-range position (your head near your right shoulder), and then return the weight under control to the starting position (your head near your left shoulder) to provide a proper stretch. After performing a set for the right side of your neck, repeat the exercise for the other side of your body (by moving your hips on the seat pad 180 degrees to the left).

Training Tips:

- Adjust the position of the seat pad so that the side part of your head is centered on the face pads when sitting upright.

- On some machines, there is an adjustable torso pad. If the machine has a torso pad, position it as far away from your torso as possible so that it does not restrict your range of motion.

- Changing the position of your torso as you perform this exercise is natural. However, movement of your torso should not be excessive or used to throw the weight — movement should only occur around your neck.

- Keep your hips on the seat pad and your feet flat on the floor as you perform this exercise.

- When performing this exercise with a selectorized machine, do not slam the weights together between repetitions; when performing this exercise with a plate-loaded machine, do not bounce the movement arm off the rubber stoppers.

Chapter 10
Manual-Resistance Exercises

Manual resistance has been referred to as a "productive alternative" for developing strength when equipment is not available. It is an extremely effective way of strength training in which another person supplies the resistance. Surprisingly, manual-resistance exercises have actually been around for quite a long time. The origins of these exercises can be traced back to the Swedish system. In one of the earliest accounts of manual-resistance exercises, Pehr Henri Ling of Sweden — who lived from 1776 - 1839 — stated that "Resistance may consist of gravity, the opposing force of antagonizing muscles, or that which is exerted by another person." In an 1862 magazine article that was written by a medical doctor named Dio Lewis, several exercises were described in which an individual pulled one or two wooden gymnastic rings that were held by another person who offered resistance. In support of these movements, Dr. Lewis wrote, "In most exercises there must be some resistance. How much better that this should be another human being, rather than a pole, ladder or bar!"

In the 1920s, Angelo Siciliano was awarded the title as "The World's Most Perfectly Developed Man" after winning a physique contest. Siciliano claimed to have used his body to provide its own resistance (although it appears as if he developed his award-winning physique using barbells and dumbbells). Siciliano called his system "Dynamic Tension," and began a lucrative mail-order service to market these self-resistive exercises under the more recognizable name of Charles Atlas.

During the late 1970s, manual resistance was refined and popularized by Dan Riley (a strength and conditioning coach who has more than 20 years of experience in the National Football League). Largely because of his earlier efforts, manual-resistance exercises have been used at the collegiate and professional levels for many years.

ADVANTAGES AND DISADVANTAGES

Manual resistance has many advantages. First, little or no equipment is required. Because of this, the exercises can be done just about anywhere without having to go to the weight room. In addition, there is little or no expense. This is an important consideration if you are trying to outfit a weight room with a limited or tight budget. Manual resistance is also a way of training large numbers of individuals in an extremely time-efficient fashion. (Regardless of the size of the group, one half of them can perform the exercises while the other half can act as spotters.)

Manual resistance has several disadvantages. The major disadvantage of manual resistance is that the resistance cannot be quantified, thereby making it impossible to monitor progress. Another drawback is that manual resistance requires a competent spotter.

GENERAL TECHNIQUE

In order for manual resistance to be productive, the exercises must be performed with proper technique. The following are general guidelines for the lifter and spotter:

The Lifter

As in lifting any weight, the lifter should perform the repetitions in a deliberate, controlled manner throughout the greatest possible range of motion that safety allows. The resistance (as applied by the spotter) should be raised in about 1 - 2 seconds and lowered in about 3 - 4 seconds. As an alternative to counting repetitions, the exercises can be performed for a pre-scribed amount of time. In this case, the lifter should reach concentric muscular fatigue within about 60 - 90 seconds for the lower body and about 40 - 70 seconds for the torso. (Muscular fatigue should occur within about 50 - 70 seconds for upper-body exercises that have a relatively short range of motion.) If counting repetitions is more preferable, muscular fatigue should be attained in 10 - 15 repetitions for the lower body and 6 - 12 repetitions for the torso. (Muscular fatigue should occur with 8 - 12 repetitions for upper-body exercises that have a relatively short range of motion.) Note that these repetition ranges are based upon a six-second repetition. The lifter must keep the muscles loaded throughout the entire exercise. Finally, the lifter must communicate to the spotter whether the resistance is too much or too little.

The Spotter

Because an individual is naturally stronger in some positions than others due to the changing biomechanical leverage of the skeletal system, the spotter is responsible for varying the resistance throughout the lifter's entire range of motion. In a lateral raise, for instance, you lose leverage as you raise your arms away from the sides of your body. As the lifter's leverage decreases, the spotter must provide less resistance. Since individuals are considerably stronger in the eccentric phase of a repetition, the spotter must apply more resistance when the lifter performs that part of the repetition. The spotter must also regulate the resistance in accordance with the lifter's momentary level of strength. In other words, the spotter must furnish less resistance as the lifter fatigues during each repetition. In addition, the spotter must control the speed with which the lifter performs the repetitions. Lastly, the spotter should motivate the lifter by providing words of encouragement.

THE EXERCISES

This chapter will describe and illustrate the safest and most productive exercises that can be performed with manual resistance. Included in the discussions of each exercise are the muscle(s) involved (if more than one muscle is involved, the first muscle listed is the prime mover), suggested repetitions (the time that the targeted muscles should be loaded is shown in parentheses), type of movement, starting position, performance description, and training tips for making the exercise safer and more productive. (In the accompanying photographs, the lifter is wearing the darker shirt.) The exercises described in this chapter are hip abduction, hip adduction, prone leg curl, leg extension, dorsi flexion, push-up, bent-arm fly, bent-over row, seated row, lat pulldown, seated press, lateral raise, front raise, internal rotation, external rotation, bicep curl, tricep extension, sit-up, neck flexion, and neck extension.

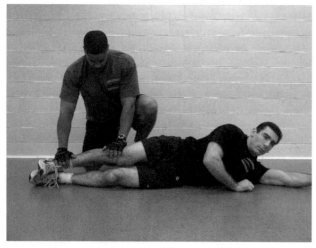 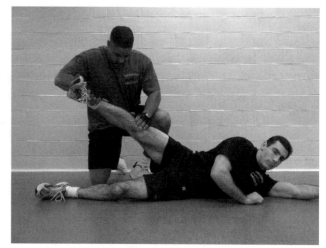

Start/Finish Position   *Mid-Range Position*

HIP ABDUCTION

Muscle Involved: gluteus medius

Suggested Repetitions: 10 - 15 (or 60 - 90 seconds)

Type of Movement: single joint

Starting Position: Lie down on the floor on the left side of your body, straighten your legs, and point your right toes toward your right knee. Extend your left arm across the floor. The spotter should kneel behind you and apply resistance against your right ankle.

Performance Description: Raise your right leg as high as possible, as the spotter provides resistance evenly throughout the full range of motion. Pause briefly in this mid-range position (your legs apart), and then resist as the spotter pushes your leg back to the starting position (your legs together) to obtain a proper stretch. After performing a set with your right leg, repeat the exercise for the other side of your body (lying on the right side of your body).

Training Tips:

• The spotter should apply resistance above your knee if you suffer from a hyperextended knee or other joint pain.

• Do not bend forward at the waist as you perform this exercise.

• Attempt to raise your leg as high as possible in the mid-range position of every repetition to ensure that you are obtaining a maximal contraction of the target muscles throughout the duration of the exercise.

• You should reach a point where you cannot lift your leg. At this time, you can overload your muscles further by having the spotter lift your leg to the mid-range position, and then push it back to the starting position as you resist for 3 - 5 negative repetitions.

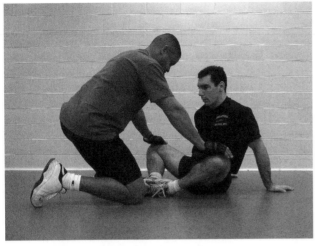
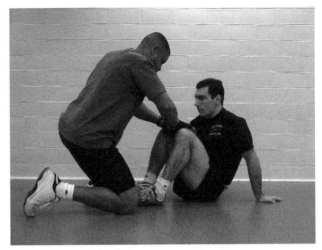

Start/Finish Position   *Mid-Range Position*

HIP ADDUCTION

Muscles Involved: hip adductors (inner thigh)

Suggested Repetitions: 10 - 15 (or 60 - 90 seconds)

Type of Movement: single joint

Starting Position: Sit down on the floor, bend your legs, and place the soles of your feet together. Position your feet close to your hips and spread your knees apart. Place your hands alongside your hips and lean back slightly. The spotter should kneel in front of you and apply resistance against the insides of your knees.

Performance Description: Bring your knees as close together as possible, as the spotter provides resistance evenly throughout the full range of motion. Pause briefly in this mid-range position (your knees together), and then resist as the spotter pushes your legs back to the starting position (your knees apart) to provide an adequate stretch.

Training Tips:

- Attempt to bring your knees as close together as possible in the mid-range position of every repetition to ensure that you are obtaining a maximal contraction of the target muscles throughout the duration of the exercise.

- You should reach a point where you cannot bring your knees together. At this time, you can overload your muscles further by having the spotter lift your legs to the mid-range position, and then push them back to the starting position as you resist for 3 - 5 negative repetitions.

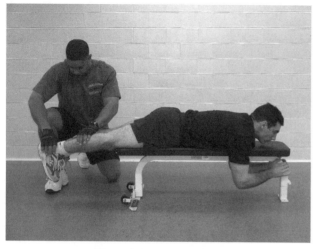

Start/Finish Position

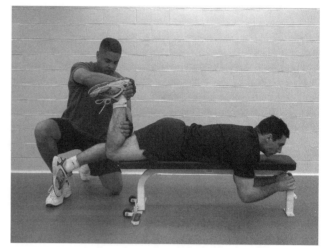

Mid-Range Position

PRONE LEG CURL

Muscles Involved: hamstrings

Suggested Repetitions: 10 - 15 (or 60 - 90 seconds)

Type of Movement: single joint

Starting Position: Lie face down on the back pad of a bench (or the floor if a bench is not available), straighten your legs, and point your right toes toward your right knee. Position the tops of your kneecaps so that they are just over the end of the back pad, not on it. The spotter should kneel behind you and apply resistance against your right heel.

Performance Description: Pull your right heel as close to your hip as possible, as the spotter provides resistance evenly throughout the full range of motion. Pause briefly in this mid-range position (your heel near your hip), and then resist as the spotter pulls your lower leg back to the starting position (your leg fully extended) to ensure a sufficient stretch. After performing a set with your right leg, repeat the exercise for the other side of your body.

Training Tips:

- The muscles of your legs are relatively strong and, therefore, you will probably have to do this exercise unilaterally (one limb at a time). However, you can perform it bilaterally (both limbs at a time) if the spotter is capable of providing you with adequate resistance.

- You can raise your hip as you perform this exercise since this actually increases your range of motion. Otherwise, movement should only occur around your knee joint.

- Attempt to bring your heel as close to your hip as possible in the mid-range position of every repetition to ensure that you are obtaining a maximal contraction of the target muscles throughout the duration of the exercise.

- The angle between your upper and lower leg should be about 90 degrees or less in the mid-range position.

- You can also perform this exercise in the seated position. In this case, sit down on the back pad of a bench, table, or chair that is high enough so that your feet do not touch the floor. Place the back of your right knee against the end of it and straighten your right leg. The spotter should kneel in front of you and apply resistance against your right heel. The exercise would be performed in the manner described above. Performing this exercise in the seated position produces less stress in the low-back region than performing it in the prone position.

- You should reach a point where you cannot lift your lower leg. At this time, you can overload your muscles further by having the spotter lift your lower leg to the mid-range position, and then pull it back to the starting position as you resist for 3 - 5 negative repetitions.

- This exercise may be contraindicated if you have low-back pain or hyperextended knees.

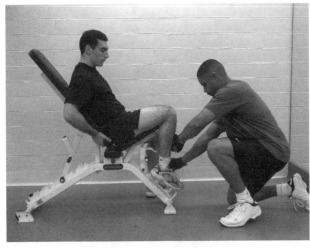

| Start/Finish Position | Mid-Range Position |

LEG EXTENSION

Muscles Involved: quadriceps

Suggested Repetitions: 10 - 15 (or 60 - 90 seconds)

Type of Movement: single joint

Starting Position: Sit down on the back pad of a bench, table, or chair that is high enough so that your feet do not touch the floor. Place the back of your right knee against the end of it. The spotter should kneel in front of you and apply resistance against your right ankle.

Performance Description: Extend your right lower leg as high as possible, as the spotter provides resistance evenly throughout the full range of motion. Pause briefly in this mid-range position (your leg fully extended), and then resist as the spotter pushes your lower leg back to the starting position (your leg flexed) to obtain a proper stretch. After performing a set with your right leg, repeat the exercise for the other side of your body.

Training Tips:

• The muscles of your legs are relatively strong and, therefore, you will probably have to do this exercise unilaterally (one limb at a time). However, you can perform it bilaterally (both limbs at a time) if the spotter is capable of providing you with adequate resistance.

• Avoid swinging your torso back and forth as you perform this exercise — movement should only occur around your knee joint.

• Attempt to extend your leg as high as possible in the mid-range position of every repetition to ensure that you are obtaining a maximal contraction of the target muscles throughout the duration of the exercise.

• You should reach a point where you cannot lift your lower leg. At this time, you can overload your muscles further by having the spotter lift your lower leg to the mid-range position, and then push it back to the starting position as you resist for 3 - 5 negative repetitions.

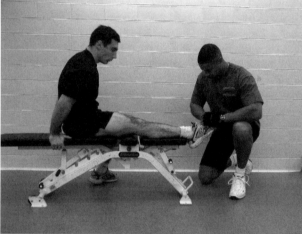

Start/Finish Position

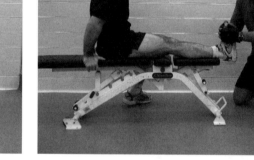

Mid-Range Position

DORSI FLEXION

Muscles Involved: dorsi flexors

Suggested Repetitions: 10 - 15 (or 60 - 90 seconds)

Type of Movement: single joint

Starting Position: Sit down on the back pad of a bench and place your right leg across the length of it. Position your right heel slightly over the end of the back pad and point your right toes away from your body. The spotter should sit or kneel in front of you and apply resistance against the lower part of your right foot.

Performance Description: Keep your right leg flat on the back pad and pull your right foot toward your knee as the spotter provides resistance evenly throughout the full range of motion. Pause briefly in this mid-range position (your ankle flexed), and then resist as the spotter pulls your foot back to the starting position (your ankle fully extended) to ensure a sufficient stretch. After performing a set with your right ankle, repeat the exercise for the other side of your body.

Training Tips:

- The muscles of your legs are relatively strong and, therefore, you will probably have to do this exercise unilaterally (one limb at a time). However, you can perform it bilaterally (both limbs at a time) if the spotter is capable of providing you with adequate resistance.

- You should reach a point where you cannot pull your foot toward your knee. At this time, you can overload your muscles further by having the spotter bring your foot to the mid-range position, and then pull it back to the starting position as you resist for 3 - 5 negative repetitions.

- This exercise may be contraindicated if you have shin splints.

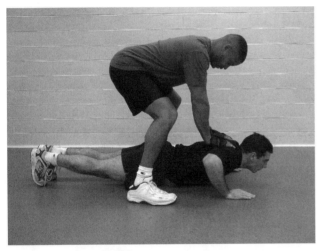

Start/Finish Position

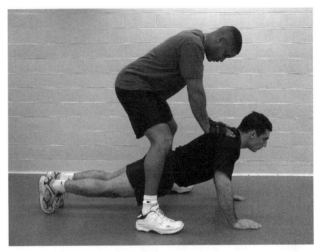

Mid-Range Position

PUSH-UP

Muscles Involved: chest, anterior deltoid, and triceps

Suggested Repetitions: 6 - 12 (or 40 - 70 seconds)

Type of Movement: multiple joint

Starting Position: Lie face down on the floor, straighten your legs, and curl your toes under your feet. Place your palms on the floor and spread your hands slightly wider than shoulder-width apart. The spotter should straddle your torso and apply resistance against your upper back.

Performance Description: Push your body up until your arms are almost fully extended (without "locking" your elbows), as the spotter provides resistance evenly throughout the full range of motion. Pause briefly in this mid-range position (your arms almost fully extended), and then resist as the spotter pushes you back to the starting position (your chest touching the floor) to obtain a sufficient stretch.

Training Tips:

- You should not use an excessively wide hand position since this will reduce your range of motion.

- Avoid arching your lower back as you perform this exercise — your torso should remain aligned with your lower body.

- You should not "lock" or "snap" your elbows in the mid-range position of a repetition. This removes the load from the target muscles and may hyperextend your elbows.

- If you are unable to do 6 repetitions in strict form using your bodyweight, you can increase your biomechanical leverage by performing this exercise in the kneeling position.

- You should reach a point where you cannot lift your body. At this time, you can overload your muscles further by having the spotter lift your body to the mid-range position, and then push it back to the starting position as you resist for 3 - 5 negative repetitions.

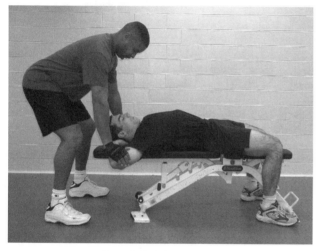

Start/Finish Position

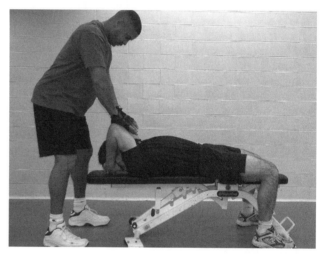

Mid-Range Position

BENT-ARM FLY

Muscles Involved: chest and anterior deltoid

Suggested Repetitions: 6 - 12 (or 40 - 70 seconds)

Type of Movement: single joint

Starting Position: Lie down on the back pad of a bench and interlock your fingers behind your head. The spotter should stand directly behind your head and apply resistance against the insides of your elbows.

Performance Description: Keep your head against the back pad and bring your elbows as close together as possible, as the spotter provides resistance evenly throughout the full range of motion. Pause briefly in this mid-range position (your elbows together), and then resist as the spotter pushes your arms back to the starting position (your elbows apart) to obtain a sufficient stretch.

Training Tips:

- Keep your head, torso, and hips against the back pad and your feet flat on the floor as you perform this exercise — movement should only occur around your shoulder joints.

- If you have low-back pain, you can place your feet on the end of the back pad or a stool. This will flatten your lumbar area against the back pad and reduce the stress in your low-back region.

- You should reach a point where you cannot bring your elbows together. At this time, you can overload your muscles further by having the spotter lift your arms to the mid-range position, and then push them back to the starting position as you resist for 3 - 5 negative repetitions.

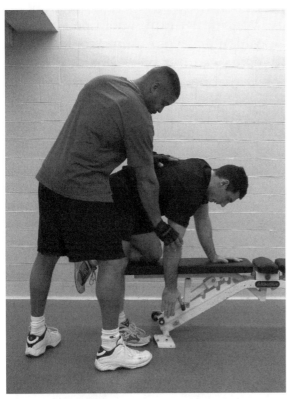

Start/Finish Position

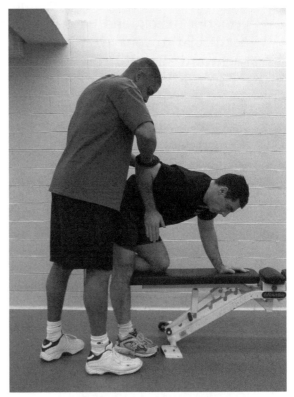

Mid-Range Position

BENT-OVER ROW

Muscles Involved: upper back ("lats")

Suggested Repetitions: 6 - 12 (or 40 - 70 seconds)

Type of Movement: single joint

Starting Position: Place your left hand and left knee on the back pad of the bench, and position your right foot on the floor at a comfortable distance from the bench. Let your right arm hang straight down and open your right hand (extending your fingers). Your right palm should be facing the bench. The spotter should stand along the right side of your torso and apply resistance against the back of your right upper arm near your elbow.

179

Performance Description: Keep your upper arm close to your torso and pull your elbow up as high as possible, as the spotter provides resistance evenly throughout the full range of motion. Pause briefly in this mid-range position (your arm flexed), and then resist as the spotter pushes your arm back to the starting position (your arm fully extended) to provide a proper stretch. After performing a set with your right arm, repeat the exercise for the other side of your body (with your right hand and right knee on the back pad for support).

Training Tips:

- Keep your hand open (with your fingers extended) as you perform this exercise.

- You can also do this exercise with your upper arm positioned farther away from your torso. Keep in mind, however, that this will produce a greater involvement of your posterior deltoid and trapezius. In this case, your upper arm would be almost perpendicular to your torso in the mid-range position and your palm would be facing backward slightly. This also dramatically increases your biomechanical leverage thereby making it more difficult for the spotter to apply adequate resistance.

- This exercise is a multiple-joint movement when performed with dumbbells, but it becomes a single-joint movement when using manual resistance because the load is applied above your elbow instead of to your hand.

- You should reach a point where you cannot lift your arm. At this time, you can overload your muscles further by having the spotter lift your arm to the mid-range position, and then push it back to the starting position as you resist for 3 - 5 negative repetitions.

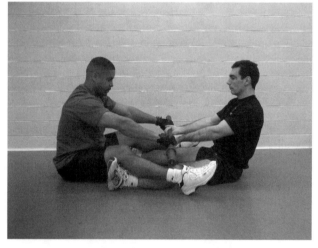

Start/Finish Position

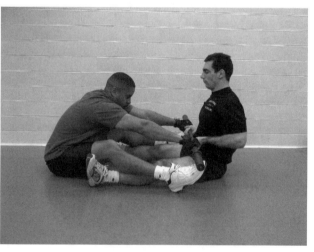

Mid-Range Position

SEATED ROW

Muscles Involved: upper back ("lats"), biceps, and forearms

Suggested Repetitions: 6 - 12 (or 40 - 70 seconds)

Type of Movement: multiple joint

Starting Position: Sit down on the floor, straighten your legs, and spread them apart. Grasp a stick (or a similar object) with your palms facing up and space your hands approximately shoulder-width apart. The spotter should sit down on the floor between your legs and grasp the stick on the outside of your grip with palms facing down. Extend your arms fully and lean back slightly.

Performance Description: Keep your upper arms close to your torso and pull the stick to your mid-section as the spotter provides resistance evenly throughout the full range of motion. Pause briefly in this mid-range position (your arms flexed), and then resist as the spotter pulls your arms back to the starting position (your arms fully extended) to ensure a sufficient stretch.

Training Tips:

- If a stick or a similar object is not available, you and the spotter can interlock each other's hands or grasp each other's wrists.

- The spotter should maintain straight arms, and supply resistance by bending forward and backward at the waist to involve the larger, more powerful muscles of the lower back.

- You should not use an excessively wide grip since this will reduce your range of motion.

- Changing the position of your torso as you perform this exercise is natural. However, movement of your torso should not be excessive or used to throw the resistance — movement should only occur around your shoulder and elbow joints.

- You can do this exercise unilaterally (one limb at a time) in the event that you have a shoulder or arm injury, or a gross difference in the strength between your limbs. You can also do it in this fashion if you desire a training variation.

- Performing this exercise with an underhand grip (your palms facing upward) is more biomechanically efficient than doing it with an overhand grip (your palms facing downward) for the same reason as described in the underhand lat pulldown exercise in Chapter 9. But this exercise is still quite productive when performed with an overhand grip in the manner described above.

- You can use wrist straps if you have difficulty in maintaining your grip on the stick.

- You should reach a point where you cannot pull the stick to your mid-section. At this time, you can overload your muscles further by having the spotter bring your arms to the mid-range position, and then pull them back to the starting position as you resist for 3 - 5 negative repetitions.

- This exercise may be contraindicated if you have hyperextended elbows.

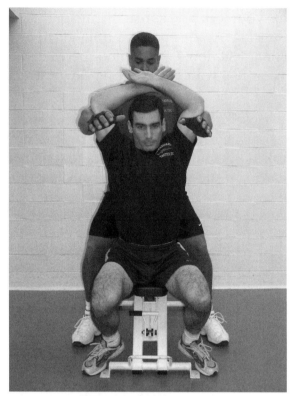

Start/Finish Position

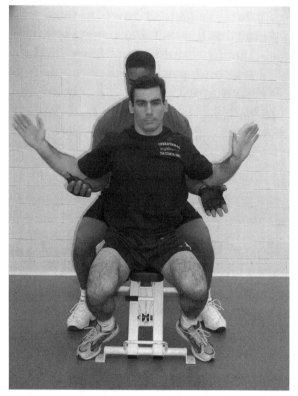

Mid-Range Position

LAT PULLDOWN

Muscles Involved: upper back ("lats")

Suggested Repetitions: 6 - 12 (or 40 - 70 seconds)

Type of Movement: single joint

Starting Position: Sit down on the back pad of a bench or a stool, and place the front part of your upper arms near the sides of your head. Cross your lower arms above your head and open your hands (extend your fingers). The spotter should stand behind you and apply resistance against the backs of your upper arms near your elbows.

Performance Description: Keep your upper arms aligned with your torso and pull your elbows down to the sides of your body as the spotter provides resistance evenly throughout the full range of motion. Pause briefly in this mid-range position (your upper arms near the sides of your body), and then resist as the spotter pulls your arms back to the starting position (your upper arms near the sides of your head) to obtain a sufficient stretch.

Training Tips:

- Your hands should not move in front of your face as you perform this exercise — they should remain out of your sight.

- Keep your hands open (with your fingers extended) as you perform this exercise.

- This exercise is a multiple-joint movement when performed with a machine, but it becomes a single-joint movement when using manual resistance because the load is applied above your elbows instead of to your hands.

- You should reach a point where you cannot perform additional repetitions. At this time, you can overload your muscles further by having the spotter bring your arms to the mid-range position, and then pull them back to the starting position as you resist for 3 - 5 negative repetitions.

- This exercise may be contraindicated if you have shoulder-impingement syndrome.

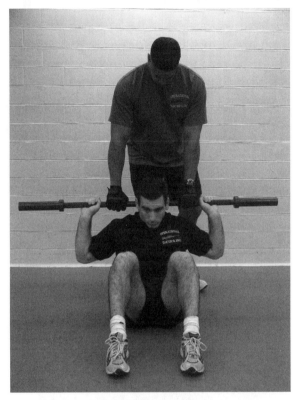

Start/Finish Position

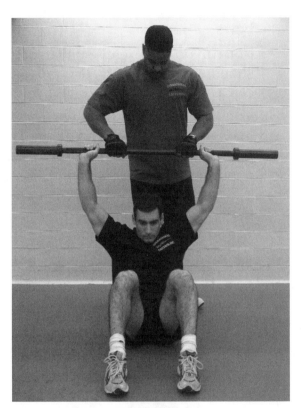

Mid-Range Position

SEATED PRESS

Muscles Involved: anterior deltoid and triceps

Suggested Repetitions: 6 - 12 (or 40 - 70 seconds)

Type of Movement: multiple joint

Starting Position: Sit down on the floor and bend your legs. Place your feet flat on the floor and lean back against the spotter's leg. Grasp a stick (or a similar object) with your palms facing up and spread your hands slightly wider than shoulder-width apart. Position the stick behind your head on the upper part of your trapezius. The spotter should grasp the stick on the inside of your grip with palms facing down.

Performance Description: Push the stick up until your arms are almost fully extended (that is, without "locking" your elbows) as the spotter provides resistance evenly throughout the full range of motion. Pause briefly in this mid-range position (your arms almost fully extended), and then resist as the spotter pushes the stick back to the starting position (your arms flexed) to provide a proper stretch.

Training Tips:

- If a stick or a similar object is not available, you and the spotter can place your palms together.

- You should not use an excessively wide grip since this will reduce your range of motion.

- You should not "lock" or "snap" your elbows in the mid-range position of a repetition. This removes the load from the target muscles and may hyperextend your elbows.

- You can do this exercise unilaterally (one limb at a time) in the event that you have a shoulder or arm injury, or a gross difference in the strength between your limbs. You can also do it in this fashion if you desire a training variation.

- You should reach a point where you cannot lift the stick. At this time, you can overload your muscles further by having the spotter lift the stick to the mid-range position, and then push it back to the starting position as you resist for 3 - 5 negative repetitions.

- This exercise may be contraindicated if you have shoulder-impingement syndrome. In this case, however, lowering the stick in front of your head rather than behind it will reduce the stress on an impinged shoulder. This exercise may also be contraindicated if you have low-back pain.

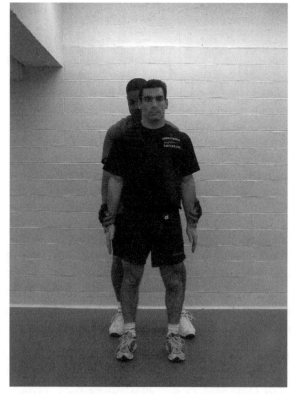

Start/Finish Position

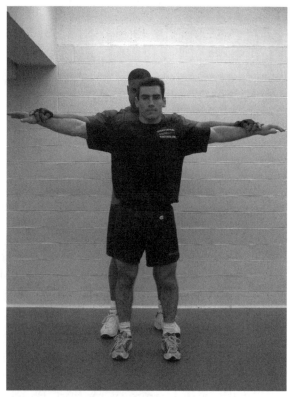

Mid-Range Position

LATERAL RAISE

Muscles Involved: middle deltoid and trapezius (upper portion)

Suggested Repetitions: 6 - 12 (or 40 - 70 seconds)

Type of Movement: single joint

Starting Position: Stand upright, let your arms hang straight down with your palms facing your legs, and open your hands (that is, extend your fingers). Spread your feet about shoulder-width apart. The spotter should stand behind you and apply resistance against your lower arms near your wrists.

Performance Description: Keep your arms fairly straight and raise them away from the sides of your body until they are parallel to the floor as the spotter provides resistance evenly throughout the full range of motion. Pause briefly in this mid-range position (your arms parallel to the floor), and then resist as the spotter pushes your arms back to the starting position (your arms at your sides) to ensure an adequate stretch.

Training Tips:

- The spotter should apply resistance above your elbows if you suffer from a hyperextended elbow or other joint pain.

- Avoid throwing your arms upward by using your legs or by swinging your torso back and forth — movement should only occur around your shoulder joints.

- You should not raise your arms beyond a point that is parallel to the floor.

- Your palms should be facing the floor in the mid-range position.

- Keep your hands open (with your fingers extended) as you perform this exercise.

- You can do this exercise unilaterally (one limb at a time) in the event that you have a shoulder or arm injury, or a gross difference in the strength between your limbs. You can also do it in this fashion if you desire a training variation.

- You should reach a point where you cannot lift your arms. At this time, you can overload your muscles further by having the spotter lift your arms to the mid-range position, and then push them back to the starting position as you resist for 3 - 5 negative repetitions.

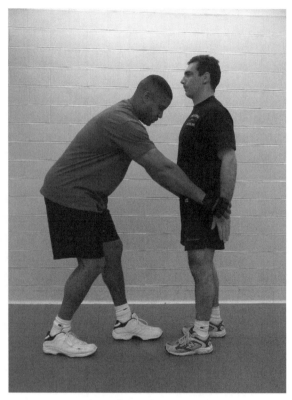

Start/Finish Position

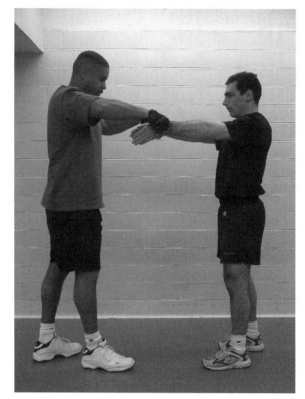

Mid-Range Position

FRONT RAISE

Muscle Involved: anterior deltoid

Suggested Repetitions: 6 - 12 (or 40 - 70 seconds)

Type of Movement: single joint

Starting Position: Stand upright, position your arms slightly past your hips with your palms facing each other, and open your hands (extending your fingers). Spread your feet a comfortable distance apart with one foot slightly in front 1of the other. The spotter should stand in front of you, place one foot to the inside of your forward foot, and apply resistance against your lower arms near your wrists.

Performance Description: Keep your arms fairly straight and raise them in front of your body until they are parallel to the floor as the spotter applies resistance evenly throughout the full range of motion. Pause briefly in this mid-range position (your arms parallel to the floor) and then resist as the spotter pushes your arms back to the starting position (your arms past your hips) to obtain a proper stretch.

Training Tips:

- The spotter should apply resistance above your elbows if you suffer from a hyperextended elbow or other joint pain.

- The spotter's front foot should slide backward as you raise your arms up to the mid-range position and forward as you lower your arms to the starting position.

- Avoid throwing your arms upward by using your legs or by swinging your torso back and forth — movement should only occur around your shoulder joints.

- You should not raise your arms beyond a point that is parallel to the floor.

- Your palms should be facing each other in the mid-range position.

- Keep your hands open (with your fingers extended) as you perform this exercise.

- You can do this exercise unilaterally (one limb at a time) in the event that you have a shoulder or arm injury, or a gross difference in the strength between your limbs. You can also do it in this fashion if you desire a training variation.

- You should reach a point where you cannot lift your arms. At this time, you can over-load your muscles further by having the spotter lift your arms to the mid-range position, and then push them back to the starting position as you resist for 3 - 5 negative repetitions.

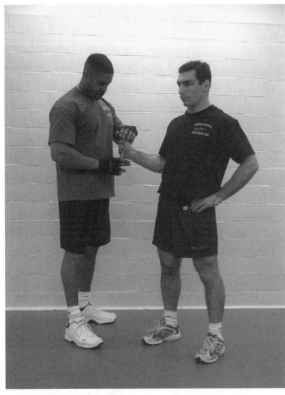

Start/Finish Position

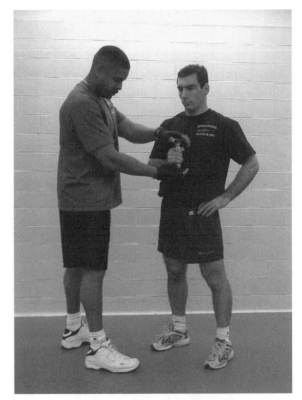

Mid-Range Position

INTERNAL ROTATION

Muscles Involved: internal rotators

Suggested Repetitions: 8 - 12 (or 50 - 70 seconds)

Type of Movement: single joint

Starting Position: Grasp a stick (or a similar object) with your right hand and stand upright. Position your left hand on your left hip and spread your feet about shoulder-width apart. Place your right elbow against the right side of your torso, and bend your right arm so that the angle between your upper and lower arms is about 90 degrees. (By doing this, your right lower arm will be approximately parallel to the floor.) Position the stick away from your mid-section. The spotter should stand alongside you and grasp the stick above and below your right hand.

Performance Description: Without moving your right elbow away from the side of your torso or changing the angle of your right arm, pull the stick to your mid-section as the spotter applies resistance evenly throughout the full range of motion. Pause briefly in this mid-range position (stick against your mid-section), and then resist as the spotter pulls the stick back to the starting position (stick away from your mid-section) to provide a proper stretch. After performing a set with your right arm, repeat the exercise for the other side of your body.

Training Tips:

- If a stick or a similar object is not available, you and the spotter can place your palms together.

- Keep your elbow against the side of your torso and your lower arm parallel to the floor as you perform this exercise.

- Do not rotate your torso as you perform this exercise — movement should only occur around your shoulder joint.

- Your palm should be facing you in the mid-range position.

- You should reach a point where you cannot pull the stick toward your mid-section. At this time, you can overload your muscles further by having the spotter bring the stick to the mid-range position, and then pull it back to the starting position as you resist for 3 - 5 negative repetitions.

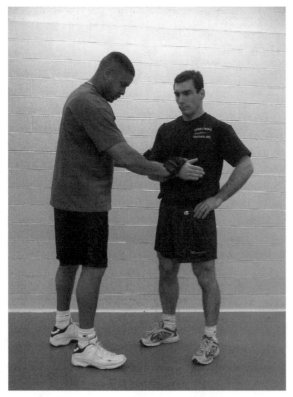

Start/Finish Position

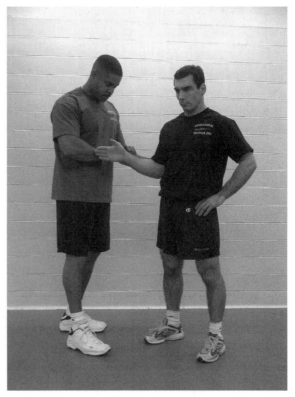

Mid-Range Position

EXTERNAL ROTATION

Muscles Involved: external rotators

Suggested Repetitions: 8 - 12 (or 50 - 70 seconds)

Type of Movement: single joint

Starting Position: Stand upright, position your left hand on your left hip, and spread your feet about shoulder-width apart. Place your right elbow against the right side of your torso, and bend your right arm so that the angle between your upper and lower arms is about 90 degrees. (By doing this, your right lower arm will be approximately parallel to the floor.) Open your right hand (extending your fingers) and position it against your mid-section. The spotter should stand alongside you and apply resistance against your right lower arm near your wrist.

Performance Description: Without moving your right elbow away from the side of your torso or changing the angle of your right arm, push your hand away from your mid-section as the spotter applies resistance evenly throughout the full range of motion. Pause briefly in this mid-range position (your hand away from your mid-section), and then resist as the spotter pushes your hand back to the starting position (your hand against your mid-section) to obtain a proper stretch. After performing a set with your right arm, repeat the exercise for the other side of your body.

Training Tips:

- Keep your hand open (with your fingers extended) as you perform this exercise.

- Keep your elbow against the side of your torso and your lower arm parallel to the floor as you perform this exercise.

- Do not rotate your torso as you perform this exercise — movement should only occur around your shoulder joint.

- Your palm should be facing you in the starting position.

- You should reach a point where you cannot push your hand away from your mid-section. At this time, you can overload your muscles further by having the spotter bring your hand to the mid-range position, and then push it back to the starting position as you resist for 3 - 5 negative repetitions.

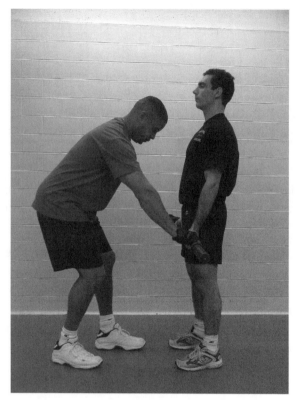

Start/Finish Position

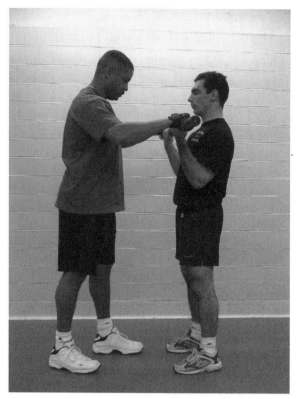

Mid-Range Position

BICEP CURL

Muscles Involved: biceps and forearms

Suggested Repetitions: 6 - 12 (or 40 - 70 seconds)

Type of Movement: single joint

Starting Position: Grasp a stick (or a similar object) with your hands spaced slightly wider than shoulder-width apart and your palms facing away from you. Stand upright and spread your feet approximately shoulder-width apart. The spotter should stand in front of you and grasp the stick on the outside of your grip with palms facing down.

Performance Description: Keep your elbows against the sides of your torso and pull the stick below your chin by bending your arms as the spotter applies resistance evenly throughout the full range of motion. Pause briefly in this mid-range position (your arms flexed), and then resist as the spotter pulls the stick back to the starting position (your arms fully extended) to obtain a sufficient stretch.

Training Tips:

- If a stick or a similar object is not available, you and the spotter can place your palms together.

- Avoid throwing the weight by using your legs or by swinging your torso back and forth — movement should only occur around your elbow joints.

- Changing the position of your elbows as you perform this exercise is natural. However, movement of your elbows should not be excessive.

- You can do this exercise unilaterally (one limb at a time) in the event that you have an arm injury or a gross difference in the strength between your limbs. You can also do it in this fashion if you desire a training variation.

- You should reach a point where you cannot lift the stick. At this time, you can overload your muscles further by having the spotter lift the stick to the mid-range position, and then pull it back to the starting position as you resist for 3 - 5 negative repetitions.

- This exercise may be contraindicated if you have hyperextended elbows.

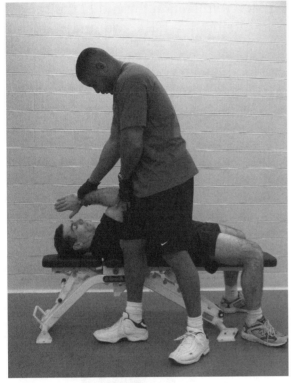

Start/Finish Position   *Mid-Range Position*

TRICEP EXTENSION

Muscle Involved: triceps

Suggested Repetitions: 6 - 12 (or 40 - 70 seconds)

Type of Movement: single joint

Starting Position: Lie down on the back pad of a bench and place your feet flat on the floor. Position the back of your right upper arm against the spotter's right thigh so that it is roughly perpendicular to the floor and point your right elbow toward your right knee. Place your right hand near the right side of your head with your palm facing your head and open your hand (that is, extend your fingers). The spotter should apply resistance against your right lower arm near your wrist.

Performance Description: Keep your right upper arm perpendicular to the floor and your right elbow pointing toward your right knee, and straighten your arm as the spotter applies resistance evenly throughout the full range of motion. Pause briefly in this mid-range position (your arm fully extended), and then resist as the spotter pushes your lower arm back to the starting position (your arm flexed) to obtain an adequate stretch. After performing a set with your right arm, repeat the exercise for the other side of your body.

Training Tips:

- Your upper arm should remain perpendicular to the floor and your elbow should be pointed toward your knee as you perform this exercise.

- Keep your hips flat on the back pad and your feet flat on the floor as you perform this exercise. If you have low-back pain, you can place your feet on the end of the back pad or a stool. This will flatten your lumbar area against the back pad and reduce the stress in your low-back region.

- Keep your hand open (with your fingers extended) as you perform this exercise.

- You can also perform this exercise while sitting or standing. In both cases, you would keep your upper arm perpendicular to the floor and raise and lower your arm behind your head.

- You should reach a point where you cannot lift your arm. At this time, you can overload your muscles further by having the spotter lift your arm to the mid-range position, and then push it back to the starting position as you resist for 3 - 5 negative repetitions.

- This exercise may be contraindicated if you have shoulder-impingement syndrome.

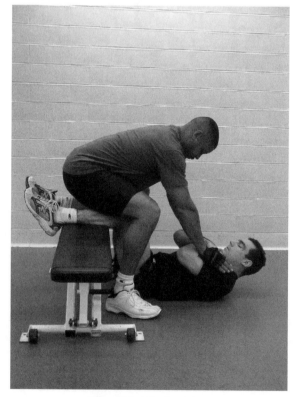 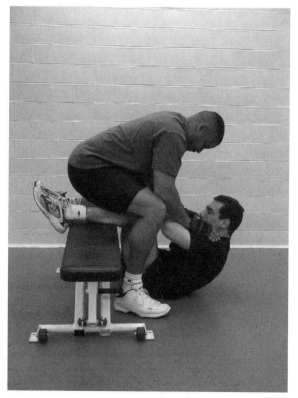

Start/Finish Position *Mid-Range Position*

SIT-UP

Muscle Involved: rectus abdominis

Suggested Repetitions: 8 - 12 (or 50 - 70 seconds)

Type of Movement: single joint

Starting Position: Lie down on the floor and place the backs of your lower legs on the back pad of a bench or a stool. Position yourself so that the angle between your upper and lower legs is about 90 degrees. Fold your arms across your chest and lift your head off the floor. (The upper portion of your shoulder blades should not be touching the floor.) The spotter should sit on your lower legs and apply resistance against the front part of your shoulders.

Performance Description: Pull your torso forward until it is just short of being perpendicular to the floor as the spotter applies resistance evenly throughout the full range of motion. Pause briefly in this mid-range position (your torso flexed), and then resist as the spotter pushes your torso back to the starting position (your torso extended) to obtain a proper stretch.

Training Tips:

- Your abdominals are used primarily during the first 30 degrees or so of this exercise. (Thereafter, your hip flexors accept most of the workload.) So, bringing your torso all the way to your upper legs is not necessary. You should stop, however, before you reach a point where your torso is perpendicular to the floor.

- You should not contact the floor with the upper portion of your shoulder blades between repetitions. This removes the load from the target muscles.

- You should always bend your knees when performing this exercise to reduce the stress on your lower back.

- Avoid throwing your torso forward by swinging your arms back and forth, or by snapping your head forward as you perform this exercise — movement should only occur around your hip joint and mid-section.

- You should reach a point where you cannot lift your torso. At this time, you can overload your muscles further by having the spotter lift your torso to the mid-range position, and then push it back to the starting position as you resist for 3 - 5 negative repetitions.

- This exercise may be contraindicated if you have low-back pain.

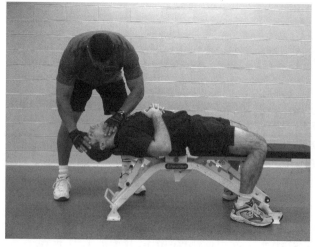

Start/Finish Position

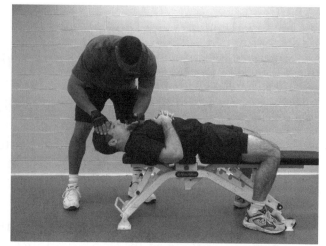

Mid-Range Position

NECK FLEXION

Muscle Involved: sternocleidomastoideus (both sides acting together)

Suggested Repetitions: 8 - 12 (or 50 - 70 seconds)

Type of Movement: single joint

Starting Position: Lie down on the back pad of a bench and place your feet flat on the floor. Position your head over the end of the back pad, interlock your fingers, and place them across your chest. The spotter should stand alongside your head and apply resistance against your chin with one hand and your forehead with the other.

Performance Description: Without moving your torso, pull your head as close to your chest as possible, as the spotter applies resistance evenly throughout the full range of motion. Pause briefly in this mid-range position (your chin near your chest), and then resist as the spotter pushes your head back to the starting position (your head hanging down) to provide an adequate stretch.

Training Tips:

- The spotter must be especially careful when applying resistance since your cervical area is involved.

- Keep your hips flat on the back pad and your feet flat on the floor as you perform this exercise. If you have low-back pain, you can place your feet on the end of the back pad or a stool. This will flatten your lumbar area against the back pad and reduce the stress in your low-back region.

- You should reach a point where you cannot lift your head. At this time, you can overload your muscles further by having the spotter lift your head to the mid-range position, and then push it back to the starting position as you resist for 3 - 5 negative repetitions.

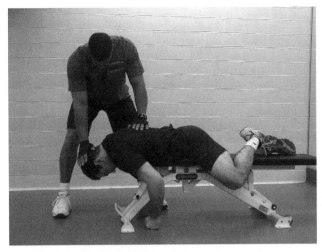

Start/Finish Position

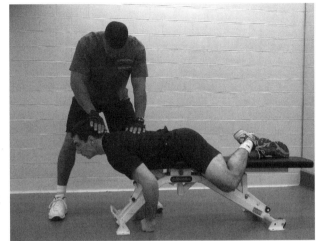

Mid-Range Position

NECK EXTENSION

Muscles Involved: neck extensors and trapezius (upper portion)

Suggested Repetitions: 8 - 12 (or 50 - 70 seconds)

Type of Movement: single joint

Starting Position: Lie face down on the back pad of a bench and place your hands and feet on the floor (or position your legs across the back pad). Position your head over the end of the back pad and place your chin near your chest. The spotter should stand alongside your head and apply resistance against the back of your head.

Performance Description: Without moving your torso, extend your head backward as far as possible, as the spotter applies resistance evenly throughout the full range of motion. Pause briefly in this mid-range position (your neck extended), and then resist as the spotter pushes your head back to the starting position (your chin near your chest) to ensure an adequate stretch.

Training Tips:

- The spotter must be especially careful when applying resistance since your cervical area is involved.

- You should reach a point where you cannot lift your head. At this time, you can overload your muscles further by having the spotter lift your head to the mid-range position, and then push it back to the starting position as you resist for 3 - 5 negative repetitions.

195

Chapter 11
Designing and Varying the Strength-Training Program

Your strength-training program should be geared toward your personal tastes in terms of exercise selection and equipment preference. You can effectively structure the framework of your program by incorporating the guidelines for strength training that are discussed in Chapter 7, in conjunction with the exercises that are detailed in Chapters 8 - 10. But first, reiterating a few concepts from Chapter 7 that are an integral part of designing your program is important.

PROGRAM DESIGN

Recall that most SWAT officers can perform a comprehensive, total-body workout in the weight room using no more than 15 exercises. You should perform one exercise for your hips, hamstrings, quadriceps, calves/dorsi flexors, biceps, triceps, forearms, abdominals, and lower back. Since your shoulder joint permits freedom of movement in numerous directions, you should perform two exercises for your chest, upper back (your "lats"), and shoulders. If you also participate in a combat sport — such as football, rugby, boxing, judo, or wrestling — your workout should include an additional 2 - 4 exercises for your neck to strengthen and protect your cervical area against possible catastrophic injury.

There is nothing inherently wrong with performing additional exercises in order to emphasize a particular muscle. But if your level of strength begins to plateau in one or more exercises, it is probably because you are overtraining — that is, you are unable to recover from the volume of your training. Also keep in mind that placing too much emphasis on one muscle may eventually produce abnormal development or create a muscular imbalance which can predispose you to injury. For instance, too much emphasis on your chest may lead to a round-shouldered appearance; too much emphasis on your quadriceps may make you susceptible to problems with your hamstrings.

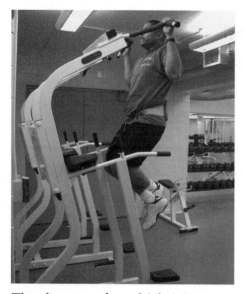

The advantage of a multiple-joint movement is that a relatively large amount of muscle mass can be trained in one exercise.

Antagonistic Muscles

How do you know if you are doing too much work for one muscle and not enough for another? All of your muscles are arranged in such a manner that they have opposing positions and functions. As an example, your biceps on the front of your upper arm flex (or bend) your elbow and your triceps on the back of your upper arm extend (or straighten) your elbow. When one muscle acts in opposition to another, it is referred to as an "antagonist." In addition to the biceps-triceps pairing, other antagonistic muscles include your hip abductors and hip adductors; hamstrings and quadriceps; calves and dorsi flexors; chest and upper back; anterior deltoid and posterior deltoid; wrist flexors and wrist extensors; and abdominals and lower back.

Providing antagonistic partnerships with an equal — or nearly equal — amount of stimulus is important. By doing this, you will ensure that a certain muscle is not overemphasized. This, in turn, will reduce your risk of producing abnormal development and of creating an imbalance between two muscles. Therefore, you should perform approximately the same volume of training — roughly the same number of exercises, sets, and repetitions — for pairs of antagonistic muscles (such as your biceps and triceps). In short, do not emphasize a particular muscle without also addressing its antagonistic counterpart with a similar volume of training.

Types of Movements

Essentially, there are two types of movements: single joint and multiple joint. A single-joint movement (also known as a "simple movement" or a "primary movement") involves a range of motion at only one joint. A good example is a pullover where the upper arm rotates at the shoulder joint. The advantage of a single-joint movement is that it usually provides muscle isolation.

A multiple-joint movement (also known as a "compound movement" or a "secondary movement") involves ranges of motion at more than one joint. A good example is a pull-up where there is rotation at both the shoulder and the elbow joints: The upper arm rotates at the shoulder joint and the lower arm rotates at the elbow joint. The advantage of a multiple-joint movement is that a relatively large amount of muscle mass can be trained in one exercise.

Whenever you perform two or more exercises for a large muscle of your torso — that is, your chest, upper back, or shoulders — at least one of them should be a single-joint movement. Why is this important?

Multiple-joint movements have a distinct disadvantage because they generally have a "weak link." When a person fatigues in a multiple-joint movement it is because the resistance has been filtered through a smaller, weaker muscle that exhausts well before the larger and stronger muscle has received a sufficient workload. In an exercise such as the aforesaid pull-up, the biceps are the smaller muscle and, therefore, will fatigue long before the upper back. In fact, the forearms may fatigue even earlier than the biceps. Therefore, the biceps and forearms get an adequate workload, but the upper back — which is really the target of the exercise — gets very little stimulus. So if all of the exercises that you do for a large muscle of your torso consist of multiple-joint movements, your smaller muscles would receive much more of the workload than your larger muscles.

By including single-joint and multiple-joint movements in your workout, you obtain the benefits of both types of movements: You get the advantage of a multiple-joint movement by addressing a relatively large amount of muscle mass in one exercise. And you get the advantage of a single-joint movement by isolating a large muscle without being hindered by the limited strength of one or more small muscles.

This does not mean that it would be totally wrong by only performing multiple-joint movements for a particular muscle. Your strength-training workouts will be more efficient and productive, however, if you do a single-joint movement to offset the limitations of a multiple-joint movement.

Sequence

Recall that you should train your muscles from largest to smallest. Specifically, the order of exercise in a total-body workout would be as follows: hips, upper legs (hamstrings and quadriceps), lower legs (calves or dorsi flexors), torso (chest, upper back, and shoulders), upper arms (biceps and triceps), lower arms (forearms), abdominals, and lower back. If you include exercises for your neck in your program, they can be done at the beginning of your workout or just after you complete your lower-body exercises.

The aforementioned order of exercise would still apply in a "split routine" (in which your muscles are "split" into several workouts instead of one total-body workout). In a workout that is designed to target only your chest, shoulders, and triceps, for example, you should still address those muscles from largest to smallest.

Exercise Options

Summaries of the exercises that are described in Chapters 8, 9, and 10 appear in Appendices E, F, and G, respectively. These chapters and appendices feature exercises that can be done with free weights (barbells and dumbbells), machines (selectorized and plate-loaded), and manual resistance. Naturally, your options will differ based upon the available equipment.

Given the wide assortment of exercise options, the design of a strength-training routine can have almost an infinite number of possibilities. The only limits are your available equipment and your imagination.

PROGRAM VARIATION

At some time in your strength training, you will undoubtedly encounter a point where your performance reaches a plateau. Quite often, this is a result of overtraining. In this case, your volume of training is so great that your muscular system is overstressed (or overworked). In effect, the demands of your training have exceeded your ability to recover. Here, you simply need to reduce your volume of training in the weight room (in terms of the number of workouts, exercises, and/or sets).

Sometimes, however, your performance will plateau because you are doing the same thing over and over again for lengthy periods of time. In this case, your program has become a form of unproductive manual labor that is monotonous, dull, and unchallenging.

You can lessen the likelihood that this situation will occur by varying your program. Chip Harrison — the Strength and Conditioning Coach at Penn State (for sports other than football) — notes, "Variety really breaks things up and allows for a different physical and mental focus."

Simply checking your workout card will reveal if you have reached a plateau. You should review your workout card carefully, however. If you think a plateau has been reached in a certain exercise, consider your performance in earlier exercises of that workout. For instance, suppose that you did 10 repetitions with 120 pounds on the leg extension for five consecutive workouts. At first glance, it may not seem as if your quadriceps have gotten any stronger. But what if the resistance that you used on the leg press increased from 250 pounds to 275 pounds during those same five workouts? This means that the load on your hips, hamstrings, and quadriceps increased by 10% — or an average of 2% per workout. In other words, your quadriceps were increasingly more pre-fatigued by the leg press in your workouts each time prior to performing the leg extension. If true, there is little doubt that your quadriceps did get stronger. In fact, simply being able to duplicate your past performances on the leg extension would actually be quite a feat — although that would not be readily apparent. Similarly, if the resistance that you used in the bicep curl reaches a plateau, it could be because your biceps are being exposed to increasingly heavier loads earlier in your workout when you do multiple-joint movements for your torso, such as the seated row or upright row. So, you must examine your entire workout in order to determine whether or not you have indeed reached a plateau.

Keep in mind that you will not be able to improve your performance in every exercise from one workout to the next. Be that as it may, you should observe gradual increases in strength in all exercises over the course of about four or five workouts. If you fail to make a progression in an exercise by this time (in the resistance and/or repetitions), you should vary some aspect of your strength-training program. There are several ways that this may be accomplished.

In general, you can vary three main components of your strength-training program: your workouts, exercises, and sets/repetitions.

Varying Workouts

There are a number of ways that your workouts can be varied. For instance, you can change your workouts on a daily basis by doing different workouts on different days, such as Workout A on Monday, Workout B on Wednesday, and Workout C on Friday. You can also vary your workouts on a weekly or monthly basis. Or you can simply change them as needed.

Regardless, the idea is to vary your workouts on a fairly regular basis. Mark Asanovich — who has been a strength and conditioning coach for several teams in the National Football League including the Minnesota Vikings, Tampa Bay Buccaneers, Baltimore Ravens, and Jacksonville Jaguars — prescribes many different workouts for his players with varying themes. For example, the players have the option of doing barbell-only, dumbbell-only, iso-lateral, no-hands, pre-exhaustion, and negative-only workouts. A few of the more high-intensity workouts even carry motivational names such as "Blood & Guts" and "Only the Strong Survive!"

Varying Exercises

There are three basic options available to vary your exercises. Specifically, you can rearrange the order, change the equipment, and alternate the exercises.

Rearrange the Order

One of the easiest ways to integrate variety into your training is to rearrange the order in which you perform your exercises for a particular muscle. Suppose, for example, that you desire a change in the way that you train your chest. If you have been doing the bench press followed by the bent-arm fly, you can incorporate variety by simply switching the two exercises. In other words, you can perform the bent-arm fly first and the bench press second.

Keep in mind that whenever you change the order in which you perform your exercises, you must adjust the levels of resistance. So if you do the bent-arm fly first (instead of second), your chest and shoulders will be fresh and, therefore, you should increase the resistance in that exercise. And if you do the bench press second (instead of first), your chest and shoulders will be fatigued and, therefore, you must decrease the resistance in that exercise.

An additional possibility is to rearrange the order in which you train your muscles. Rather than go from chest to upper back ("lats") to shoulders, you might start with your shoulders, proceed to your upper back and then finish with your chest. So a six-exercise sequence for your torso of bench press, bent-arm fly, seated row, pullover, seated press, and shoulder shrug could be changed to shoulder shrug, seated press, pullover, seated row, bent-arm fly, and bench press. In fact, these six exercises alone could be rearranged for 720 different sequences. [Six exercises can be placed in six different ordered positions. The first exercise that is chosen can be put in six possible spots, the second exercise can be put in one of the five remaining spots, a third exercise can be put in one of the four remaining spots and so on. Therefore, the total number of possible arrangements for six exercises is $6 \times 5 \times 4 \times 3 \times 2 \times 1 = 720$.] Once again, remember that you will need to adjust the levels of resistance any time that you rearrange the order of exercises.

Change the Equipment

Another way that you can vary the exercises is to change the equipment that you use. Say that you have been doing the bicep curl with a barbell for quite some time and, consequently, desire a change of pace. In this situation, you can perform a bicep curl with another type of equipment such as dumbbells, machines (selectorized and plate-loaded), or manual resistance. There is even variety within selectorized machines since some have one movement arm while others have independent movement arms (meaning that they function separately). Obviously, the extent to which you can change the equipment depends upon what is available.

Alternate the Exercises

A third means of varying exercises is to alternate them with other ones that employ the same muscles. Consider this: The seated row is a multiple-joint movement that involves your upper back, biceps, and forearms. And so do other rowing, chinning, and pulling movements such as the bent-over row, chin, pull-up, underhand lat pulldown, and overhand lat pulldown. Therefore, any of these exercises are potential substitutes for the seated row. Once again, the availability of equipment will determine how much you can alternate your exercises.

Besides providing for variety, periodically alternating your exercises and/or equipment has another advantage: It allows you to train your muscles through different ranges of motion. In this way, you can target your muscles in a more complete and comprehensive manner.

Varying Sets/Repetitions

A final component of your strength-training program that you can vary is the way that you perform a set which essentially is the way that you do a repetition. Ordinarily, repetitions are performed in a bilateral manner — that is, with both limbs at the same time. You can, however, do at least six other variations including negative-only, negative-accentuated, duosymmetric-polycontractile, unilateral, modified-cadence, and extended-pause repetitions.

But a few words of caution: Although the forthcoming ways of varying a repetition may sound simple, a reasonably high level of skill is required to do them in a manner that is safe and effective. Because of this, you should not attempt to implement these advanced applications in your program until you can demonstrate proper technique when you perform repetitions in a bilateral fashion.

Negative-Only Repetitions

You can perform your repetitions in a negative-only manner by having a partner raise the resistance and you lower it. Essentially, the partner does the positive (or concentric) work and the lifter does the negative (or eccentric) work. As an example, here is how you would do negative-only repetitions on the leg curl: With no help from you, your partner brings the movement arm to the mid-range position (your heels near your hips). Then, your partner releases the movement arm and you slowly lower the resistance to the stretched position (your legs fully extended). Repeat the procedure for the desired number of repetitions.

As noted in Chapter 7, your eccentric (or negative) strength is always greater than your concentric (or positive) strength in the same exercise. In other words, you can always lower a greater amount of resistance than you can raise (again, in the same exercise). This means that you can use more resistance for repetitions done in a negative-only manner than you can for repetitions done in a traditional manner. How much more? If you are performing negative-only repetitions for the first time, start with about 10% more resistance than you are normally capable of handling. So if you most recently used 150 pounds on an exercise in the traditional manner, increase the resistance by about 15 pounds — that is, to 165 pounds — for your first attempt at a set of negative-only repetitions. If you attain the maximum number of negative-only repetitions, you should increase the resistance for your next workout.

To obtain the best results, negative-only repetitions should be done slowly. In general, each negative-only repetition should be performed in about 6 - 8 seconds. But the duration of the repetition depends upon the range of motion in the exercise. An exercise with a large range of motion should take longer to complete than an exercise with a short one. Chapter 7 discusses different time frames for training your muscles. Ranges of time that will work well for most SWAT officers are about 90 - 120 seconds for a hip exercise, 60 - 90 seconds for a leg exercise, and 40 - 70 seconds for an upper-body exercise. Based upon these windows of time, then, an eight-second negative-only repetition would translate into repetition ranges of about 11 - 15 for the hips, 8 - 11 for the legs, and 5 - 9 for the upper body.

Performing negative-only repetitions is extremely demanding. For this reason, they should not be done in any given exercise more than once per week.

Negative-Accentuated Repetitions

The major disadvantage of negative-only repetitions is that at least one other person is almost always required to lift the weight. For the most part, you can only do negative-only repetitions without needing assistance from someone else in a handful of exercises that involve your bodyweight as resistance, such as push-ups, dips, chins, pull-ups, and sit-ups. As an example, you can do negative-only chins by stepping or climbing up to the mid-range position (your arms flexed), and lowering your body under control to the stretched position (your arms fully extended). Stated otherwise, your lower body does the positive work and your upper body does the negative work.

The value of negative-accentuated repetitions is that they emphasize the eccentric component of an exercise, yet they can be performed without any assistance from another individual. When doing negative-accentuated repetitions, the positive work is shared by both limbs, but the negative work is done by only one limb. In other words, the resistance is raised with both arms or legs, and then lowered with only one arm or leg. As a result, the resistance is literally twice as high during the negative phase as it is during the positive phase.

Although performing negative-accentuated repetitions with a barbell is impossible, most machines permit you to do so. To illustrate, you would perform negative-accentuated repetitions on the leg extension as follows: Using both legs, raise the resistance to the mid-range position (your legs fully extended) and pause briefly. Move your left leg away from the roller pad and hold the resistance momentarily with your right leg. Lower the resistance slowly and steadily to the starting position (your leg flexed) with your right leg. Raise the resistance to the mid-range position with both legs, and continue the preceding sequence using your left leg to lower the resistance. Repeat the procedure for the desired number of repetitions.

Similar to negative-only repetitions, the resistance should be lowered in about 6 - 8 seconds. As a starting point, use about 70% of the resistance that you normally handle in the traditional fashion. So if you last used 100 pounds on an exercise, begin with 70 pounds for negative-accentuated repetitions. In the case of negative-accentuated exercise, appropriate repetition ranges for most SWAT officers are about 15 - 20 for the hips, 10 - 15 for the legs, and 6 - 12 for the upper body. (Note that these are the total repetitions for both limbs, not the total repetitions for each limb.)

One final point: Maintaining a stable position when doing negative-accentuated repetitions is important. In particular, you should avoid twisting or turning your torso.

Duosymmetric-Polycontractile Repetitions

The term "duosymmetric-polycontractile" — or "duo-poly," for short — was first introduced in the mid-1970s as a style of performing repetitions with equipment that was fairly unique at the time because it had independent movement arms. Nowadays, many pieces of equipment are available with independent movement arms, thereby giving you the option of executing duo-poly repetitions.

If you have access to a bicep-curl machine with independent movement arms, you can perform duo-poly repetitions in this manner: Using both arms, raise the resistance to the mid-range position (your arms flexed) and pause briefly. Lower the resistance to the starting position (your arm fully extended) with your right arm while keeping your left arm in the mid-range position. Raise the resistance to the mid-range position with your right arm and

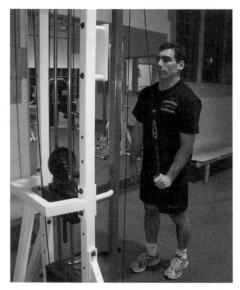

As a variation in the repetition style, many exercises can be done unilaterally — that is, with one limb at a time.

pause briefly. Lower the resistance to the starting position with your left arm while keeping your right arm in the mid-range position. Repeat the procedure for the desired number of repetitions. Incidentally, you can also perform duo-poly repetitions for your biceps with dumbbells in the manner described here.

Unilateral Repetitions

As a variation in the repetition style, many exercises can be done unilaterally — that is, with one limb at a time. Dr. Ken Leistner — who has been an authority in strength training for several decades — states, "One-limb work is effective because, in almost all cases, it is more intense than the same exercise done with two limbs working simultaneously."

Besides making the exercise more intense, unilateral repetitions are advisable for those who have a strength imbalance between one side of their body and the other. They are also recommended for individuals with hypertension.

Modified-Cadence Repetitions

Another option is to vary the cadence or speed with which you normally perform your repetitions. One cadence that has received a great deal of national attention is the SuperSlow® Protocol which was introduced by Ken Hutchins in the early 1980s. The basic cadence for SuperSlow® repetitions is to raise the resistance in 10 seconds and lower it in 5 seconds (or 10/5). Other popular variations of repetition speed include 4/4, 8/8, and 10/10. A single set consisting of one 30/30 repetition can also be done — in other words, one repetition that takes 60 seconds to complete. Keep in mind that you will need to adjust your repetition ranges any time that you modify the duration of a repetition.

Extended-Pause Repetitions

As pointed out in Chapter 7, pausing briefly in the mid-range position of each repetition is important. There are at least three reasons for emphasizing the mid-range position. First, it enables you to strengthen an otherwise weak position in your range of motion. Second, it allows you to focus attention on your muscles when they are most fully contracted. Third, it permits a smooth transition between the raising and lowering of the weight, thereby helping to reduce the influence of momentum.

As a repetition variation, the brief pause in the mid-range position can be done for a slightly longer duration — perhaps in three or four seconds. Using this technique is also an excellent tool to incorporate in the initial stages of training in order to understand the concept — and value — of pausing in the mid-range position. Once again, remember that repetition ranges will need to be adjusted any time that you modify the duration of a repetition.

Note that an extended pause in the mid-range position essentially involves a mild isometric muscular contraction that tends to elevate blood pressure beyond that which is normally encountered. As such, individuals who have hypertension should not use this technique.

WORKOUT A	WORKOUT B	WORKOUT C
Neck Flexion (MR)	Neck Lateral Flexion/R (SM)	Neck Extension (SM)
Neck Extension (MR)	Neck Lateral Flexion/L (SM)	Neck Flexion (MR)
Leg Press (PM)	Hip Adduction (SM)	Hip Abduction (MR)
Prone Leg Curl (SM)	Seated Leg Curl (SM)	Prone Leg Curl (PM)
Leg Extension (MR)	Leg Extension (PM)	Leg Extension (SM)
Standing Calf Raise (DB)	Dorsi Flexion (MR)	Seated Calf Raise (PM)
Dip (BW)	Bent-Arm Fly (DB)	Incline Press (BB)
Bent-Arm Fly (MR)	Bench Press (BB)	Bent-Arm Fly (MR)
Chin (BW)	Pullover (SM)	Bent-Over Row (DB)
Pullover (SM)	Seated Row (PM)	Pullover (DB)
Seated Press (BB)	Internal Rotation (MR)	Shoulder Shrug (TB)
Lateral Raise (SM)	External Rotation (MR)	Upright Row (BB)
Bicep Curl (MR)	Bicep Curl (BB)	Tricep Extension (MR)
Tricep Extension (SM)	Tricep Extension (SM)	Bicep Curl (DB)
Wrist Flexion (BB)	Wrist Extension (DB)	Wrist Flexion (DB)
Side Bend (DB)	Sit-Up (MR)	Rotary Torso (SM)
Back Extension (BW)	Back Extension (SM)	Back Extension (BW)

FIGURE 11.1: SAMPLE TOTAL-BODY WORKOUTS
Equipment Codes: BB = Barbell; BW = Bodyweight; DB = Dumbbells; MR = Manual Resistance; PM = Plate-loaded Machine; SM = Selectorized Machine; TB = Trap Bar

WORKOUT A	WORKOUT B
Deadlift (TB)	Neck Flexion (MR)
Seated Leg Curl (PM)	Neck Extension (PM)
Leg Extension (SM)	Chest Press (SM)
Seated Calf Raise (PM)	Bent-Arm Fly (DB)
Pullover (SM)	Seated Press (BB)
Pull-Up (BW)	Bent-Over Raise (MR)
Bicep Curl (DB)	Tricep Extension (DB)
Wrist Flexion (BB)	Rotary Torso (SM)
	Back Extension (SM)

FIGURE 11.2: SAMPLE TWO-DAY SPLIT ROUTINE
Equipment Codes: BB = Barbell; BW = Bodyweight; DB = Dumbbells; MR = Manual Resistance; PM = Plate-loaded Machine; SM = Selectorized Machine; TB = Trap Bar

APPLICATIONS

Based on the information contained here and in Chapter 7, three sample total-body work-outs are shown in Figure 11.1; similarly, a sample two-day split routine is shown in Figure 11.2. These sample workouts will give you some ideas for designing and varying your strength-training program.

How often should you vary your strength-training program? For the most part, this depends upon the individual. But in general, SWAT officers who are just initiating a strength-training program or have not been doing one for too long probably will not require much variety. Those who are more experienced will need to vary their programs on a regular basis.

Chapter 12
Metabolic Training

Most people typically perform their strength training separate from their aerobic training. Yet, many individuals — including SWAT officers — are required to integrate their muscular strength with their aerobic fitness. Great examples of this are participating in a realistic tactical operations training program or deploying on an actual mission. During training and on most operations, you must move continuously for more than three minutes which has an aerobic component, while intermittently performing tasks or activities that have a strength component (such as possibly carrying a one-person ram, climbing on top of a roof, scaling a fence or wall, and/or carrying an injured teammate — all of which will probably be done while wearing full SWAT gear). Being able to merge your muscular strength with your aerobic fitness is a true measure of your metabolic fitness.

Metabolic training integrates strength training with aerobic training. This directly relates to performing a dynamic entry on a tactical operation where SWAT officers must run to the scene carrying a ram, shield, and all operational equipment. They must then breach the door and quickly move throughout the building, carrying out their assignments.

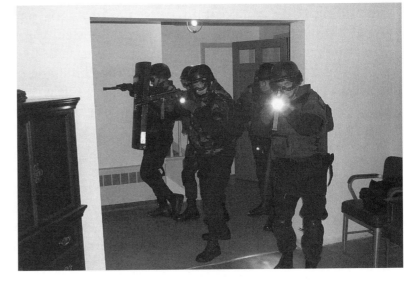

Essentially, metabolic training is a combination of intense strength training (or other anaerobic efforts) and aerobic training. It involves three major biological systems: the musculoskeletal, respiratory, and circulatory systems. In order to improve your metabolic fitness, these three systems must share the physiological demands.

Unfortunately, training the metabolic system is rarely emphasized or even addressed. However, a thorough understanding of metabolic training and an application of specific training techniques can enhance your performance in activities that involve the collective efforts of your muscular strength and aerobic fitness.

PROJECT TOTAL CONDITIONING

In the early 1970s, research designated as "Project Total Conditioning" was conducted at the United States Military Academy in New York. The research used members of several athletic teams at the academy as test subjects. Project Total Conditioning actually consisted of a number of different studies. For instance, one study examined the effects of a strength-training program on the neck size and strength of rugby players. Another study investigated the effects of two different training protocols on the vertical jumping ability of volleyball players.

However, the main portion of Project Total Conditioning was a six-week study that examined metabolic training. An experimental group consisted of 18 varsity football players from the academy (a nineteenth subject was injured during spring football practice). This group performed a strength-training workout three times per week on alternate days with two days of recovery after the third workout of the week. Each workout consisted of 10 exercises and took an average of about 30 minutes to complete. (The subjects also performed six neck exercises twice per week.) Each subject was required to perform as many repetitions as possible using proper technique in every exercise of every workout. One set of each exercise was performed to the point of muscular fatigue within a repetition range of 5 - 12. The group took a minimum amount of recovery time between exercises.

In order to minimize the influence of the "learning effect," the experimental group followed the training protocol for two weeks prior to the study. (The "learning effect" refers to the dramatic increases that are often attained by individuals in the initial stages of a training program that are attributable to improvements in their neurological function rather than their muscular function.) Prior to the six-week study, the subjects were pre-tested in several areas — including body composition, muscular strength, aerobic fitness, the 40-yard dash, the vertical jump, and flexibility — and were re-tested following the study.

The study produced very compelling results. After six weeks of training, the subjects increased the resistance they used between their first and seventeenth workouts by an average of 58.54%. The minimum improvement in strength was 45.61% while the maximum increase in strength was 69.70%. (Incidentally, the average increase in the resistance that was used between the second and sixteenth workouts was 43.06%.) The subjects also increased the number of repetitions they performed between their first and seventeenth workouts by an average of 6.59%.

Interestingly, the time that the subjects needed to complete their workouts decreased substantially. Comparing the first workout to the seventeenth, the experimental group reduced the average duration of their workouts by 24.09% — from an average of 37.73 minutes to an average of 28.64 minutes. Two individuals almost literally cut their workout times in half —

one from 49 to 25 minutes and the other from 43 to 22 minutes — yet increased their strength levels by 68.32% and 65.59%, respectively. A third individual reduced his workout time from 42 to 27 minutes and increased his strength by 66.32%.

Besides the tremendous improvements in muscular strength, the subjects also reduced their average time in the two-mile run by 88 seconds — from an average of 13:18 to an average of 11:50. This represented an average improvement of 11.03% — without having performed any running except during the course of spring football practice (which occurred during the first four weeks of training). Following the six weeks of training, the subjects also had lower resting heart rates and lower training heart rates at various workloads on a stationary cycle. Moreover, they were able to perform more work before reaching heart rates of 170 beats per minute.

At the end of the six-week study, the experimental group had reduced their average time in the 40-yard dash from 5.1467 seconds to 5.0933 seconds — a 1.04% improvement. Their vertical jump had increased from an average of 22.6 inches to an average of 24.067 inches — an average improvement of 6.49%. Finally, their average improvement in three flexibility measures was 10.92%.

These striking results are even more impressive when you consider that they were accomplished in such a time-efficient manner. In fact, the total amount of actual training time performed by each individual during the six-week program averaged less than 8.5 hours — which is less than 30 minutes per workout. Note that the test subjects were highly conditioned football players who were already quite strong and fit at the start of the program. Nonetheless, the study demonstrated the far-reaching effects of short-duration, high-intensity strength training on metabolic fitness.

Your metabolic fitness may be improved by simply performing your strength training with a high level of intensity while taking very little recovery between your exercises.

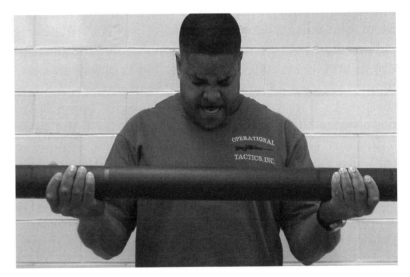

TYPES OF METABOLIC WORKOUTS

Your metabolic fitness may be improved by simply performing your strength training with a high level of intensity while taking very little recovery between your exercises. Performed in this fashion, the shared demands that are placed on your major biological systems create metabolic improvements that cannot be approached by traditional methods of training. The two most popular types of metabolic workouts are high-intensity training and circuit training.

High-Intensity Training (HIT)

One form of metabolic training that has seen a renewed interest is high-intensity training or, simply, HIT. The term "high-intensity training" appears in trade publications as early as 1973. (The acronym "HIT" became fashionable in 1988 with the publication of the *HIT Newsletter*.) HIT can be effective for anyone — regardless of lifting experience or aspiration — as long as it encourages progressive overload and allows sufficient recovery. The past three decades have provided literally tens of thousands of examples of individuals — both male and female with various levels of experience ranging from "untrained" beginners to "highly trained" athletes — as empirical evidence that HIT can be extremely efficacious.

Since it was first popularized more than three decades ago, there have been endless interpretations, variations, and applications of HIT. Nevertheless, most versions of HIT have several common denominators. As the name implies, HIT is characterized by intense, aggressive efforts: Each exercise is typically performed to the point of muscular fatigue or "failure." A minimum number of sets are usually performed — often only one set of each exercise, but sometimes several sets. Another characteristic of HIT is the emphasis on progressive overload: Whenever possible, an attempt is made to increase either the repetitions that are performed or the resistance that is used from one workout to the next. With safety as a major concern, HIT does not include fast-speed (or "explosive") movements or exercises so that momentum does not play a significant role in raising the resistance: All repetitions are performed with a controlled speed of movement. Additionally, HIT is comprehensive — training all of the major muscle groups is a priority.

In general, HIT also involves very brief workouts with a minimum amount of recovery time between exercises. The short recovery interval between exercises enables you to maintain a fairly high training heart rate for the duration of your workout. Like other forms of metabolic training, the length of the recovery i1nterval that is taken between exercises depends upon your present level of metabolic fitness. The recovery period is not usually structured, timed, or predetermined. Initially, however, a recovery time of perhaps three minutes may be necessary between efforts; with improved fitness, your pace should be quickened to the point where you are moving as rapidly as possible between exercises. (These and other concepts of HIT are described in greater detail in Chapter 7.)

In short, HIT places an incredible workload upon every major muscle in your body and, at the same time, stresses your circulatory and respiratory systems. Furthermore, this type of workout can be used to improve your metabolic fitness in a safe and time-efficient manner.

The 3x3 Workout. One of the most strenuous of all HIT workouts is sometimes referred to as a "3x3" — that is, a "three by three" — and, for this reason, deserves special note. A 3x3 Workout simply means that you do a series of three exercises a total of three times. For example, one of the most popular and demanding versions of a 3x3 Workout looks like this: leg press, dip, chin, leg press, dip, chin, leg press, dip, and chin. But this routine is just one of many possible versions of a 3x3 Workout. This form of metabolic training can actually be modified in a countless number of ways.

Essentially, a 3x3 Workout consists of a multiple-joint hip movement followed by a multiple-joint chest movement followed by a multiple-joint upper-back movement, and repeated two more times with as little recovery as possible between exercises. These three types of movements address virtually every major muscle in your body including your hips, hamstrings, quadriceps, chest, upper back, shoulders, biceps, triceps, and forearms.

The most demanding multiple-joint exercises for your hips (along with your hamstrings and quadriceps) are some type of leg press, squat, or deadlift (with an Olympic bar, a trap bar, or dumbbells). Dips and chins certainly represent the most challenging selections for your chest and upper back, respectively. Those who cannot perform dips and/or chins with their bodyweight can do alternative multiple-joint movements that incorporate the same muscles. Any type of multiple-joint movement that involves a pushing motion — such as the bench press, incline press, or push-up — can be used to target the muscles of your chest (as well as those of your shoulders and triceps); any type of multiple-joint movement that involves a pulling motion — such as a lat pulldown, seated row, or bent-over row — can be used to target the muscles of your upper back (along with your biceps and forearms).

The first time that the three movements are done, you should reach muscular fatigue at about 20 repetitions for the hip exercise, 12 for the chest exercise, and 12 for the upper-back exercise. When the sequence is repeated the second time, the repetition goals would be 15 for the hip exercise, 10 for the chest exercise, and 10 for the upper-back exercise. The third time through the movements should have goals of 12 for the hip exercise, 8 for the chest exercise, and 8 for the upper-back exercise. In summary, the repetition goals for these movements should be 20, 15, and 12 for the hip exercise and 12, 10, and 8 for the chest and upper-back exercises.

A 3x3 Workout is extremely time-efficient — most variations can be performed in about 20 minutes or less. The simplicity of this specific type of HIT workout can be deceptive. Though it may not appear to be challenging, a 3x3 Workout — if done as outlined here — can place Herculean demands upon your physiological systems that translate into a tremendous metabolic workload.

Circuit Training

One of the oldest and most popular forms of metabolic training has been dubbed "circuit training." The birth of circuit training can be traced back to England in the 1950s. With circuit training, the idea is to perform a series of exercises (or activities) in a sequence (or "circuit") with a very brief recovery interval between each "station." In a sense, therefore, circuit training is a form of interval training. (Chapter 6 discusses interval training as it applies to anaerobic training.)

Circuit Weight Training. The merger of circuit training with weight training is known as "circuit weight training" or, simply, CWT. Usually, CWT is performed on a multi-station apparatus. This offers several advantages. First, the exercises of multi-station equipment are in close proximity to each other which allows you to move quickly around the circuit. Secondly, the selectorized weight stacks of multi-station equipment enable you to make quick and easy adjustments in the resistance. But CWT can also be performed with single-station equipment and/or free weights provided that the distance between the exercises is not too great.

CWT is very versatile — you can manipulate the number of exercises in the circuit, the number of repetitions for each exercise, and the amount of recovery between exercises. The number of exercises you do in the circuit and the amount of recovery that you take between the exercises is a function of your level of fitness. However, a comprehensive session of CWT involves a series of about 12 - 14 exercises that address each of your major muscle groups. A total-body circuit on a typical piece of multi-station equipment might be as follows: leg press, leg curl, leg extension, bench press, dip, pull-up, lat pulldown, seated press, shoulder shrug, bicep curl, tricep extension, wrist flexion, and sit-up. (Several other productive exercises can be performed on most multi-station equipment including the upright row, knee-up, and side bend.)

At each station, you can either perform a given number of repetitions or do as many repetitions as possible during a specified time frame (with a controlled speed of movement). At a pace of 60 seconds per exercise (the work interval) with 30 seconds of recovery between stations including the set-up for the next exercise (the recovery interval), a circuit of 12 - 14 exercises can be completed in as little as 18 - 21 minutes. Note that the resistance you use at each station should permit you to reach muscular fatigue by the end of the allotted work interval.

To ensure that you obtain continued metabolic improvements from CWT, you can progressively overload your metabolic system by (1) increasing the resistance you use at a given station; (2) increasing the length of the work interval (thereby doing more repetitions); (3) decreasing the length of the recovery interval taken between stations; or (4) any combination of the three previous options.

To summarize CWT: You begin at a particular station and complete one set of an exercise. After this, you move to the next station in the circuit where you set up for your next exercise and recuperate for the remainder of your recovery period. This cycle is repeated over and over again until the entire circuit is complete.

Circuit Aerobic Training. Since the term "cross training" came into vogue in the mid-1990s, there has been a growing interest in circuit aerobic training (CAT) which involves a series of aerobic activities or stations. The circuit can be designed a number of different ways — you can vary the number of aerobic activities, the duration and intensity of each activity, and the amount of recovery taken between stations. As with all other types of training, most of these variables are dependent upon your level of fitness. Your goal, however, is to perform the equivalent of about 20 - 60 minutes of aerobic activity with an appropriate level of effort. Keep in mind that 30 minutes of exercise can be done as one 30-minute session, two 15-minute sessions, three 10-minute sessions, or even six 5-minute sessions. So, you can exercise for 10 minutes on a stationary cycle, 10 minutes on a rower, and 10 minutes on a stair-climbing machine for a total of 30 minutes of aerobic activity. Or, you might perform each of those same three activities for five minutes, but repeat the circuit twice for a total of 30 minutes. Regardless, your level of intensity should be as high as possible during each of your efforts. (Monopolizing a group of activities for intervals of less than five minutes per station in a commercial facility would probably not be practical or permissible.)

Other Variations. Yet another version of circuit training is to integrate strength-training exercises with one or more aerobic-training activities. For instance, you might perform a strength-training exercise, pedal a stationary cycle for 1 - 3 minutes, perform another strength-training exercise, pedal a stationary cycle for another 1 - 3 minutes, and so on. Along these lines, you can do a simple albeit brutal form of metabolic training by alternating dips and chins with running. In other words, you might perform a set of dips, run a specified distance, perform a set of chins, run a specified distance, and repeat this circuit several times. (If done indoors, you can run on a motorized treadmill.)

The "Fitness Trail" is a form of circuit training that originated in several of the Scandinavian countries. This method of circuit training is performed outdoors in a natural environment such as a park. A typical fitness trail consists of numerous stations that are positioned several hundred yards apart and arranged along a circuitous route. You would walk, jog, or run to a station, stop and perform some type of exercise or activity that may be for agility (such as hurdles, log walks, and vaults), strength (such as push-ups, sit-ups, chins, and dips) or flexibility, and then proceed to the next station.

METABOLIC DYNAMICS

At rest, your body does not consume much oxygen and your energy (and metabolic) needs are easily satisfied by your Aerobic System. As your metabolic demands increase during activity, you require more energy immediately. Your Aerobic System cannot transport and deliver oxygen fast enough to address this physiological urgency. Therefore, you must rely upon your anaerobic pathways to provide energy until your aerobic pathway is able to meet your needs.

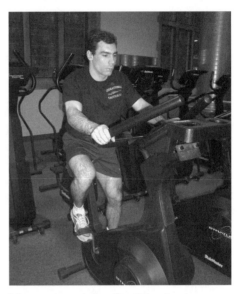

For the most part, metabolic training involves intense efforts that last about 60 - 90 seconds (though the time of activity can approach 120 seconds when performing strength-training exercises for your hips). In the early stages of intense activity, a limited amount of energy can be supplied rapidly by your two anaerobic pathways: the ATP-PC System and Anaerobic Glycolysis. During intense efforts, your ATP-PC System exhausts your phosphagen

You can exercise for 10 minutes on a stationary cycle, 10 minutes on a rower, and 10 minutes on a stair-climbing machine for a total of 30 minutes of aerobic activity.

stores in a matter of seconds; as a result of Anaerobic Glycolysis, the glycogen content of your working muscles drops progressively. As additional oxygen becomes available, your Aerobic System is used to a greater degree. After a few minutes, your Aerobic System is able to furnish all of the energy that is needed for mild activity.

Metabolic training presents an enormous physiological challenge to your musculoskeletal, respiratory, and circulatory systems. In response to this metabolic stress, your systems make a number of sudden, temporary adjustments that return to resting levels once you complete your effort. The degree of your metabolic response increases in direct proportion to your intensity and the duration of the activity, and is also related to other factors such as your body size, gender, and level of fitness. Therefore, detailing your precise biological reaction to metabolic training is impossible. However, your metabolic adjustments can be estimated with a reasonable degree of accuracy. When going from a resting state to an exercising state, your predicted physiological responses include:

Musculoskeletal Responses

When you perform a strength-training exercise, your intensity is lowest during the first repetition. At this point, only a small percentage of your available muscle fibers is innervated (or recruited) by your nervous system — just enough to move the weight. When your muscular intensity is low, your metabolic needs are met by your slow-twitch fiber population. As you perform each repetition, your intensity increases progressively and deeper inroads are made into your muscles. Some of your muscle fibers fatigue and are no longer able to keep up with the increasing metabolic demands. Fresh fibers are simultaneously called upon to assist the fatigued fibers in generating ample force. Your fast-twitch fibers are recruited by your nervous system only when your fatigue-resistant slow-twitch fibers have depleted their energy stores to the point where they cannot meet the force requirements. This process continues until the last repetition when you reach concentric muscular fatigue and your intensity is at its highest. Now, the collective efforts of your remaining fibers cannot produce enough force to raise the weight. During this final repetition, the cumulative effect of each preceding repetition has fatigued your muscles thereby providing a sufficient — and efficient — stimulus for muscular growth. Note that your first few repetitions of a set are the least productive because your intensity is very low; on the other hand, your very last repetition of a set is the most productive because your intensity is very high.

Respiratory Responses

The most obvious respiratory response to intense metabolic training is an increase in the frequency and depth of your breathing. Indeed, rapid and deep breathing is an unmistakable indicator of intense activity. Your labored breathing leads to a heightened sense of respiratory distress, general discomfort, and widespread fatigue. Specifically, your number of breaths per minute (breaths/min) may increase from a resting rate of about 10 - 12 breaths/min to about 40 - 50 breaths/min.

"Tidal volume" refers to the amount of air entering or leaving your lungs during a single breath and is measured in liters per breath (L/breath). During intense activity, your tidal volume may rise to more than six times its resting level — from about 0.5 L/breath to about 3.0 L/breath or more.

The amount of air you inhale or exhale each minute is known as your "pulmonary ventilation." It is measured in liters per minute (L/min) and is calculated by multiplying the frequency of your breathing (in breaths/min) by your tidal volume (in L/breath). Because of the combined increases in the rate and depth of your breathing, your pulmonary ventilation may increase from 5.0 L/min [such as 10 breaths/min x 0.5 L/breath] to more than 150.0 L/min [such as 50 breaths/min x 3.0 L/breath]. To aid in forced expiration during intense efforts, there is also a greater involvement of your respiratory muscles — that is, your abdominal and internal intercostal muscles (which lie between your ribs). In fact, your respiratory muscles may demand 8 - 10% of your oxygen intake during intense activity.

Circulatory Responses

During physical training, your heart beats faster to meet the demands of your muscles for more blood and oxygen. Specifically, your heart rate may climb from a resting level of about 60 - 70 beats per minute (bpm) to as much as 80 - 90% of your age-predicted maximum or more for brief periods. (Your heart rate actually increases above resting levels prior to your efforts due to the so-called anticipatory response.) The greater the intensity of your effort, the faster the beat of your heart. The increase in your heart rate is greatest when you perform exercises involving your larger muscle groups — particularly your hips and legs. Monitoring your heart rate while training provides a very accurate reflection of the metabolic intensity of the activity.

"Stroke volume" refers to the volume of blood pumped by your heart and is measured in liters per beat (L/beat). During intense efforts, your stroke volume may rise from about 0.08 L/beat to perhaps 0.2 L/beat or more. As a result of the combined increases in your stroke volume and heart rate, your cardiac output may increase from about 5.0 L/min [such as 0.08 L/beat x 60 bpm] to more than 30.0 L/min [such as 0.2 L/beat x 150 bpm]. Once your stroke volume reaches your physiological limit, further increases in your cardiac output are only possible through increases in your heart rate.

Your cardiac output is distributed to your organs and tissues according to their functions and needs at any given moment. During intense activity, your blood flow is redistributed from areas where it is not very critical to areas where it is absolutely essential. Specifically, there is a diminished blood flow to your inactive muscles and less active tissues such as your liver, kidneys, and digestive organs (that is, your stomach and intestines). At rest, 15 - 20% of your systemic blood flow is to your muscles — the majority of the blood goes to your digestive organs and brain. During intense activity, your blood flow is redirected to your working muscles. In fact, your exercising muscles may receive 85 - 90% of the total blood flow. This means that for a cardiac output of 30.0 L/min, more than 25.0 liters of blood can be delivered to your active muscles every minute. Your heart also receives an increased supply of blood during intense efforts — from a resting level of about 0.25 L/min to about 0.75 L/min. (The blood flow to your brain is unchanged.)

Your blood pressure is measured in millimeters of mercury (mmHg). Your systolic blood pressure increases in proportion to your training intensity and can rise from a normal resting level of 120 – 129 mmHg to more than 200 mmHg. During intense activity, the diastolic blood pressure remains the same as a normal resting level of 80 – 84 mmHg or drops slightly. Maximum blood pressure usually occurs at maximum heart rate.

Your body temperature rises during intense activity — especially in hot, humid conditions. Your body has a temperature-regulatory mechanism and, like a thermostat, tries to maintain its temperature at a relatively constant value of roughly 98.6 degrees Fahrenheit (or about 37 degrees Celsius). During intense activity, your body temperature may exceed 102 degrees Fahrenheit (or about 39 degrees Celsius). As your body temperature rises, there is an increased blood flow from your warmer core to the surface of your skin. This process facilitates heat dissipation and allows heat loss. Unfortunately, this also reduces the amount of blood available to supply your working muscles with oxygen. (Guidelines for exercising in hot, humid environments are given in Chapter 19.)

General Responses
Short-term, high-intensity activity increases the production of carbon dioxide and lactic acid. This, in turn, lowers your pH. Your muscle pH may briefly decrease from a resting value of about 7.0 to as low as 6.4. The lactate spreads from your muscles into the surrounding tissues and eventually spills into your blood. This causes your blood pH to temporarily drop from a resting value of perhaps 7.4 to as low as 6.8. As the lactic acid begins to accumulate, it irritates your nerve endings and causes feelings of muscular pain, discomfort, distress, and fatigue. As lactic acid accumulates, it also causes your breathing to become labored.

During intense metabolic training, your oxygen intake may increase from about 3.5 ml/kg/min at rest to about 26.0 ml/kg/min or more. For a 198-pound person, this equates to an increase from a resting level of roughly 0.315 L/min to about 2.34 L/min or more. Compared to pure aerobic training, these values for oxygen intake are somewhat low. Such low values are primarily due to the intermittent nature of metabolic training. At any given heart rate, the metabolic demands — in terms of oxygen intake — are lower for strength training compared to aerobic training. Research has shown that the oxygen intake during strength training averages 68% of that seen during aerobic training at the same exercising heart rate. Expressed in different terms: At a given level of oxygen intake, heart rates are higher during strength training compared to aerobic training. For instance, an oxygen intake of 25.0 ml/kg/min elicits a heart rate of about 180 bpm during strength training compared to a heart rate of about 155 bpm for aerobic training. During strength training, the heart rate is disproportionately elevated relative to oxygen intake.

Your expenditure of calories per minute (cal/min) is also elevated during intense activity. Like most of your other metabolic responses, the rate of your caloric expenditure largely depends upon your intensity and your bodyweight. The rate of caloric expenditure for a 198-pound individual may increase from about 1.575 cal/min to perhaps 11.7 cal/min or more. Finally, note that your oxygen intake and caloric expenditure is greatest when you train the larger muscles in your body such as your hips and legs.

Chapter 13
Rehabilitative Training

Injuries are an unforeseen, inevitable, and unfortunate fact of life as a SWAT officer. In spite of how much you prepare, many injuries are purely the result of being in the wrong place at the wrong time.

In general, injuries can be either traumatic or non-traumatic. Traumatic injuries are more serious and severe such as fractures of bones, and tears of muscle or connective tissue. Quite often, these types of injuries require surgical intervention. On the other hand, non-traumatic injuries are less serious and severe such as tendinitis and bursitis. Sometimes, these kinds of injuries simply result from overuse. Regardless of the type of injury, consulting with a qualified sports-medical specialist such as an orthopedic physician, physical therapist, or athletic trainer is important.

In many instances, an individual who suffers an injury ends up eliminating all forms of physical training — even those that involve uninjured bodyparts. Yet, it is extremely important to continue some type of physical training whenever possible — even in the event of an injury. Many authorities have suggested that a muscle begins to lose size and strength if it does not receive an adequate amount of stimulation within 48 - 96 hours of a previous workout. There is some anecdotal evidence suggesting that it may be a bit longer than this time frame — at least for some individuals. But it is clear that a loss of muscular size and strength will occur after some period of extended inactivity. Moreover, the rate of strength loss is most rapid during the first few weeks. Because of this, rehabilitative training can prevent a significant loss of not only muscular size and strength, but also aerobic, anaerobic, and metabolic fitness. This, of course, is provided that the training can be done in a pain-free — or nearly pain free — fashion.

Whether the injury is traumatic or non-traumatic, it will have some degree of impact on your physical training. In fact, some injuries — especially those that are traumatic — might not permit any physical activity whatsoever. Nevertheless, you can often train parts of your body that are not related to the afflicted area. And in many cases, you may even be able to address the injured bodypart directly.

PRUDENT METHODS

There are several different options and adjustments that can be used to continue training an injured area or bodypart in a safe, sensible, and pain-free manner. Note that these methods are not intended for those injuries that are viewed as being very serious or extremely painful. As such, you should receive approval from a certified sports-medical authority before initiating any prescription for rehabilitative training.

Rehabilitative training can be performed by considering and then applying the following guidelines:

1. Lighten the weight.

If you want to continue training an injured bodypart in the weight room, your first step is to decrease the amount of resistance that you normally use in exercises that involve the afflicted area. This is usually the easiest and most straightforward recommendation. Suppose you had a knee injury and, as a result, you experienced pain in your patellar tendon when performing the leg extension with your usual level of resistance. Decreasing the amount of weight will produce less stress on your tendon and perhaps allow you to perform the exercise in a pain-free — or nearly pain-free — manner. The amount that you reduce the weight depends upon the extent and the nature of your injury.

2. Slow the speed of movement.

Often done in conjunction with decreasing the amount of resistance for an exercise is using a slower speed of movement. Slowing the repetition speed will decrease the orthopedic stress placed on a given joint. John Thomas, the Strength and Conditioning Coach for the Penn State Football Team, sometimes has his players do repetitions that are 20 seconds long when training their injured areas: They raise the weight in 10 seconds and lower it in 10 seconds.

As the injury heals, you can gradually return to your preferred speed of movement. Then again, you may find that the extra-slow speed of movement is more appealing and continue using it after you complete your rehabilitative training. Or perhaps you may even adopt the slower speed of movement to train other bodyparts that are not injured. Incidentally, slowing the speed of movement will also necessitate using a reduced amount of weight, thereby lowering the stress even further.

3. Change the exercise angle.

If pain persists during certain exercises that involve an injured bodypart, it may be possible for you to change the angle of the exercise. This essentially alters — and restricts — the angle through which your limb is moved.

This option can be used with many exercises for your torso — particularly those that involve your shoulder joint. This is especially important because the mobility and instability of the shoulder joint make it highly prone to injury. In fact, one of the most frequently injured bodyparts for SWAT officers is the shoulder joint. A common problem in this joint is known as "shoulder-impingement syndrome" — a general term used to describe pain that is often characterized as tightness or pinching in the shoulder.

Suppose you have slight shoulder impingement when doing a bench press. In some cases, if you change the angle of the exercise from flat to decline — in other words, change from the bench press to the decline press — there is significantly less orthopedic stress on your shoulder joint.

Likewise, some people experience pain due to shoulder impingement when moving the bar behind their heads during the seated press and overhand lat pulldown. Generally speaking, the discomfort in both of these exercises can be lessened considerably by changing the angle of the push and pull. This can be done by performing the exercises with the bar traveling in front of the head rather than behind the neck.

This option has limited — but useful — applications for aerobic and anaerobic training. If you have low-back pain, for example, you can pedal a cycle in a recumbent position rather than an upright one. This angle offers greater support for your lower back thereby decreasing the amount of stress in your lumbar area.

4. Use a different grip or hand position.

Many times there is less orthopedic stress when you use a different grip or hand position. Once again, this is extremely relevant when addressing the shoulder joint. If you have a slight pain in your shoulder when performing an exercise such as the bench press, it is quite possible that there will be a significant reduction in pain by simply changing the position of your hands from that used with a barbell to a "parallel grip" (that is, your palms facing each other) with dumbbells. In exercises for your torso, changing the position of your hand in this manner causes the head of your humerus (your upper-arm bone) to rotate laterally which may relieve the stress in your shoulder joint.

Note that every exercise that can be performed with a barbell can also be performed with dumbbells. These exercises include the bench press, incline press, decline press, seated press, upright row, shoulder shrug, bicep curl, tricep extension, and wrist flexion. As such, you have an option for varying the position of your hands that you use in exercises for just about every major muscle in your torso. Additionally, many machines allow you to vary the position of your grip/hand at your convenience without any major loss of technique or function.

5. Perform different exercises.

Yet another option for rehabilitative training in the weight room is to perform different exercises that require the same muscle groups. For instance, if you simply cannot perform

If you have low-back pain, you can pedal a cycle in a recumbent position rather than an upright one.

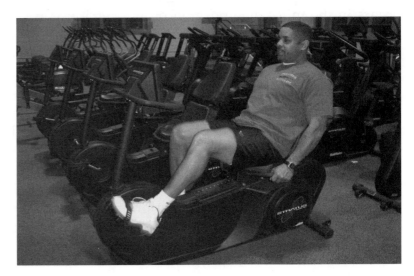

any type of lat pulldown without experiencing shoulder pain or discomfort, then perhaps you can implement another exercise that addresses the same muscles albeit in a pain-free fashion. In this situation, a seated row or bent-over row can be substituted for the lat pulldown. All of these exercises involve the same major muscles, namely your upper back (or "lats"), biceps, and forearms.

This guideline can also be applied to aerobic and anaerobic training. If you cannot run due to a bruised or sprained ankle, for example, you may be able to perform aerobic and anaerobic training with a non-weightbearing activity such as an upright or recumbent cycle.

6. Bypass the injured area.

One of the biggest advantages of machines and manual resistance is that they allow you to apply the resistance above a joint, so that it does not involve an injured area. Presume that you sprained your wrist and, consequently, exercises for your torso were difficult or uncomfortable — if not impossible — to perform with conventional equipment such as barbells and dumbbells. In this case, however, you could still use machines and manual resistance to perform a variety of exercises that target the major muscles of your torso without involving your wrist joint. Among the machine exercises that bypass the wrist area are the pec fly (a.k.a. the "pec dec"), pullover, and lateral raise; many other exercises that avoid the wrist area can be done with manual resistance. Actually, you could still perform the aforementioned exercises — and others — with machines and manual resistance even if your wrist was immobilized with a cast.

Also consider this: If your leg was placed in a cast from your mid-thigh to your ankle, performing any multiple-joint movements that address your hips such as the deadlift and leg press would not be possible. However, it would be possible to bypass your knee joint, and train your hips in a safe and effective fashion — despite the cast — by doing a single-joint movement with machines or manual resistance such as hip abduction or hip adduction.

7. Limit the range of motion.

There is a good possibility that pain only occurs at certain points in your range of motion (ROM) such as the starting or the mid-range position of the repetition. In either case, you can restrict your ROM for the exercise. For example, an injury such as a hyperextended elbow or knee is especially painful in the starting (or stretched) position of an exercise. In this instance, you should stop short of lowering the weight all the way down; by the same token, if pain occurs in the mid-range position of an exercise, you should stop short of fully flexing or extending your muscles. As the injured area heals over a period of time, you can gradually and carefully increase your ROM until it is possible for you to perform repetitions that are pain-free throughout a full ROM.

Nowadays, many machines offer range-limiting devices. This enables you to restrict your ROM in a precise, repeatable manner. As a matter of fact, the ROM can sometimes be adjusted in fractional increments without exiting the machine. Documenting your ROM (as well as the resistance and repetitions) that you use during rehabilitative training is also a good idea.

Sometimes, your pain-free ROM may be restricted to a specific joint angle plus or minus a few degrees. In this case, you can perform an isometric (or static) contraction of varying durations to train your muscles at pain-free positions. One way to accomplish this is to use your good limb to raise the weight to the pain-free position of your injured limb. At this point,

For rehabilitative training, machines offer the ability to train injured and healthy limbs seperately by creating independent workloads.

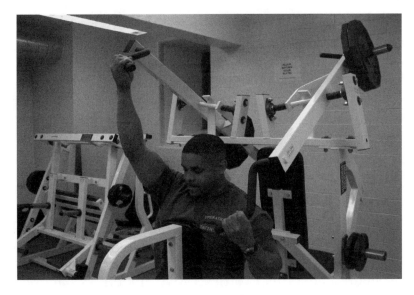

you would "hand off" the weight to your injured limb. Then, you would exert force against this resistance without changing the angle of your injured limb. You can also exert force isometrically against another person who is applying manual resistance.

This option can be implemented during aerobic and anaerobic training. If you have knee pain while cycling, you can lower the height of the seat thereby reducing the ROM of your knee joint.

8. Exercise the good limb.

If all else fails, you can still train your unaffected limb. Here is an example: Suppose you had surgery and, as a result, your left ankle was casted. Obviously, the cast would not allow you to perform any exercises that involved any ROM whatsoever for your left ankle. Even so, you could still do exercises with your right ankle. This has important ramifications in rehabilitation because some scientific studies have shown that training a muscle on one side of your body will actually benefit the contralateral muscle (that is, the same muscle that is on the opposite side of your body). This phenomenon has been dubbed "indirect transfer" or "cross transfer." Researchers are not exactly sure why this occurs, but the fact of the matter is that it does occur.

Many exercises can be performed unilaterally (that is, with one limb at a time) on machines in a safe and comfortable fashion. Indeed, numerous machines are equipped with independent movement arms that allow you to train your limbs separately if needed. Essentially, the independent movement arms create an independent workload. According to Coach Thomas, "Each side of the body is forced to work independently of the other without the threat of losing balance or attaining an awkward position from favoring one side." If you do not have access to machines, you can use dumbbells and manual resistance for unilateral (single-limb) training.

9. Exercise unaffected bodyparts.

In the event that you cannot train an injured area due to an unreasonable amount of pain or discomfort, you can still perform exercises for your uninjured bodyparts. So, if you have a knee injury that prohibits activity for your lower body, you can still do exercises or activities for your entire torso — as long as they are done while you are sitting or lying, and not standing. Likewise, if you have a dislocated shoulder or a torn rotator cuff that does not allow you to do exercises or activities for the major muscles of your torso, you can still do exercises for your lower body along with your arms and mid-section — provided that they do not indirectly produce shoulder pain.

Once again, this guideline is also appropriate for aerobic and anaerobic training. Suppose that you have a hip, leg, or ankle injury that prohibits you from doing any aerobic or anaerobic training with your lower body. There are a few commercial devices that enable you to do aerobic and anaerobic training exclusively with the muscles of your torso such as an upper-body ergometer.

PRUDENT CHOICES

In many instances, you can exercise an injured area or bodypart in a safe, prudent, and pain-free manner. This will prevent a significant loss in muscular size and strength as well as aerobic, anaerobic, and metabolic fitness. And even though you may not be able to exercise an injured area due to an excessive amount of pain or discomfort, you can still train your uninjured bodyparts. Once the injured area heals, you can reintroduce exercises that were previously painful to perform.

Remember that the critical factor in the prudent administration of rehabilitative training is pain-free — or nearly pain-free — exercise and activity. However, understanding that there is a distinct difference between muscular pain and joint pain is important. Muscular pain is not necessarily cause for alarm. It is an indication that you are doing high-intensity work and your muscles are being fatigued. Joint pain, however, is of great concern. Localized pain in a joint usually means that there is some type of structural problem. If you experience pain in your joints while exercising, you are merely aggravating your condition and perhaps even causing further damage by brutalizing the joint infrastructure. Simply, an exercise that produces joint pain must be avoided or altered.

For chronic pain or serious injuries always consult a sports-medical specialist. If surgery is required to repair an injury, physical therapy is recommended both prior to, and after surgery. By performing as many of the post-surgical physical-therapy exercises as possible prior to surgery, the muscles and tendons around the injured area will get stronger and adapt, thereby facilitating a shorter recovery period. Under these circumstances physical therapy will play a vital role in the recovery process.

Appropriate rehabilitative training is absolutely essential for SWAT officers. Most SWAT teams function with less than an ideal number of team members available for deployment on critical incidents. If you are not able to participate on a tactical operation due to an injury, the likelihood of injury to your fellow officers is increased and your team's ability to successfully resolve the situation is decreased. Rehabilitative training allows SWAT officers the opportunity to recover from an injury faster and to continue as part of the team.

How important is rehabilitative training? According to Ken Mannie, the Strength and Conditioning Coach at Michigan State University, "Our philosophy . . . has always been that strength training is a vital constituent in the rehab process and that all training options for an injured area will be considered before deciding not to address the area."

Chapter 14
Power Training

An important aspect of your performance potential is power. Performing the so-called "quick lifts" — such as the power clean, push press, snatch, and/or their derivatives — and doing fast-speed repetitions has long been thought necessary in order to improve power. When individuals use a program that does not incorporate these methods, they are sometimes criticized because they do not "train for power" or do "power training." The fact of the matter is that individuals can "train for power" and do "power training" — but not by implementing the quick lifts or fast-speed repetitions. How is it possible for you to improve your power without using these methods?

UNDERSTANDING POWER

Before discussing how you can improve your power, understanding the meaning of the term is important. In physics, a mathematical definition of "power" is "work divided by time." Since "work" is defined as "force times distance," it follows that power is also "force times distance divided by time."

Another definition of "power" is "force times velocity." The term "velocity" is defined as "distance divided by time." Once again, it follows that "power" is "force times distance divided by time."

So power has three variables: force, distance, and time. Manipulating any of these three variables will affect power.

METHODS FOR IMPROVEMENT

Based upon the equation "power equals force times distance divided by time," you can improve your power output three different ways: (1) increase the amount of force; (2) increase the distance of application; and (3) decrease the time of application.

Increase the Amount of Force

If you increase the amount of force that you apply and keep the other two variables in the equation the same — namely, the distance over which you apply the force and the time that it takes you to apply the force — you will produce more power. Here is an example: If you can bench press 160 pounds a distance of 18 inches (1.5 feet) in 2 seconds, your power output is 120 foot-pounds per second [160 lbs x 1.5 ft ÷ 2 sec = 120 ft-lbs/sec]. Suppose that at some point in the future, you increased your bench press to 180 pounds. Assuming that the distance you moved the resistance (18 inches) and the time it took you to move the resistance (2 seconds) remained the same, your power output is now 135 foot-pounds per second. So, by increasing the amount of force that you applied, you have improved your power output.

How do you increase the amount of force that you apply? The short answer is to increase the strength of your muscles. If you increase the strength of your muscles, they can produce more force; if your muscles produce more force, you will have the potential to produce more power.

How do you improve your strength so that you can produce more force? While there is no shortage of opinions, any strength-training program will be productive if — and only if — it incorporates the Overload Principle. Arguably, this principle is the most important underlying construct for improving physical performance — whether it is strength, endurance, or even flexibility. As far as strength training is concerned, the principle states that in order for a muscle to increase in strength (and size) it must be stressed — or "overloaded" — with a workload that is beyond its present capacity.

You can overload your muscles by using a double-progressive technique. When implementing this technique, overload is accomplished by two means. One way is to make the resistance — or the "load" — progressively more challenging over time; another way is to do more repetitions with the same resistance. Your muscles will adapt to the "overload" — from using a heavier amount of resistance or performing a greater number of repetitions — by increasing in strength. Without imposing greater demands, there will not be any compensatory adaptation because your muscles will literally have no reason to get stronger. Stated otherwise, your muscles must be exposed to demands that they have not experienced previously.

Also remember that it matters little whether your muscles are loaded with resistance from machines, barbells, dumbbells, elastic cords, sandbags, bricks, or even other human beings. Your muscles do not possess the ability to distinguish between different modes of resis-

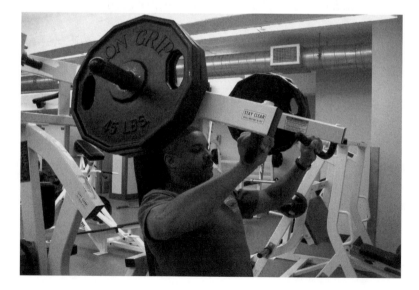

Your muscles do not possess the ability to distinguish between different modes of resistance.

tance. They simply respond to being loaded. (Chapter 7 contains detailed information about strength training.)

Increase the Distance of Application

If you increase the distance over which you apply the force and do not change the other two variables in the equation — specifically, the amount of force that you apply and the time that it takes you to apply the force — you will produce more power. Consider this example: If you can squat 300 pounds a distance of 21 inches (1.75 feet) in 2 seconds, your power output is 262.5 foot-pounds per second [300 lbs x 1.75 ft ÷ 2 sec = 262.5 ft-lbs/sec]. Suppose that at some point in the future, you increased your range of motion in the squat so that you are now displacing the resistance a distance of 24 inches. Assuming that the resistance you lifted (300 pounds) and the time it took you to move the resistance (2 seconds) did not change, your power output is now 300 foot-pounds per second. So, by increasing the distance over which you applied the force, you have improved your power output.

How do you increase the distance over which you apply force? One way is to become more flexible. If you become more flexible, you can increase the ranges of motion of your joints; if you increase the ranges of motion of your joints, you will have the potential to produce more power.

How do you improve your flexibility in order to apply force over a greater distance? Like strength training, there is no one optimal program for improving flexibility. Successful flexibility programs, however, have several commonalities. To reduce your risk of injury, you should stretch under control without any bouncing, bobbing, or jerking movements. Moreover, you should hold the stretched position for about 30 - 60 seconds. Similar to strength training, you must make your flexibility training progressively more challenging. You can do this by attempting to stretch a little bit farther than the last time. Finally, stretching each of your major muscle groups on a regular basis is important. (Chapter 3 contains detailed information about flexibility training.)

Decrease the Time of Application

If you decrease the time that it takes you to apply the force and keep the other two variables in the equation the same — namely the amount of force that you apply and the distance over which you apply the force — you will produce more power. Here is an example: If you can deadlift 400 pounds a distance of 18 inches (1.5 feet) in 2 seconds, your power output is 300 foot-pounds per second [400 lbs x 1.5 ft ÷ 2 sec = 300 ft-lbs/sec]. Suppose that at some point in the future, you increased your speed of movement in the deadlift to 1.5 seconds (that is, you did the repetition faster). Assuming that the resistance you lifted (400 pounds) and the distance you moved the resistance (18 inches) remained constant, your power output is now 400 foot-pounds per second. So, by increasing the speed at which you applied force, you have improved your power output.

How do you decrease the time that it takes you to apply force? One alternative is to perfect your technique (in your chosen sport). If you perfect your technique, you can perform the skill more quickly; if you can perform the skill more quickly, you will have the potential to produce more power.

How do you improve your technique so that you can decrease the time that it takes you to apply force? The motor-learning literature is in general agreement as to how this can be best achieved. Learning how to perform the skill correctly is important. In addition, you must perform the skill repeatedly and consistently, until you can execute it without conscious effort. The skill must be practiced in a flawless manner. Remember, practice makes perfect ... but only if you practice perfect.

Lastly, the skill should be practiced exactly as you would use it in competition. Tim Wakeham, an Assistant Strength and Conditioning Coach at Michigan State University, offers this insight: "Students do not study algebra to take a geometry test even though those are similar subjects. Both subjects are under the umbrella of mathematics, and because of their similarities, studying one may positively affect test results in the other. But it should be obvious that the *best* results would come from preparing for an algebra test by studying algebra." (Chapter 15 contains detailed information about skill training.)

SWAT APPLICATIONS

Examples in the weight room were given to illustrate how the three variables in the power equation — that is, force, distance, and time — can be manipulated to improve power output. Several applications of those concepts can also be illustrated during tactical operations:

- If you apply more force over the same distance in the same amount of time, you will have the potential to pull down a suspect with increased power.

- If you move a greater distance with the same amount of force in the same amount of time, you will have the potential to use a one-person ram with more power.

- If you move in less time with the same amount of force over the same distance, you will have the potential to run up a flight of stairs with more power.

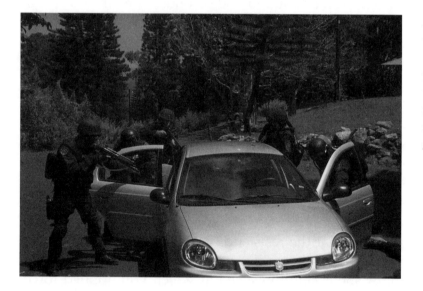

Power requirements necessary to remove a suspect from a vehicle must be trained differently than power requirements inside the weight room, although both types of power are important for SWAT officers. The same is true for athletes who must train for skill-specific power.

POWER INSIDE AND OUTSIDE THE WEIGHT ROOM

So an individual who is powerful can apply a large force over a long distance in a short period of time. As demonstrated earlier, your power output can be improved by three different means: (1) increase the amount of force that you apply; (2) increase the distance over which you apply the force; and (3) decrease the amount of time that it takes you to apply the force. This can be accomplished by improving your strength, flexibility, and technique.

Be forewarned, however, that just because you can produce more power during a given exercise inside the weight room does not mean that you will automatically produce more power during a given skill outside the weight room. Simply stated, there is no legitimate, scientific evidence that the ability to produce power transfers from one activity to another.

For example, if performing the power clean or another explosive-type movement improves your vertical jump, then doing the vertical jump should improve your power clean. But it does not. The bottom line is that producing power inside the weight room is only advantageous inside the weight room, and producing power outside the weight room is very different and requires skill-specific training.

Chapter 15
Skill Training

The science of motor learning is the study of muscular movement or, simply, "motor skills." Research in this discipline promotes an understanding of how skills are learned, applied, and refined. The intent to expedite the acquisition of skills has given rise to a number of practices that are well meaning, but are generally unsupported by the motor-learning literature.

SKILLS AND ABILITIES

Though the terms are often used interchangeably and are somewhat related, skills are vastly different from abilities. A skill refers to the level of performance in one specific action. Examples of specific skills include shooting a pistol, climbing a chain-link fence, and hitting a speed bag. Skills can be modified and improved through practice. On the other hand, an ability refers to a general trait. This includes dynamic strength, static strength, explosive strength, speed of limb movement, quickness, coordination, dynamic balance, static balance, and stamina. Abilities are thought to be genetically determined and, unlike skills, cannot be changed by practice or experience. Abilities are not specific skills in themselves. However, abilities are factors that determine performance potential and form the foundation of a number of specific skills. For example, performing a distinct skill such as firing a submachine gun at a target from a kneeling position requires the general underlying abilities of static strength and static balance.

Each ability is responsible for only a very limited number of movements — and even slightly different movements require that different abilities come into play. For instance, shooting a pistol and shooting a submachine gun would involve different motor abilities. Further, abilities are thought to be independent of each other — the quality of any one ability is not dependent upon the quality of another. Stated otherwise, individuals who perform well in one task do not necessarily perform well in another.

Quickness and Balance Exercises

General "quickening" and "balancing" drills are frequently used with the expectation that the movement patterns learned in those exercises will transfer to specific skills and thus improve performance. Numerous studies have investigated the possibility of transferring quickness and balance to other skills. According to Richard Schmidt, Ph.D., there is little evidence that practicing a skill that requires a certain ability — such as quickness or balance — will improve another skill that requires the same abilities.

Being "quick" is advantageous in many physical activities (and sports). Dr. Schmidt suggests that there are at least three separate abilities that are used to act quickly: (1) reaction time (the interval of time between an unanticipated stimulus and the start of the response); (2) response orientation (where one of many stimuli is presented, each of which requires its own response); and (3) speed of movement (the interval of time between the start of a movement and its completion). Each of these three abilities involves quickness. However, these three abilities are separate and independent of each other. Studies have reported no transfer effect from quickening exercises to a motor task requiring quickness. Other research has shown that reaction time and speed of movement have essentially no correlation — that is, the abilities have very little in common. Therefore, being "quick" depends upon the circumstances under which speedy responses are required.

Balance is an ability that is important for the performance of a wide range of skills. As with quickness, the balance required for one activity is not related to the balance needed in another. In a study that involved 320 subjects, the researcher found no underlying ability for balance, and noted that two balance tasks were dependent upon separate and independent abilities. The author concluded that the correlation between the two balance tasks was "little more than zero." Researchers in another study examined six tests of static and dynamic balance, and found that the abilities supporting one test of balance were separate from those supporting another. Their study suggests that there is no general ability for balance and that even skills that appear quite similar usually correlate poorly.

Similar findings have been reported in a number of other studies. With very few exceptions, the correlations among motor tasks are very low. In short, there is no general ability for quickness, balance, or anything else. No one should expect that an ability such as quickness and balance could be improved by practice anyway. However, skills involving quickness and balance can be improved. For example, running up a flight of stairs or performing a ranger crawl across a rope can be improved with practice, as long as these specific skills are practiced. But, perfecting the skill of walking across a narrow balance beam will not improve your balance when crawling across a rope.

Open and Closed Skills

Skills can be classified as either "open" or "closed." Both types of skills differ in several areas and demand entirely different learning strategies. Designations of "open" and "closed" actually mark the extreme points of a spectrum, with skills residing between them having varying degrees of environmental variability and predictability.

Open skills are performed in an environment that is variable and unpredictable. A SWAT operator must react to a situation and produce a response that can match the constantly changing environmental conditions. Since environmental conditions may vary from one response to another, the operator must have a variety of responses available to accomplish the skill. Examples of open skills are clearing a room and reacting to an individual's movement. (Basketball, soccer, and baseball are sports in which open skills dominate.)

Conversely, a closed skill occurs in an environment that is stable and predictable. Because the environment does not fluctuate, a SWAT officer can plan or predict a response well in advance. Ken Mannie, the Strength and Conditioning Coach at Michigan State University, notes that in a closed skill, an object waits to be acted upon by the performer. Further, the performer is not required to begin action until ready to do so. Closed skills depend upon strength, endurance, and technique for performance. An example of a closed skill is shooting at a stationary target from a prone position. (Gymnastics, diving, and golf are sports in which closed skills dominate. Weightlifting — whether it is competitive or recreational — is also an activity in which closed skills dominate.)

THE TRANSFER OF LEARNING

The transfer of learning refers to the effects of past learning upon the acquisition of a new skill. Many individuals take the transfer of learning for granted. They assume that movements for the execution of one skill always and automatically transfer or "carryover" to the learning of another.

Types of Transfer

The acquisition of skills can be enhanced or impaired depending upon the correct use of the transfer of learning principles. Prior to incorporating skill training into an overall training program, an analysis of each skill must first occur. The transfer of learning from one skill to another may be positive, negative, or absent altogether.

Positive transfer occurs when the influence of prior learning facilitates the learning of a new skill. Learning to free-rappel off of a water tower or catwalk would facilitate learning to rappel out of a helicopter. Both skills have many exact qualities, but primarily differ by a moving vs. stationary platform. By becoming proficient in the first skill, a transfer of ability would occur, benefiting the learning process and application of the second skill.

Negative transfer happens when the learning of a new skill inhibits the learning of a second skill. For instance, after shooting a revolver, shooting a 9mm semi-automatic pistol will likely create *initial* motor confusion. In this case, shooting hundreds of rounds or more may be required before the new skill can be ingrained in muscle memory. For this reason, many law enforcement agencies designate a transition period when switching to new weapon systems.

No transfer occurs if the learning of one skill has a negligible influence on the learning of a second skill. As an example, learning to shoot a shotgun would have no effect on learning to climb a rope. Obtaining a high level of proficiency in either of these skills would not enhance proficiency in the other.

THE USE OF WEIGHTED OBJECTS

People widely believe that using weighted implements contributes to the learning of specific motor patterns and sports skills. This has led to the practice of trying to simulate skills in the weight room using a variety of weighted objects. In the motor-learning literature, practicing a particular motor skill with weighted implements is known as "overload training." Barbells, dumbbells, medicine balls, and other weighted objects are used during overload training with the expectation of improving performance.

The basis for mimicking skills with weighted implements is entirely anecdotal, having very little support from the motor-learning literature. There is no research evidence suggesting that basic movement patterns can be transferred from task to task. Yet, many individuals still insist that the use of certain weightlifting movements encourages a positive transfer of motor ability to other skills. If there was a correlation between weightlifting skills and other skills, then highly successful weightlifters would excel at literally every sports-related movement that they attempted. And we know that this is not true.

The Kinesthetic Aftereffect

Motor-learning research refers to a "kinesthetic aftereffect" which is defined by George Sage, Ph.D., as a "perceived modification in the shape, size or weight of an object . . . as a result of experience with a previous object." Individuals experience the kinesthetic aftereffect during overload training. This phenomenon is exemplified by a person who runs with a weighted vest and after removing it, has the perceived ability to run faster. Essentially, the kinesthetic aftereffect is nothing more than a sensory illusion.

Research indicates that the kinesthetic aftereffect is not accompanied by a measurable improvement in performance in the skills that have been practiced using weighted objects. One study reported no significant changes in the speed of movement during elbow flexion immediately following the application of overload. Another study had subjects perform vertical jumps with a weighted vest followed by jumps without the weight. The researchers found no improvements in vertical jump performance after the overload practices. Nearly identical results have been reported in many other studies.

Dr. Sage suggests that "any attempt to improve performance by utilizing objects that are slightly heavier than normal while practicing gross motor skills that will be later used in sports competition seems to be hardly worth the time spent and the money paid for the weighted objects." Dr. Schmidt adds, "Teaching a particular Skill A simply because you would like it to transfer to Skill B, which is of major interest, is not very effective, especially if you consider the time spent on Skill A that could have been spent on Skill B instead."

Problems with Using Weighted Objects

According to Wayne Westcott, Ph.D., four problems occur when practicing sports skills with weighted objects. The problem areas relate to neuromuscular confusion, incorrect movement speed, orthopedic stress, and insufficient workload.

Neuromuscular confusion. Attempting to duplicate a skill with a weight or a weighted implement is a gigantic step in the wrong direction. Each time that you perform a given skill, there is a specific neuromuscular pattern involved that is unique to that movement alone. Introducing anything foreign to the "pattern" — such as weighted vests, ankle weights, barbells, or medicine balls — will only serve to confuse your original neuromuscular pathways, actually creating a negative transfer and a resultant decrease in performance. Watch someone attempt to mimic a skill with a weighted object and you will quickly notice that the effort used to direct the unfamiliar weight results in a different movement pattern that is labored and awkward. In reality, it is a very different motion altogether.

Incorrect movement speed. If a skill is to be performed at a given speed, it should be practiced at that speed in order to facilitate the learning of the skill. Practicing a skill at a slower or a faster speed than actually would be used in the performance of the skill will cause a momentary negative transfer. On a related note, Thomas Pipes, Ph.D., suggests that running with ankle weights will train the neuromuscular system at slower speeds and can cause a person to actually run slower. The same negative effects are produced when running with a parachute or while pulling a sled.

Orthopedic stress. Another problem associated with practicing a skill with a weighted object pertains to the stresses that are placed on the joints. Practicing with implements that are heavier than usual can place considerable orthopedic stress on the bodyparts involved and, as a result, is dangerous. Structural stress is most evident in the shoulder, elbow, and wrist.

Insufficient workload. Another reason why weighted objects do not enhance performance is that they do not increase strength in the involved musculature. The added resistance provided by a weighted object is not sufficient enough to surpass the "threshold" for strength development. The added resistance is a mere fraction of what is necessary to overload your muscles.

SPECIFICITY VERSUS GENERALITY

The Principle of Specificity states that activities must be specific to an intended skill in order for a maximal transfer of learning — or carryover — to occur. Specific means "exact" or "identical," not "similar" or "just like." Indeed, one researcher has stated that "transfer is highly specific and occurs only when the practiced movements are identical."

Movement patterns for different skills are never executed exactly alike. One researcher has noted that very similar-appearing motor skills are based upon very different patterns of muscular activity. According to Dr. Schmidt, some movement patterns — although they outwardly appear to use the same muscular actions — are actually quite different and require learning and practicing of each task separately.

In one study, subjects performed elbow flexion (that is, a bicep curl) in the standing position. After training, elbow flexion strength had increased considerably when measured in the standing position. However, similar movements in an unfamiliar position (supine) revealed only a slight increase in strength. In other words, a standing bicep curl is not even specific to a nearly identical exercise such as a supine bicep curl. Exercises that are performed in the weight room are even less similar to other skills and, therefore, are not specific to other skills.

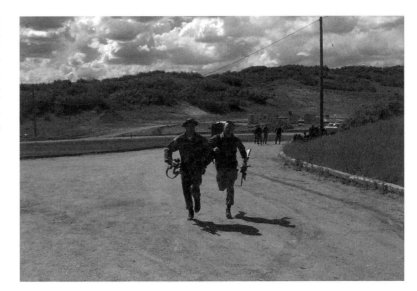

A SWAT sniper team running 100 yards with their rifles, carrying all operational equipment, and then taking a shot under time constraints involves muscle, movement, speed, and resistance specificity. It is directly related to performing operational skills under these circumstances.

So, doing power cleans may be similar to performing a vertical jump and doing lunges may be just like using a one-person ram, but the truth is that power cleans will only help you get better at doing power cleans and lunges will only help you get better at doing lunges. Similarly, heaving medicine balls around is great for improving your skill at heaving medicine balls around and nothing else. Also, jumping off boxes will only perfect your skill at jumping off boxes. There are no exercises that can be performed in the weight room — with barbells or machines — that will expedite the learning of other skills.

A lot of time and patience is required to master the specific neuromuscular patterns of complex exercises such as the power clean. This valuable time and energy could be used more effectively elsewhere such as perfecting specific skills and techniques that will actually be used during tactical operations or a particular competitive event.

Elements of Specificity

There are four elements of specificity that define the rules for determining whether two movements are specific or not:

- *Muscle specificity*. The exact muscle(s) used in the exercise must also be used in the skill.

- *Movement specificity*. The exact movement pattern used in the exercise must be the same as the skill.

- *Speed specificity*. The speed of movement used in the exercise must be identical to the skill.

- *Resistance specificity*. The precise resistance used in the exercise must be identical to the external resistance encountered in the skill.

In order for a weight-training exercise to be specific to another skill, all four of these elements would have to be true. One skill may resemble another in terms of identical muscle(s), movement pattern, speed of movement, and resistance used. However, at best a weight-training exercise can only approximate another skill . . . it cannot duplicate it.

IMPROVING SKILLS

The acquisition and improvement of skills is a process in which an individual develops a set of responses into an integrated and organized movement pattern. Depending upon the skill, three requirements are necessary in order for you to increase your efficiency: practicing the skill, strengthening the muscles, and increasing aerobic capacity.

Practicing the Skill

The first requirement for improving a skill is to literally practice the intended skill for thousands and thousands of task-specific repetitions. Each repetition must be done with perfect technique so that its specific movement pattern becomes firmly ingrained in your "motor memory." The skill must be practiced perfectly and ex-

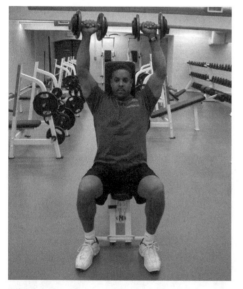

There are no excercises that can be performed in the weight room that will directly or automatically improve operational skills.

actly as it would be used during a tactical operation or competitive event. Further, the skill should not be practiced with weighted implements.

Strengthening the Muscles

The next requirement for improving a skill is to strengthen the major muscle groups that are used during the performance of the skill. However, strength training should not be done in a manner that mimics or replicates a particular skill, so as not to confuse or impair the intended movement pattern. A stronger muscle can produce more force; if you can produce more force, you will require less effort and be able to perform the skill more quickly, more accurately, and more efficiently. But again, this is provided that you have practiced enough in a correct manner, so that you will be more skillful in applying that force. Remember, practice makes perfect ... but only if you practice perfect.

Increasing Aerobic Capacity

The final requirement for improving a skill is to improve your aerobic capacity. This is not applicable for all skills, but is related to skills involving aerobic exertion. However, it must still be applied during the execution of the specific skill. Reducing the onset of fatigue can enhance the ability to perform certain skills, as long as they are being practiced correctly.

While there are benefits of cross training with similar exercises to enhance strength and aerobic conditioning, the best way to improve operational skills is to practice the specific skills required in an identical manner during training. Otherwise, carryover will be minimal at most. And in some cases, the carryover (or transfer) will be negative (or detrimental). A runner will perform better in fitness tests that involve running than a cyclist (and vice versa), even though they have both progressively challenged their aerobic systems. Training has to be as *identical* as possible for maximum benefits relating to specific skill performance.

However, this should not be confused with cross training to improve overall physical fitness. The benefits of exercise are numerous whether they specifically relate to a skill or not. But exercise will only improve a skill when the aforementioned requirements are met. Skill training must be practiced correctly to enhance effectiveness on tactical operations and in competitive events. For SWAT officers, in order to properly practice skill training, an understanding of operational requirements is essential.

An analysis of your SWAT team's operational tasks should be conducted. Once completed, practicing these specific skills in training is the best way to increase each team member's skill level. Skill training, as it relates to physical fitness should then be incorporated into an overall fitness training program. Ensure that the skills are practiced while wearing all operational gear and under as close to operational conditions as possible. Improving your speed at running a 60-yard dash in shorts and a t-shirt is not going to improve your speed while running the same distance wearing a gas mask, all operational gear, and carrying a ram. For these reasons, an operationally-related physical fitness test should be implemented for all SWAT officers.

Chapter 16
Operational Fitness Standards for SWAT Team Personnel

Operationally-related fitness standards for all SWAT team candidates and current officers must be established by every law enforcement agency employing a SWAT team. The courts have overwhelmingly held that any mandatory standard must be reflective of essential job-related tasks. In *Thomas v. City of Evanston* 610 F.Supp. 422, 42 Fair Empl.Prac.Cas. (BNA) 1795 (N.D.Ill., Feb 26, 1985) (NO. 80 C 4803), the court held that, "To be *content valid* the test must satisfy several attributes. First, the test makers must have done a proper *job analysis*, that is, a study of important work behaviors required for successful performance and their relative importance. Second, the test must be related to and representative of the content of the job. In other words, the test must measure ability to perform competently on the specific job. Third, the test must be scored so that it properly discriminates between those who can and cannot perform the job well."

While legal issues relating to legal liability are important concerns, an even greater concern is the relationship between an individual's level of physical fitness, and his or her ability to perform on a tactical operation. Will a team member be able to carry out the duties of a SWAT officer in an operational situation? A comprehensive fitness test must be able to address liability and operational concerns.

To better understand this issue and to provide a solution, Operational Tactics, Inc., and the authors examined fitness standards currently in use by SWAT teams throughout the United States. Most current standards were found to be inadequate. For example, exercises such as push-ups and sit-ups are used by many teams throughout the country; however they are not job-related. When was the last time a SWAT officer was required to perform either of these exercises on a tactical operation? Many standards in use are gender or age based, providing preferential treatment for female or older officers. Flexibility tests such as the "sit-and-reach" test, favor individuals with long arms and/or short legs. A significant number of teams use a rope-climb test performed at a local school or military base, even though they do not have a rope in their inventory that can be used for climbing on a tactical operation. And even tests such a 1.5-mile run are conducted in gym shorts and running shoes, neither of which are typical SWAT attire for tactical operations.

The ability to accomplish all assignments on a tactical operation is non-discriminatory. Carrying a 90-pound ram or the ability to move/rescue a 230-pound injured teammate are examples of tasks that may have to be performed on a tactical operation. Neither the ram nor the 230-pound officer becomes any lighter for officers who receive preferential treatment based on gender or age. Discrimination or preferential treatment should not be a part of any fitness test. The same standards must be applied to everyone, since the requirements of a SWAT officer are the same for all team members.

Operational Tactics, Inc., and the authors conducted a case study to develop practical, operationally-related fitness standards, as well as methodology to implement these new standards. SWAT teams throughout the United States were selected to participate in our study testing the newly developed standards. The SWAT teams selected were comprised of full-time and part-time SWAT officers from large metropolitan, as well as small rural areas. Team size varied from an eight-member part-time team to a 30-member full-time team. The purpose of the study was to develop one standardized test that reflects an appropriate level of operational fitness for all SWAT officers, regardless of team size and status (full/part-time).

Three testing phases were conducted, with modifications made at the conclusion of each phase. A final test was determined and is now being implemented by many SWAT teams throughout the United States and abroad. The following test is the result of this study and is recommended by Operational Tactics, Inc., and the authors as operational fitness requirements for all SWAT officers.

OPERATIONAL FITNESS REQUIREMENTS FOR SWAT OFFICERS

1. One-mile run in 12 minutes or less, carrying an assigned unloaded shoulder-fired weapon system[1] while wearing full SWAT gear[2] including tactical footwear. For safety reasons, the run may be conducted at a school track.

2. 60-yard run carrying a 45-pound dumbbell[3] or a one-person ram, in full SWAT gear wearing a gas mask, within 15 seconds.

3. 30-yard low-crawl in full SWAT gear wearing a gas mask, within 60 seconds. The elbows and knees must touch the ground at all times.

4. Climb over a six-foot fence, unassisted within 10 seconds in full SWAT gear.

5. Five vertical raises (pull-ups) in full SWAT gear. Using a bar or a beam, start in a hanging position with the palms facing away from the body and the arms fully extended. For the repetition to be counted, the chin must be completely seen over the bar or beam at the conclusion of the upward motion.

6. Five vertical pushes (dips) in full SWAT gear. Using two parallel bars or beams, start in the down position with the arms bent such that the upper arms are approximately parallel to the ground. Then push up the body until both arms are almost completely extended at the top (without "locking" the elbows). Prior to beginning the next repetition, a "one-one-thousand" pause count at the top must occur.[4]

7. Run up eight flights of stairs (four floors) in full SWAT gear carrying a 45-pound dumbbell or a one-person ram, within 30 seconds.

8. Move the heaviest team member 20 yards, both in full SWAT gear, within 40 seconds. Any safe carrying, pulling, or dragging technique may be used, but the officer being moved may not offer any assistance. The heaviest team member will move the next heaviest team member on his/her turn.

    Notes are found at the end of this chapter

The test is to be performed in the order as shown. Team members should begin the next event after the last team member has completed the previous one. Breaks should not be taken between events, except for possible travel time if the run was conducted at a different location from the rest of the test. All team members must pass the test according to the requirements as given, regardless of gender, age, height, and weight. Participants should properly hydrate throughout the test, but not consume so much fluid that bloating and cramping occur. Anyone experiencing dizziness, nausea, or physical illness should not take part in the testing.

Rationale and Justification

In addition to the testing phases, Operational Tactics, Inc., conducted a survey of SWAT team personnel from throughout the United States and several foreign countries to determine relevant job-related standards based on actual tactical operation deployments conducted over the past five years. The rationale and justification of each phase is the following (the term "reasonable" refers to the results of this survey combined with Operational Tactics, Inc., instructor cadre's vast operational experience):

1. The one-mile run was determined to be a reasonable distance SWAT officers could be expected to run on a tactical operation. For example, when deploying from the command post to an entry or perimeter position, the distance is rarely, if ever, more than one mile, but could in fact equal one-mile. And while most deployments are less than this distance, a standard that reflects a *maximum*, yet operationally-related requirement, needs to be instituted. The time limit of 12 minutes or less was established as a reasonable time period to arrive in position, and still be able to perform the duties of a SWAT officer, as well as the remaining requirements of this operational fitness test. Officers taking the test must carry their assigned shoulder-fired weapon system that they would primarily use on a tactical operation. SWAT teams throughout the United States utilize a variety of shoulder-fired weapon systems, so this requirement offers the flexibility to adapt to your individual team's primary weapon system. By wearing full SWAT gear[2] including tactical footwear, you are able to assess this requirement with the actual attire that is worn and equipment that is carried on a tactical deployment. The run may be conducted at any location that accounts for officer safety such as a school track.

2. The 60-yard run carrying a 45-pound dumbbell[3] or a one-person ram is a reasonable task that any SWAT officer could be required to perform on a tactical operation in order to breach a door or to bring the ram to someone designated to breach a door. Successful completion of this requirement would allow for the opportunity of an im-

mediate entry by SWAT team personnel. If you have the available facilities to include a door that can be breached, then this skill can also be tested in conjunction with the physical requirements of carrying the ram to the door in a timely manner. Officers taking the test must wear full SWAT gear[2] including tactical footwear and a gas mask to simulate the actual attire that is worn on a tactical deployment in an environment where chemical agents have been deployed. A time limit of 15 seconds represents a reasonable duration to arrive in position with the ram.

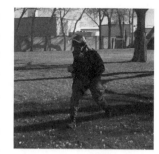

3. Oftentimes, SWAT officers are required to low-crawl into a perimeter position or a position to gather intelligence on a tactical operation. A distance of 30 yards reflects a practical distance requirement to achieve this objective. The elbows and knees must touch the ground at all times to ensure officers are low enough to the ground. Officers taking the test must wear full SWAT gear[2] including tactical footwear and a gas mask to simulate the actual attire that is worn on a tactical deployment in an environment where chemical agents have been deployed. A time limit of 30 seconds represents a reasonable duration to arrive in position.

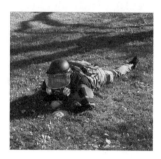

4. Most fences throughout the United States are six feet high or less. The ability to climb over a six-foot fence, unassisted, represents a SWAT officer's ability to perform this task, so that he or she may not be unduly delayed while responding to the scene. Officers taking the test must wear full SWAT gear[2] including tactical footwear to simulate the actual attire that is worn on a tactical deployment. The time limit of 10 seconds allows sufficient opportunity for multiple attempts to traverse the fence should an officer lose his or her footing.

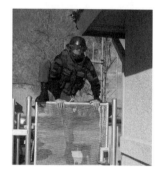

5. In researching tactical operations involving displays of physical fitness skills, many SWAT officers were required to pull themselves onto ledges, balconies, and rooftops on multiple occasions during a critical incident. The five vertical raises while using a bar or a beam represents a method of testing this operational requirement as closely as possible. By starting in a hanging position with the palms facing away from the body and the arms fully extended, and the chin being completely seen over the bar or beam at the conclusion of the upward motion, the maximum range of motion is required to complete this skill. Officers taking the test must wear full SWAT gear[2] including tactical footwear to simulate the actual attire that is worn on a tactical deployment.

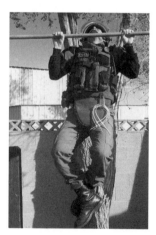

6. In researching tactical operations involving displays of physical-fitness skills, many

SWAT officers were required to push themselves onto barriers, small fences, ledges, decks, and balconies on multiple occasions during a critical incident. The five vertical pushes while using two parallel bars or beams represents a method of testing this operational requirement as closely as possible. By starting in the down position with the arms bent such that the upper arms are approximately parallel to the ground, then pushing up until both arms are almost completely extended at the top (without "locking" the elbows), and pausing at the top for a "one-one-thousand" count, the maximum range of motion without an excessive amount of momentum is required to complete this skill. Officers taking the test must wear full SWAT gear[2] including tactical footwear to simulate the actual attire that is worn on a tactical deployment.

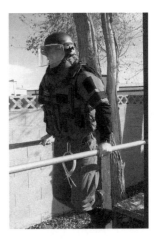

7. On deployment for critical incidents as well as high-risk search and arrest warrants, oftentimes, elevators are not available or will not hold an entire entry team for transport to the designated floor where the target is located. Running up eight flights of stairs (four floors) carrying a 45-pound dumbbell[3] or a one-person ram is a reasonable task that any SWAT officer could be required to perform on a tactical operation in order to breach a door or to bring the ram to someone designated to breach a door. Successful completion of this requirement would allow for the opportunity of an immediate entry by SWAT team personnel. If you have the available facilities to include a door that can be breached, then this skill can also be tested in conjunction with the physical requirements of carrying the ram to the door in a timely manner. Officers taking the test must wear full SWAT gear[2] including tactical footwear to simulate the actual attire that is worn on a tactical deployment. A time limit of 30 seconds represents a reasonable duration to arrive in position with the ram.

8. The most critical skill that could be required on a tactical operation is the rescue of a fellow officer. Many teams have implemented a fitness test where a 160- or 180-pound dummy made of cloth or fire hose must be moved a certain distance to simulate the rescue of an injured officer. There are several problems with using a weight other than the heaviest member of your SWAT team. First, moving a human is different than moving a bag, dummy, or fire hose configuration of a human. Next, and most important, if your team consists of officers who weigh more than the dummy, then they, too, deserve the opportunity to be rescued. By moving the heaviest team member 20 yards, you have ensured that every member of your team can individually rescue any other member. Any safe carrying, pulling, or dragging technique may be used, but the officer being moved may not offer any assistance. This part of the requirement is to assess a situation where a completely incapacitated, critically injured officer is in need of rescue. The heaviest team member will move the next heaviest team member on his/her turn. A time limit of 40 seconds represents a reasonable duration to move an injured team member to safety. Officers taking the test must wear full SWAT gear[2] including tactical footwear to simulate the actual attire that is worn on a tactical deployment.

The order that the Operational Fitness Requirements for SWAT Officers is performed is also important. The established order reflects the hierarchy of fitness skills that are most likely to be performed on a tactical operation. The instruction that team members begin the next event after the last team member completes the previous one offers some, but not excessive, rest between requirements. It also helps develop and enhance team camaraderie.

If your SWAT team has additional deployment responsibilities such as waterborne operations, then an operationally-related swimming standard should also be incorporated within these requirements. In this regard, your team's specific deployment concerns should determine the exact swimming standard to implement.

When initiating fitness requirements for a newly formed or established SWAT team, officers should be afforded a 90-day period to prepare for the new standards before successful completion becomes mandatory. This allows officers the opportunity to properly train to perform these skills. After this time period, department policy will dictate repercussions for failure to successfully complete the fitness requirements.

Operationally-related fitness requirements also serve as skill-training exercises. As previously mentioned, the best way to become proficient at a specific skill is to practice that skill. The Operational Fitness Requirements for SWAT Officers represent many critical skills that could be performed on a tactical operation. Practicing these skills in training will not only provide fitness standards for your SWAT team, but will also improve operational preparedness and efficiency.

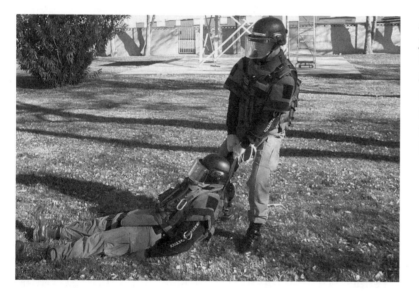

Any safe carrying, pulling, or dragging technique may be used, but the officer being moved may not offer any assistance. Note that during testing it was found the straps attached to most vests would break off even though they were designed to be a means to rescue injured officers.

Notes

1. Officers should carry their assigned shoulder-fired weapon system that they would primarily use on a tactical operation. These weapons should always be checked to ensure they are unloaded prior to the run.

2. Full SWAT gear consists of the following items: Highest level ballistic vest assigned to team members, web gear with holster (no weapon) and equipment pouches, fully loaded magazines, ballistic helmet, gas masks, and any additional equipment normally carried by an officer on a tactical operation. All weapons (except the shoulder-fired weapon system which is only carried on the one-mile run), diversionary devices, and chemical agents may be excluded for safety reasons.

3. A 45-pound dumbbell reflects one-half of the weight of a 90-pound two-person ram and may be carried in any position. If your two-person ram is a different weight, divide by two and select the corresponding dumbbell weight.

4. A "one-one-thousand" pause count at the top will eliminate the opportunity to use excessive momentum, instead of strength to complete the repetition.

Chapter 17
Nutritional Training

Nutrition is the process of selecting, consuming, digesting, absorbing, and utilizing food. Unfortunately, this important aspect of overall training is either inadequately addressed or entirely overlooked.

Nutritional training has several purposes. First, proper nutrition plays a critical role in your capacity to perform as a SWAT officer or athlete at optimal levels, in addition to expediting your recovery. Clearly, your ability to fully recuperate after an exhaustive activity directly affects future performances and the intensity of your physical training. Your nutritional habits are also a factor in the development of physical attributes such as muscular strength and aerobic fitness.

The knowledge base for nutritional training is very critical. You can improve nutritional skills by recognizing the desirable food sources, understanding the recommended intakes of those food sources, and realizing the caloric contributions of the various nutrients. In addition, becoming familiar with your caloric needs can provide support for your nutritional planning. Moreover, knowing what foods/fluids to consume before and after intense activity will facilitate your objective to maximize your physical performance. Finally, good nutritional skills will help you determine whether or not supplementation is warranted.

THE NUTRIENTS

Everything that you do requires energy. The energy is obtained through the foods (or nutrients) that you consume and is measured in calories (which, technically, are units of heat). Essentially, the foods that you eat serve as a fuel for your body. Food is also necessary for the growth, maintenance, and repair of your biological tissues such as muscle and bone.

Foods are composed of six nutrients: carbohydrates, protein, fat, water, vitamins, and minerals. These main constituents of food can be grouped as either macronutrients or micronutrients. In order to be considered nutritious, your food intake must contain the recommended

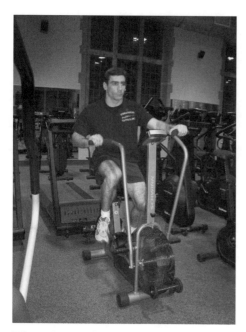

The primary function of carbohydrates (or "carbs") is to furnish you with energy, especially during intense activity.

amounts of the macronutrients as well as appropriate levels of the micronutrients. No single food satisfies this requirement. As a result, variety is the key to a balanced diet. (Here and in other discussions that follow, the term "diet" simply refers to your normal food intake, not a specialized regimen of eating.)

The Macronutrients

As the name implies, macronutrients are needed in relatively large amounts. Three macronutrients — carbohydrates, protein, and fat — provide you with calories and, therefore, a supply of energy. Although it has no calories, water is also categorized as a macronutrient because it is needed in considerable quantities.

Carbohydrates

The primary function of carbohydrates (or "carbs") is to furnish you with energy, especially during intense activity. Your body breaks down carbohydrates into glucose (or "blood sugar"). Glucose can be used as an immediate form of energy during a physical activity or stored as glycogen in your liver and muscles for future use. Highly conditioned muscles can stockpile more glycogen than poorly conditioned muscles. If your glycogen stores are depleted, you will feel overwhelmingly exhausted. For this reason, having greater glycogen stores can give you a significant physiological advantage. Therefore, having a carbohydrate-based diet makes a great deal of sense, especially for physically active individuals. In fact, at least 65% of your daily calories should be in the form of carbohydrates.

Carbohydrates are classified as either "simple" (which are sugars such as table sugar and honey) or "complex" (which are starches such as the starch in bread). Carbohydrate-rich foods include potatoes, cereals, pancakes, breads, spaghetti, macaroni, rice, grains, fruits, and vegetables.

Protein

Protein is necessary for the growth, maintenance, and repair of your biological tissues, particularly muscle tissue. Additionally, protein regulates your water balance and transports other nutrients. Protein can also be used as an energy source in the event that adequate carbohydrates are not available.

When proteins are ingested as foods, they are broken down into their basic building blocks: amino acids. Your body can manufacture most of the 22 known amino acids. Eight (or nine in the case of children and certain adults) *must* be provided in your diet and are termed "essential amino acids" (or "indispensable amino acids"). When a food contains all of the essential amino acids in amounts that facilitate the growth and repair of muscle tissue, it is deemed a "complete protein." In addition, such foods are considered to have a high "biological value" meaning that a large portion of the protein is absorbed and retained. The biological value is an index in which all protein sources are compared to egg whites because they are the most complete protein. (Egg whites have a biological value of 100.) All animal proteins — with the exception of gelatin — are complete proteins and, as a result, have a high biological value. Conversely, the protein found in vegetables and other sources is considered to be an "incomplete protein" — having a low biological value — because it does not include all of the essential amino acids. A white potato, for instance, has a biological value of 34.

Approximately 15% of your daily calories should be from protein. Good sources of this macronutrient are beef, pork, fish, poultry, egg whites, liver, dry beans, and dairy products.

Fat

It may be difficult to believe, but fat is actually vital to a balanced diet. First, fat serves as a major source of energy during low-intensity activities such as sleeping, reading, and walking. Second, fat helps in the transportation and the absorption of certain vitamins. Third, fat adds substantial flavor to foods. This makes food more appetizing — and also explains why fat is craved so much.

Foods that are high in fat include butter, cheese, margarine, meat, nuts, dairy products, and cooking oils. Animal fats — such as butter, lard, and the fat in meats — are referred to as "saturated fats" and contribute to heart disease; vegetable fats — such as corn, olive, and peanut oils — are dubbed "unsaturated fats" and are less harmful. (At room temperature, saturated fats tend to be solid while unsaturated fats are usually liquid.)

There is really no need to add extra fatty food to your diet in order to obtain adequate fat. If anything, far too much fat is often consumed. The fact is that fat often accompanies carbohydrate and protein choices. In addition, foods are often prepared in such a way that the fat content is elevated. For example, baked potatoes have a negligible amount of fat — barely a trace of their calories; french-fried potatoes, on the other hand, have a considerable amount of fat — nearly one half of their calories.

At most, 20% of your daily calories should be composed of fat. Keep in mind that this allotment of fat — as well as that of carbohydrates and protein — is to be distributed over the course of the day. So, there is nothing wrong with eating a food that is more than 20% fat as long as this particular choice is offset by other foods consumed throughout the day that have a lower fat content.

Obviously, any fat that is not used as energy is stored in your body as fat. If not used for energy, however, carbohydrates and protein are converted into fat and stored in that form as well.

Water

Since it is needed in rather large quantities, water is usually classified as a macronutrient. Water does not have any calories or provide you with any energy, but it does play major roles in your body. Water lubricates your joints and regulates your body temperature. It also helps carry nutrients to your cells and waste products from your cells. Incredibly, almost two thirds of your bodyweight is water.

The best sources of water are milk, fruits, fruit juices, vegetables, soup, and, of course, water. You should consume about 16 ounces of water for every pound of bodyweight that you lose while training.

The Micronutrients

Vitamins and minerals are classified as micronutrients because they are required in somewhat small amounts. Neither of these nutrients supplies you with any calories or energy. But vitamins and minerals have many other important functions. (Providing you with an extensive overview of the functions and sources of vitamins and minerals is well beyond the scope of this chapter. For more detailed information, you are encouraged to pursue other sources.)

Vitamins

The Polish chemist Casimir Funk coined the term "vitamine" in 1912. Vitamins are potent compounds that are required in very minute quantities. They occur in a wide variety of foods, especially in fruits and vegetables. You can obtain an adequate intake of vitamins from a balanced diet that contains a variety of foods. Even though vitamins are not a source of energy, they perform many different functions that are vital to an active lifestyle. Vitamins can be grouped as either fat-soluble or water-soluble.

Fat-Soluble Vitamins

The four fat-soluble vitamins — vitamins A, D, E, and K — require proper amounts of fat to be present before transportation and absorption can take place. Excessive amounts of fat-soluble vitamins are stored in your body. Here is a brief listing of their functions and sources:

- *Vitamin A (retinol)* is required for normal vision (especially at night) and promotes bone growth, healthy hair, skin, and teeth. Organ meats, dairy products, fish, eggs, carrots, spinach, and sweet potatoes are good sources of this vitamin.

- *Vitamin D (calciferol)* enhances calcium absorption, and is vital for strong bones and teeth. The "sunshine vitamin" can be found in fish, fortified milk products and cereals, dairy products, and egg yolks.

- *Vitamin E (tocopherol)* acts as an antioxidant, aids in the formation of red blood cells, and helps to maintain your muscles and other biological tissues. Once known as "the vitamin in search of a disease," good sources of it are poultry, seafood, eggs, vegetable oils, nuts, fruits, vegetables, and meats.

- *Vitamin K* assists in blood clotting and bone metabolism. It is found in green leafy vegetables, brussel sprouts, cabbage, potatoes, plant oils, oats, and organ meats.

Water-Soluble Vitamins

The eight B vitamins — biotin, cobalamin, folate, niacin, pantothenic acid, pyridoxine, riboflavin, and thiamine — and vitamin C are considered to be water-soluble vitamins because they are found in foods that have a naturally high content of water. There is minimal storage of water-soluble vitamins in your body — excess amounts are generally excreted in your urine. Their functions and sources are summarized as follows:

- *Biotin* helps to synthesize glycogen, amino acids, and fat. Rich sources of biotin are liver, fruits, vegetables, nuts, eggs, poultry, and meats.

- *Cobalamin (B_{12})* forms and regulates red blood cells, prevents anemia, and maintains a healthy nervous system. This vitamin can be found in fortified cereals, meats, fish, poultry, and dairy products.

- *Folate (folic acid and folacin)* is needed to manufacture red blood cells and aids in the metabolism of amino acids. Enriched cereal grains, fruits, dark green leafy vegetables, meats, fish, liver, poultry, enriched and whole-grain breads, and fortified cereals are good sources of folate.

- *Niacin (B_3)* promotes normal appetite, digestion, and proper nerve function and is required for energy metabolism. It is found in meats, fish, poultry, eggs, potatoes, enriched and whole-grain breads and bread products, orange juice, peanuts, and fortified cereals.

- *Pantothenic acid (B_5)* helps in the metabolism of carbohydrates, protein, and fat. Good sources of this vitamin are chicken, beef, potatoes, oats, cereals, tomato products, liver, kidney, yeast, egg yolks, broccoli, and whole grains.

- *Pyridoxine (B_6)* assists in the formation of red blood cells and the metabolism of carbohydrates, protein, and fat. Fortified cereals, organ meats, lean meats, poultry, fish, eggs, milk, vegetables, nuts, and bananas are rich sources of this vitamin.

- *Riboflavin (B_2)* aids in the maintenance of your skin, mucous membranes, and nervous structures. This vitamin is found in organ meats, poultry, beef, lamb, fish, milk, dark green leafy vegetables, bread products, and fortified cereals.

- *Thiamine (B_1)* maintains a healthy nervous system and heart, and helps to metabolize carbohydrates and amino acids. Good sources of thiamine are enriched, fortified, and whole-grain products, bread and bread products, ready-to-eat cereals, meats, poultry, fish, liver, and eggs.

- *Vitamin C (ascorbic acid)* promotes healing, helps in the absorption of iron, and the maintenance and repair of connective tissues, bones, teeth, and cartilage. Citrus fruits, tomatoes, tomato juice, potatoes, brussel sprouts, cauliflower, broccoli, strawberries, watermelon, cabbage, and spinach are rich sources of vitamin C.

Minerals

Minerals are found in tiny amounts in foods. Like vitamins, nearly all of the minerals that you need can be obtained with an ordinary intake of foods. Minerals can be divided into two subcategories: macrominerals and microminerals.

Macrominerals

As the name implies, macrominerals are required in relatively large amounts — specifically, more than 250 milligrams per day. The macrominerals are calcium, chloride, magnesium, phosphorus, potassium, sodium, and sulfur. Here is a brief overview of their functions and sources:

- *Calcium* is essential in blood clotting, muscle contraction, nerve transmission, and the formation of bones and teeth. Rich sources of this mineral are milk, cheese, yogurt, oysters, broccoli, and spinach.

- *Chloride* is an electrolyte that regulates body fluids into and out of your cells, and helps to maintain a proper acid-base (pH) balance. It is found in table salt, milk, canned vegetables, and animal foods.

- *Magnesium* is essential for healthy nerve and muscle function, and bone formation. Green leafy vegetables, nuts, meats, poultry, fish, oysters, starches, milk, and beans are good sources of magnesium.

- *Phosphorus* maintains pH, helps in energy production, and is essential for every metabolic process in your body. Good sources are milk, yogurt, ice cream, cheese, peas, meats, poultry, fish, and eggs.

- *Potassium* is an electrolyte that regulates body fluids into and out of your cells, and promotes proper muscular contraction and the transmission of nerve impulses. This mineral is found in citrus fruits, bananas, deep yellow vegetables, and potatoes.

- *Sodium* is an electrolyte that regulates body fluids into and out of your cells, transmits nerve impulses, maintains normal blood pressure, and is involved in muscle contraction. Table salt, milk, canned vegetables, and animal foods are good sources of sodium.

- *Sulfur* is needed to make hair and nails. It is found in beef, peanuts, clams, and wheat germ.

Microminerals

As you might suspect, microminerals are needed in relatively small amounts — specifically, less than 20 milligrams per day. The microminerals are chromium, copper, fluoride, iodine, iron, manganese, molybdenum, selenium, and zinc. (A number of other minerals — including arsenic, boron, cobalt, lithium, nickel, silicon, tin, and vanadium — are probably essential in very small amounts, but their roles in the human body are unclear and Recommended Dietary Allowances have not been established.) This is a brief description of the functions and sources of the microminerals:

- *Chromium* functions in the metabolism of carbohydrates and fat, and helps to maintain blood-glucose levels (homeostasis). Meats, poultry, fish, and peanuts are good sources of chromium.

- *Copper* stimulates the absorption of iron and has a role in the formation of red blood cells, connective tissues, and nerve fibers. Good sources are organ meats, seafood, nuts, beans, whole-grain products, and cocoa products.

- *Fluoride* prevents dental caries and stimulates the formation of new bones. This mineral is found in fluoridated water, teas, and marine fish.

- *Iodine* is necessary for proper functioning of your thyroid gland, and prevents goiter and cretinism. Seafood, processed foods, and iodized salt are good sources of this mineral.

- *Iron* is involved in the manufacture of hemoglobin and myoglobin (two proteins that transport oxygen to your tissues), and has a role in normal immune function. It is found in liver, fruits, vegetables, fortified bread and grain products, meats, poultry, and shellfish.

- *Manganese* is involved in the formation of bones and the metabolism of carbohydrates. Good sources of manganese are nuts, legumes, coffee, tea, and whole grains.

- *Molybdenum* helps to regulate the storage of iron. Dark green leafy vegetables, legumes, grain products, nuts, and organ meats are good sources of this mineral.

- *Selenium* protects cell membranes. It is found in organ meats, chicken, seafood, whole-grain cereals, and milk.

- *Zinc* has a role in the repair and growth of your biological tissues. Good sources of this mineral are fortified cereals, meats, poultry, eggs, and seafood.

DAILY SERVINGS

Consuming an assortment of foods helps to ensure that you have obtained adequate amounts of carbohydrates, protein, and fat along with sufficient quantities of vitamins and minerals. According to the U. S. Department of Agriculture and Department of Health and Human Services, a variety of daily foods should include an appropriate number of servings from these six food groups (with the servings in parentheses):

- Bread, Cereal, Rice, and Pasta (6 - 11)
- Vegetable (3 - 5)
- Fruit (2 - 4)
- Milk, Yogurt, and Cheese (2 - 3)
- Meat, Poultry, Fish, Dry Beans, Eggs, and Nuts (2 - 3)
- Fats, Oils, and Sweets (use sparingly)

The exact number of servings that are suitable is contingent upon your caloric (or energy) needs. Your caloric needs depend upon a number of factors, including your age, gender, size, body composition, metabolic rate, and level of activity. For example, less active individuals will not require as many servings of bread, cereal, rice, and pasta, as active individuals such as SWAT officers and athletes.

The recommendations for daily servings are based upon the Food Guide Pyramid which was introduced by the U. S. Department of Agriculture and Department of Health and Human Services in 1992. Dr. Meir Stampfor, Professor in the Departments of Epidemiology and Nutrition, and Chair of the Department of Epidemiology at the Harvard School of Public Health, has suggested a new pyramid with different daily servings. While his proposal is interesting, it has yet to gain wide acceptance by the scientific and medical communities.

The type of food that you consume from these food groups is also important. Dr. Stampfor recommends that whole grains are preferred over refined grains because they still have their outer (bran) layer and inner (germ) layer. During the milling and production of refined grains (such as white flour), the healthful bran and germ layers are removed — and with them go many important nutrients, such as vitamins, minerals, and fiber. Eating too many refined-grain foods has been linked to diabetes as well as heart disease. The intake of red meat has been associated with increased risk for colon cancer. Also, within the category of meat, some types are especially bad for your overall health, including processed and preserved meats, such as bacon, sausage, and luncheon (salami-type and cured) meats. These meats are high in salt and preservatives and are generally higher in saturated fat. There is also considerable evidence that replacing red meat with nuts, legumes, chicken, and fish reduces the risk of developing heart disease. Dried beans, peas, and other legumes are very low in saturated fat, yet they are high in dietary fiber and are good sources of protein.

RECOMMENDED DIETARY ALLOWANCES

First published in 1943 and updated regularly, the Recommended Dietary Allowances (RDAs) were developed by the Food and Nutrition Board of the National Academy of Sciences/National Research Council. The RDAs are set by first determining the "floor" below which deficiency occurs and then the "ceiling" above which harm occurs. A margin of safety is included in the RDAs to meet the requirements of nearly all healthy people. In fact, the

VITAMIN (units)	Males				
	9-13	14-18	19-30	31-50	51-70
Vitamin A (mcg)	600	900	900	900	900
Vitamin D (mcg)	5	5	5	5	10
Vitamin E (mg)	11	15	15	15	15
Vitamin K (mcg)	60	75	120	120	120
Biotin (mcg)	20	25	30	30	30
Choline (mg)	375	550	550	550	550
Folate (mcg)	300	400	400	400	400
Niacin (mg)	12	16	16	16	16
Pantothenic Acid (mg)	4	5	5	5	5
Riboflavin (mg)	0.9	1.3	1.3	1.3	1.3
Thiamin (mg)	0.9	1.2	1.2	1.2	1.2
Pyridoxine (mg)	1.0	1.3	1.3	1.3	1.7
Cobalamin (mcg)	1.8	2.4	2.4	2.4	2.4
Vitamin C (mg)	45	75	90	90	90

VITAMIN (units)	Females					Pregnancy		Lactation	
	9-13	14-18	19-30	31-50	51-70	19-30	31-50	19-30	31-50
Vitamin A (mcg)	600	700	700	700	700	770	770	1,300	1,300
Vitamin D (mcg)	5	5	5	5	10	5	5	5	5
Vitamin E (mg)	11	15	15	15	15	15	15	19	19
Vitamin K (mcg)	60	75	90	90	90	90	90	90	90
Biotin (mcg)	20	25	30	30	30	30	30	35	35
Choline (mg)	375	400	425	425	425	450	450	550	550
Folate (mcg)	300	400	400	400	400	600	600	500	500
Niacin (mg)	12	14	14	14	14	18	18	17	17
Pantothenic Acid (mg)	4	5	5	5	5	6	6	7	7
Riboflavin (mg)	0.9	1.0	1.1	1.1	1.1	1.4	1.4	1.6	1.6
Thiamin (mg)	0.9	1.0	1.1	1.1	1.1	1.4	1.4	1.4	1.4
Pyridoxine (mg)	1.0	1.2	1.3	1.3	1.5	1.9	1.9	2.0	2.0
Cobalamin (mcg)	1.8	2.4	2.4	2.4	2.4	2.6	2.6	2.8	2.8
Vitamin C (mg)	45	65	75	75	75	85	85	120	120

TABLE 17.1: RECOMMENDED DIETARY ALLOWANCES (RDAs) OF SELECTED VITAMINS FOR MALES AND FEMALES AGED 19 - 70

MINERAL (units)	Males				
	9-13	14-18	19-30	31-50	51-70
Calcium (mg)	1,300	1,300	1,000	1,000	1,200
Chromium (mcg)	25	35	35	35	30
Copper (mcg)	700	890	900	900	900
Fluoride (mg)	2	3	4	4	4
Iodine (mcg)	120	150	150	150	150
Iron (mg)	8	11	8	8	8
Magnesium (mg)	240	410	400	420	420
Manganese (mg)	1.9	2.2	2.3	2.3	2.3
Molybdenum (mcg)	34	43	45	45	45
Phosphorus (mg)	1,250	1,250	700	700	700
Selenium (mcg)	40	55	55	55	55
Zinc (mg)	8	11	11	11	11

MINERAL (units)	Females					Pregnancy		Lactation	
	9-13	14-18	19-30	31-50	51-70	19-30	31-50	19-30	31-50
Calcium (mg)	1,300	1,300	1,000	1,000	1,200	1,000	1,000	1,000	1,000
Chromium (mcg)	21	24	25	25	20	30	30	45	45
Copper (mcg)	700	890	900	900	900	1,000	1,000	1,300	1,300
Fluoride (mg)	2	3	3	3	3	3	3	3	3
Iodine (mcg)	120	150	150	150	150	220	220	290	290
Iron (mg)	8	15	18	18	8	27	27	9	9
Magnesium (mg)	240	360	310	320	320	350	360	310	320
Manganese (mg)	1.6	1.6	1.8	1.8	1.8	2.0	2.0	2.6	2.6
Molybdenum (mcg)	34	43	45	45	45	50	50	50	50
Phosphorus (mg)	1,250	1,250	700	700	700	700	700	700	700
Selenium (mcg)	40	55	55	55	55	60	60	70	70
Zinc (mg)	8	9	8	8	8	11	11	12	12

TABLE 17.2: RECOMMENDED DIETARY ALLOWANCES (RDAs) OF SELECTED MINERALS FOR MALES AND FEMALES AGED 19 - 70

RDAs are designed to cover the biological needs of *97.5% of the population*. In other words, the RDAs exceed what most people require in order to meet the needs of those who have the highest requirements. So, the RDAs do not represent minimum standards. And failing to consume the recommended amounts does not necessarily indicate that you have a dietary deficiency. (The RDAs of selected vitamins and minerals for males and females aged 19 - 70 are given in Tables 17.1 and 17.2.)

CALORIC CONTRIBUTIONS

As mentioned previously, three macronutrients — carbohydrates, protein, and fat — furnish you with calories, albeit in different amounts. Carbohydrates and protein yield four calories per gram (cal/g). Fat is the most concentrated form of energy, containing nine cal/g. Armed with this information, you can determine the caloric contributions for each of the three energy-providing macronutrients in any food — provided that you know how many grams of each macronutrient are in a serving.

As an example, consider a snack food such as Fritos® Brand Original Corn Chips (Frito-Lay, Inc.). Examining the nutrition label reveals that a one-ounce serving of this product contains 15 grams of carbohydrates, 2 grams of protein, and 10 grams of fat. To find the exact number of calories that are supplied by each macronutrient, simply multiply its number of grams per serving by its corresponding energy yield. In this example, each serving of the food has 60 calories from carbohydrates [15 g x 4 cal/g], 8 calories from protein [2 g x 4 cal/g], and 90 calories from fat [10 g x 9 cal/g]. Therefore, this food has a total of 158 calories per serving (which is rounded up to 160 on the nutrition label). As you can see, this product has 50% more grams of carbohydrates than fat (15 compared to 10) — yet nearly 57% of the calories (90 of the 158) are furnished by fat. Moreover, consuming the entire contents of the 2.5-ounce bag will contribute 25 grams of fat — or 225 calories from fat — to your caloric budget.

Compare this to Baked Lays® Potato Crisps, another snack food by the same manufacturer. A one-ounce serving of this product has 23 grams of carbohydrates, 2 grams of protein, and 1.5 grams of fat. Each serving of this food contains 92 calories from carbohydrates [23 g x 4 cal/g], 8 calories from protein [2 g x 4 cal/g], and 13.5 calories from fat [1.5 g x 9 cal/g]. So, this food has a total of 113.5 calories per serving (which is rounded down to 110 on the nutrition label). This particular product, then, has more than 15 times as many grams of carbohydrates than fat (23 compared to 1.5) — and only 11.9% of the calories (13.5 of the 113.5) are supplied by fat. Furthermore, consuming 2.5 ounces of this product will add a mere 3.75 grams of fat — or 33.75 calories from fat — to your caloric budget.

Knowing the different caloric contributions of the macronutrients is also helpful in understanding information about fat content on the packaging of a product that could easily be misinterpreted. Case in point: A package that proclaims a product to be "99 percent fat free" means that it is 99% fat free by *weight*, not by *calories*. This is a very critical distinction. Placing one gram of fat into 99 grams of water forms a product that — in terms of weight — is "99 percent fat free." But since water has no calories, this particular "99 percent fat free" product would actually be — in terms of calories — 100% fat.

Although the preceding example was hypothetical, the fact is that this discrepancy actually occurs on the packaging of many products. Here are four illustrations of real products:

- A package of Hershey®'s Chocolate Drink (Hershey® Foods Corp.) states that it is "99% fat free." As would be expected, this leads many consumers to believe that a mere 1% of its calories come from fat. In reality, one serving of this product (eight ounces) has 129 calories of which 9 are from fat — meaning that it is 6.98% fat. (The numbers on the nutrition label are rounded up to 130 calories per serving with 10 calories from fat.)

- A package of Black Bear of the Black Forest™ Gourmet Cooked Ham (Black Bear Enterprises, Inc.) notes that it is "98% fat free." Naturally, this prompts many consumers to think that only 2% of its calories are derived from fat. In actuality, one serving of this product (two ounces) has 49 calories of which 9 are from fat — meaning that it is 18.37% fat. (The values on the nutrition label are rounded up to 50 calories per serving with 10 calories from fat.)

- A package of Black Bear of the Black Forest™ Barbeque Flavor Breast of Chicken (Black Bear Enterprises, Inc.) states that it is "96% fat free." This, of course, leads many consumers to conclude that only 4% of its calories come from fat. In reality, one serving of this product (two ounces) has 66 calories of which 18 are from fat — meaning that it is 27.27% fat. (The numbers on the nutrition label are rounded up to 70 calories per serving with 20 calories from fat.)

- A package of Oscar Mayer® Dinner Ham (Oscar Mayer Foods) notes that it is "96% fat free." Again, this leads many consumers to believe that only 4% of its calories are from fat. In actuality, one serving of this product (three ounces) has 83 calories of which 27 are from fat — meaning that it is 32.53% fat. (The values on the nutrition label are rounded down to 80 calories per serving with 25 calories from fat.)

While the percentages of fat calories for these four products are not terribly bad, it is certainly a far cry from how the percentages on the packages can be interpreted.

ESTIMATING YOUR CALORIC BUDGET

As previously mentioned, your caloric needs are determined by several factors such as your age, gender, size, body composition, metabolic rate, and level of activity. During a resting state, your caloric requirements can be established precisely by both direct and indirect calorimetry. Direct calorimetry measures the heat produced by the body in a small, insulated chamber; indirect calorimetry calculates the heat given off by the body based upon the amount of oxygen that is consumed and carbon dioxide that is produced. Unfortunately, both of these methods can be expensive and impractical for most people. For a quick and reasonably accurate estimate of your daily caloric needs, the U. S. Department of Agriculture suggests that you multiply your bodyweight by a number that corresponds to your approximate level of activity. Essentially, this number represents your energy requirements in calories per pound of bodyweight (cal/lb). For a woman, the values are 14 if she is sedentary, 18 if she is moderately active, and 22 if she is very active; for a man, the values are 16, 21, and 26, respectively. To illustrate, a 200-pound man who is very active requires approximately 5,200 calories per day (cal/day) to meet his energy needs [200 lb x 26 cal/lb]. Although this calculation has gray areas — such as the characterization of the term "moderately active" — it still results in a fairly good approximation.

Once you have estimated your caloric budget, you can determine how many of these calories should come from carbohydrates, protein, and fat. Using the previous example, someone who requires about 5,200 cal/day should consume roughly 845 grams of carbohydrates

[5,200 cal/day x 0.65 ÷ 4 cal/g], 195 grams of protein, [5,200 cal/day x 0.15 ÷ 4 cal/g], and 116 grams of fat [5,200 cal/day x 0.20 ÷ 9 cal/g]. Note that these numbers are based upon a diet that consists of 65% carbohydrates, 15% protein, and 20% fat.

PRE-ACTIVITY FOODS/FUELS

A meal that is consumed prior to an activity — whether it be some type of physical training or a competition — should accomplish several things such as removing your hunger pangs, readying your body with fuel for the upcoming activity, and relaxing your psychological state. There is no food that you can consume before an activity that will directly improve your performance. But there are certain foods that you can consume before an activity that can impair your performance and, for that reason, should be avoided. For instance, fats and meats are digested slowly, and should not be eaten prior to training or competing. Other foods to omit include those that are greasy, highly seasoned, and flatulent (gas-forming) along with any specific foods that you may personally find distressful to your digestive system. If anything, the choices for your pre-activity meal should be almost bland, yet appetizing enough so that you want to eat it.

Prior to an activity, you should also avoid eating foods that cause a sharp increase in your levels of blood glucose. Here is why: In response to highly elevated blood-glucose levels, your body increases its blood-insulin levels to maintain a stable internal environment (known as "homeostasis"). As a result of this biochemical balancing, your blood glucose is sharply reduced. This leads to hypoglycemia (or "low blood sugar") which decreases the availability of blood glucose as a fuel and causes you to feel severely fatigued. Although this condition is usually temporary, it remains an important consideration.

The idea, then, is to consume foods that elevate or maintain your blood glucose without triggering a dramatic response by blood insulin. At one time, it was thought that simple carbohydrates (sugars) increase blood glucose more rapidly than complex carbohydrates (starches). A more recent trend of thought has been to consider the Glycemic Index (GI) of a food. The GI dates back to 1981 when it was conceptualized by a group of scientists as a way to help determine which foods were best for people with diabetes. The GI is a system of quantifying the carbohydrates in foods based upon how they affect blood glucose. A value is assigned to a food that correlates to the magnitude of the increase in blood glucose. For instance, a food with a GI of 25 means that it elevates blood glucose to a level that is 25% as great as consuming the same amount of pure glucose. Incidentally, the GI is not related to portion size. So, the GI is the same whether you consume 10 grams of a particular food or 110 grams. (The number of calories, of course, would differ according to the size of the portion.)

Before an activity, consuming foods that are easy to digest and high in carbohydrates — specifically, those with a low GI is best. These foods help to keep your blood-glucose levels within a desirable range.

Do not simply assume that a sugary food raises blood glucose more than a starchy food. Indeed, honey (58) has a lower GI than a bagel (78) and, given these two options, would be a better choice for a pre-activity food. Foods with a relatively low GI include roasted peanuts (14), cherries (22), pure fructose (23), grapefruit (25), milk (34), pears (36), plain pizza (36), apples (38), apple juice (40), spaghetti (40), oranges (43), grapes (43), macaroni (46), oatmeal (55), and orange juice (55).

Water is perhaps the best liquid for you to drink before training or competing. Your fluid intake should be enough to guarantee optimal hydration during the activity. In addition, depending upon the duration of the activity, continual hydration may be necessary.

The timing of your pre-activity meal is also crucial. To ensure that your digestive process does not impair your performance, you should eat your pre-activity meal at least three hours prior to training or competing. In short, your pre-activity meal should include foods that are familiar to you and are well tolerated — preferably carbohydrates with a low GI.

POST-ACTIVITY FOODS/FLUIDS

After an intense activity, proper nutrition accelerates your recovery and better prepares you for your next physical challenge. The idea is to replenish your depleted glycogen stores and to expedite the recovery process as soon as possible after you train or compete.

Following an activity, consuming foods that are high in carbohydrates — specifically, those with a high GI is best. These foods will help to restore your muscle glycogen in the quickest fashion. Foods with a relatively high GI include bananas (60), table sugar (65), watermelon (72), waffles (76), rice cakes (77), Rice Krispies® (82), pretzels (83), corn flakes (84), white rice (88), baked potatoes (93), white bread (95), glucose (100), and buckwheat pancakes (103).

Because your appetite is suppressed immediately after intense efforts, initially consuming fluids that are high in carbohydrates rather than solid food or a meal may be more practical. Cold fluids also help to cool your body. Commercial sports drinks can be excellent post-activity fluids. In terms of recovery, there are two important components of a sports drink: carbohydrates and electrolytes (sodium and potassium). Since all sports drinks are different, you should read the nutrition labels to be sure of their exact contents. As an example, 12 ounces of Gatorade® Energy Drink (The Gatorade Co.) has 78 grams of carbohydrates which provide 312 calories; the same amount of Gatorade® Thirst Quencher contains 21 grams of carbohydrates which provide 84 calories. Both products have adequate amounts of electrolytes and a high GI but vastly different levels of carbohydrates and calories.

According to Nancy Clark, M.S., R.D. — an internationally known sports nutritionist and author — you should consume 0.5 grams of carbohydrates per pound of your bodyweight (g/lb) within two hours of completing an intense activity. This should be repeated again within the next two hours. For instance, the 200-pound individual in our continuing example needs to ingest about 100 grams of carbohydrates — or 400 calories of carbohydrates — within two hours after an intense activity and another 100 grams of carbohydrates during the next two hours [0.5 g/lb x 200 lb].

There is some evidence to suggest that combining the carbohydrates with a small amount of protein can expedite recovery by improving the rate at which the glycogen stores are replenished. However, simply increasing the quantity of post-activity carbohydrates appears to have the same results. Nonetheless, consuming a small amount of protein following an intense activity may aid in the repair of muscle tissue.

Finally, rehydrating after an activity is also important. You should consume about 16 ounces of water for every pound of bodyweight that you lose during physical activity.

NUTRITIONAL SUPPLEMENTS

Skillful promoters regularly tout nutritional supplements — including protein, vitamins, and minerals — with almost supernatural powers, having the ability to do practically everything imaginable. People are frequently tempted, teased, and seduced by their brilliant promises to "lose flab," "gain muscle," "get stronger," and "improve performance." Because of this, many individuals spend huge sums of money on a never-ending parade of nutritional supplements — or the more trendy buzzword "neutraceuticals." Unfortunately, most of the claims concerning nutritional supplements are purely speculative and anecdotal with little or no scientific or medical basis.

Protein Supplements

Many individuals think that they need to consume additional protein in order to increase their muscular strength and lean-body mass and, for that reason, take protein supplements. A number of studies have shown that the protein needs of active individuals may be higher than those of their inactive counterparts. But this need has been drastically exaggerated and overrated by health-food manufacturers and promoters.

The fact is that individuals who consume adequate calories generally obtain sufficient protein. Recall that your caloric requirements are determined by several factors including your size and level of activity. Larger, more active individuals require and consume more calories than the average person. With these additional calories come additional protein. In other words, the increased protein need of active individuals is met by an increased caloric intake. According to Dr. Gail Butterfield, a registered dietician and fellow of the American College of Sports Medicine, "I am not convinced that even with the initiation of a [strength-training] program that protein requirement is increased as long as [caloric] intake is increased."

For adults, the RDA for protein is 0.8 grams per kilogram of bodyweight per day (g/kg/day). Assuming a sufficient caloric intake, 1.2 - 2.0 g/kg/day (about 150 - 250% of the RDA for adults) is present in any mixed diet that contains 15% of its calories as protein. Recall the 200-pound man in the ongoing example who must consume 5,200 cal/day to maintain his bodyweight. If 15% of these calories came from protein, he would be receiving 780 calories from protein or 195 grams [780 cal ÷ 4 cal/g]. Based upon the RDA of 0.8 g/kg/day, this person would be consuming enough protein to meet the daily needs of a man who weighed a little more than 536 pounds [195 g/day ÷ 0.8g/kg/day x 2.2 lb/kg = 536.25 lb]. This amount of protein is actually about 2.15 g/kg/day — or about 2.5 times the RDA. And remember, this is without the individual making any effort to consume extra protein. So even if the requirement for active individuals may be greater, it is likely that they are already consuming enough protein to ensure proper levels of consumption. If you are concerned that you are not getting enough protein in your diet, you can obtain sufficient amounts by simply consuming more foods that are high in protein.

While on the subject, understand that an excessive intake of protein carries the potential for numerous unwanted side effects. An intake of protein that is in excess of your needs for growth, maintenance, and repair of tissue is either stored as fat or excreted in the urine. When excessive protein is urinated, it places a heavy burden on the liver and kidneys, and may damage those organs. An excessive intake of protein also increases the risk of dehydration which, in turn, increases the risk of developing a heat-related disorder such as heat exhaustion, heat stroke, or heat cramps. Other potential side effects from a high intake of protein include an excessive loss of calcium in the urine, diarrhea, cramps, and gastrointestinal upset.

Vitamin and Mineral Supplements

Many individuals believe that their foods do not supply sufficient micronutrients and, therefore, they take vitamin and mineral supplements. There is no unbiased, scientific evidence to suggest that those who consume a balanced diet need vitamin and mineral supplementation in excess of the RDA; likewise, there is no unbiased, scientific evidence to suggest that an increased consumption of vitamins and minerals improves performance. Recall that active individuals typically require and consume more calories than the average person. With these additional calories come additional vitamins and minerals. In truth, even a marginal diet provides adequate vitamins and minerals. Understand, too, that your liver is a storehouse for vitamins and minerals. This organ can quickly compensate for a temporary dietary shortfall by releasing its stored nutrients as needed and then replenishing its reservoirs when the opportunity arises.

That being said, vitamin and mineral supplements may be needed by those who do not consume adequate diets. For example, a multi-vitamin and -mineral supplement may be warranted for vegetarians, and women who are pregnant or lactating. Supplementation may also be appropriate for athletes who restrict their caloric intake in order to reach a certain weight class to compete in activities such as competitive weightlifting and combat sports (that is, boxing, judo, wrestling, etc.). And since women are at an increased risk for iron and calcium deficiency, supplementation may be justified for those two minerals.

Whenever possible, getting vitamins and minerals from foods rather than pills is better because the high concentration of these micronutrients in pill form may interfere with the absorption of some other nutrients. Also keep in mind that supplements containing more than 150% of the RDA are for disease treatment and should never be used unless a competent health professional has diagnosed their need. Professional advice concerning nutritional supplementation should be sought from a registered dietitian (R.D.) or a sports nutritionist.

When consumed in reasonable doses, vitamins and minerals pose no health or safety risks. The American Dietetic Association — the largest and most established organization that is devoted to both practice and research in nutrition — reports that high doses of vitamins and minerals pose a risk of toxicity that can create adverse side effects and may lead to serious medical complications. When taken in megadoses — any dose greater than 10 times the RDA — the vitamins that are in excess of those needed to saturate the enzyme systems function as free-floating drugs instead of receptor-bound nutrients. Like all drugs, high doses of vitamins and minerals have the potential for adverse side effects.

Of greatest concern is excessive intake of the fat-soluble vitamins — particularly vitamins A and D — which can be extremely toxic and may have undesirable side effects. Consuming large doses of vitamin A can result in decalcification of the bones (resulting in fragile bones), an increased susceptibility to disease, enlargements of the liver and the spleen, muscle and joint soreness, vomiting, cessation of menstruation (amenorrhea), stunted growth, loss of appetite, loss of hair, irritability, double vision, skin rashes, headaches, nausea, drowsiness, and diarrhea. Consuming large doses of vitamin D can result in nausea, loss of hair, loss of weight, vomiting, decalcification of the bones (resulting in fragile bones), drowsiness, diarrhea, headaches, hypertension, elevated cholesterol, and loss of appetite.

Excess amounts of the B vitamins and vitamin C are generally excreted in the urine (which prompts many authorities to suggest that supplementation with water-soluble vitamins leaves a person with nothing more than expensive urine). This action places an inordinate amount of stress on the liver and kidneys. Though mainly excreted, excess amounts of the water-soluble vitamins may still have toxic effects. For example, megadoses of vitamin C can be harmful while in the body. Potential side effects from an excessive intake of vitamin C include kidney stones, diarrhea, bladder irritation, intestinal problems, destruction of red blood cells, nausea, stomach cramps, an increase in plasma cholesterol, ulceration of the gastric wall, leaching of calcium from the bones, and gout.

FOOD FOR THOUGHT

As long as you consume a variety of foods that provide adequate calories and nutrients, there is no need to take nutritional supplements unless you have a specific health-related problem diagnosed by a medical professional. Nutritional supplements are not currently regulated by the Food and Drug Administration (FDA). Many do not contain ingredients listed or contain "extra" ingredients not listed. In addition, the combination of ingredients as well as additives in many nutritional supplements can even be harmful and outweigh their potential benefits.

Investing your money in high-quality foods instead of purchasing expensive nutritional supplements will allow you to achieve greater success in maximizing your physical potential in a much safer manner. Remember, there are no shortcuts on the road to proper nutrition.

Chapter 18
Weight Management

Managing your bodyweight consists of gaining, losing, or maintaining your weight. Consider it as a simple matter of arithmetic, similar to managing your savings account. If you deposit (consume) more calories than you withdraw (expend), you have produced a caloric profit and will gain weight; if you withdraw (expend) more calories than you deposit (consume), you have produced a caloric deficit and will lose weight; and lastly, if you deposit (consume) the same amount of calories that you withdraw (expend), you have produced a caloric balance and you will not affect any change in your bodyweight.

A CLOSER LOOK

Despite its conceptual simplicity, a closer look should be taken at weight management. Specifically, an examination of gaining and losing weight in greater detail is an important compliment to following proper nutritional guidelines.

Gaining Weight

Some SWAT officers will be healthier — and more effective — if they increase their bodyweight. The potential to gain weight is determined by a number of factors, the most important of which is a person's inherited characteristics. An individual whose ancestors had ectomorphic tendencies — that is, lean features with little in the way of muscular size — has the genetic destiny for that type of physique. This does not mean that a person with those inherited characteristics — who would be categorized as an "ectomorph" — is incapable of gaining weight. But it will be difficult for those who have a high degree of ectomorphy to achieve a significant increase in their bodyweight.

The primary goal of gaining weight is to increase lean-body (or muscle) mass. One pound of muscle has about 2,500 calories. Therefore, if you consume 250 calories per day (cal/day) above your caloric budget — a 250-calorie profit — it will take you 10 days to gain one pound of lean-body mass [2,500 cal ÷ 250 cal/day = 10 days]. So if a 200-pound man who is very active requires 5,200 cal/day to maintain his bodyweight [200 lb x 26 cal/lb], he must consume 5,450 cal/day — 250 calories above his need — to gain one pound of lean-body mass in 10 days. Keep in mind that this estimate must be recalculated on a regular basis to account for changes in bodyweight. After increasing his bodyweight to 201 pounds, for example, he will now require 5,226 cal/day to meet his energy needs [201 lb x 26 cal/lb]. In order to gain another pound of lean-body mass in 10 days, he must increase his caloric consumption to 5,476 cal/day — 250 calories above his need.

The daily caloric profit should not be more than about 350 - 700 calories above the normal daily needs. If the weight gain is more than about 1% of your bodyweight per week, it is likely that some excess calories will be stored in the form of fat. However, if the weight gain is less than about 1% of your bodyweight per week and is the result of a demanding strength-training program in conjunction with a balanced nutritional intake, then it will probably be in the form of increased lean-body mass.

Gaining weight for ectomorphic individuals requires total nutritional dedication. Additional calories must be consumed daily on a regular basis until the desired gain in weight is achieved. The best way for the body to absorb food is when it is divided into several regular-sized meals intermingled with a few snacks. The body does not absorb one or two large meals as well — most of these calories are simply jammed through the digestive system. As a matter of fact, when consuming a large number of calories at one time, some of them will be diverted to fat deposits because of the sudden demand on the metabolic pathways. (This has been referred to as "nutrient overload.")

Besides what has been discussed, the following are additional tips for gaining weight:

- Set short-term goals that are realistic
- Keep a food/activity log or diary
- Eat at least three meals per day (five to six are preferable)
- Eat at least three nutritious snacks per day
- Consume foods that are high in calories (but not high in fat)
- Eat dense fruit (such as bananas, pineapples, and raisins)
- Eat dense vegetables (such as peas, corn, and carrots)
- Drink juice and milk
- Increase the size of portions

Losing Weight

Some SWAT officers will be healthier — and more effective — if they decrease their bodyweight. Similar to gaining weight, the potential to lose weight is primarily determined by a person's inherited characteristics. An individual whose ancestors had endomorphic tendencies — that is, round features with little in the way of muscular definition — has the genetic destiny for that type of physique. This does not mean that a person with those inherited characteristics — who would be categorized as an "endomorph" — is incapable of losing weight. But it will be difficult for those who have a high degree of endomorphy to achieve a significant decrease in their bodyweight.

Understand that the numbers on height/weight charts and bathroom scales are poor indicators of whether or not someone should lose weight. The need for weight loss should be determined by body composition rather than bodyweight, especially in the case of an active individual. For the most part, active individuals tend to be larger and have more lean-body mass than the general population. To illustrate, think about two men who stand five feet, nine inches tall and weigh 200 pounds. If you consider their height and weight without regard for their body composition, you might conclude that they are both a bit overweight. But what if one man had 15% body fat and the other had 30% body fat? If this was the case, then only one man might need to lose weight — the one with the higher percentage of body fat. As such, determining the need to lose weight should be based upon body composition.

A variety of methods can be used to measure body composition such as air displacement plethysmography (ADP), bioelectrical impedance analysis (BIA), computerized tomography (CT), dual energy x-ray absorptiometry (DEXA), hydrostatic (underwater) weighing, and near infrared reactance. But perhaps the most popular method of assessing body composition is to use skinfold calipers. In general, this is considered to be the most practical and least expensive method of assessment without sacrificing much in the way of accuracy (assuming that the tester is reasonably skilled and the formula is reliable). For the most part, active individuals tend to have percentages of body fat that are lower than their inactive counterparts. In most sports, a low percentage of body fat is desirable; in some sports, however, a high percentage of body fat is actually advantageous. For instance, long-distance swimmers obtain increased buoyancy and thermal insulation from higher levels of body fat.

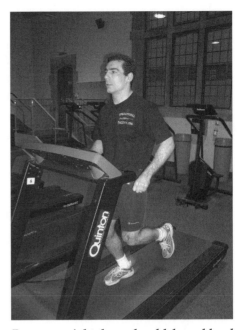

Proper weight loss should be a blend of consuming less calories and expending more calories.

The primary goal of losing weight is to decrease body fat. One pound of fat has about 3,500 calories. As such, if you consume 250 cal/day below your caloric budget — a 250-calorie deficit — it will take you 14 days to lose one pound of fat [3,500 cal ÷ 250 cal/day = 14 days]. So if the 200-pound man in the ongoing example requires 5,200 cal/day to maintain his bodyweight, he must consume 4,950 cal/day — 250 calories below his need — to lose one pound of fat in 14 days. Remember that this estimate must be recalculated on a regular basis to account for changes in bodyweight. After decreasing his bodyweight to 199 pounds, for example, he will now require 5,174 cal/day to meet his energy needs [199 lb x 26 cal/lb]. In order to lose another pound of fat in 14 days, he must decrease his caloric consumption to 4,924 cal/day — 250 calories below his need.

Actually, a caloric deficit can be achieved by decreasing caloric consumption, increasing caloric expenditure (through additional activity), or a combination of the two. In fact, proper weight loss should be a blend of consuming less calories and expending more calories.

The daily caloric deficit should not be more than about 500 - 1000 calories below the normal daily needs. If the weight loss is more than about 1% of your bodyweight per week, it is likely that some of this weight reduction will be the result of decreased lean-body mass and/

or water rather than body fat. However, if the weight loss is less than about 1% of your bodyweight per week and is the result of a rigorous training program in conjunction with a reduced caloric intake, then it will probably be in the form of decreased body fat.

Losing weight must be a carefully planned activity. Skipping meals — or all-out starvation — is not a desirable method of weight loss, since sufficient calories are still needed to fuel an active lifestyle. Oddly enough, losing weight should be done in a fashion similar to that of gaining weight: Frequent — but smaller — meals spread out over the course of the day will suppress the appetite. Drinking plenty of water before, during, and after meals is also a good idea. This creates a feeling of fullness without providing any calories.

Besides what has been discussed, the following are additional tips for losing weight:

- Set short-term goals that are realistic
- Keep a food/activity log or diary
- Read the nutrition labels
- Eat a moderate/reduced amount of sugars
- Add water to juice drinks to further reduce sugar intake
- Eat foods that are low in fat
- Reduce the intake of saturated fats
- Eat more fruits and vegetables
- Chew your food slowly
- Decrease the size of portions
- Eat five to six smaller meals throughout the day
- Refrain from eating before bedtime, especially foods high in fats and complex carbohydrates such as pasta, rice, and bread.

WEIGHT-LOSS SUPPLEMENTS

Ephedra

Ephedra, with its principal active ingredient — "ephedrine" — is an over-the-counter herbal stimulant derived from the Chinese herbal Ma Huang. It is found in many cold and flu medications as well as supplements that are marketed for weight loss and improved performance. Ephedrine is an amphetamine-like compound that has many adverse side effects to include heart arrhythmia, elevated blood pressure, seizures and strokes, dizziness, and headaches. In addition, it can interfere with the body's ability to combat and regulate heat causing the potential for dehydration.

Since the mid-90s, the Food and Drug Administration has received *more than 800 reports* of adverse side effects from ephedrine — including *at least 50 deaths*. In 2001, the National Football League banned the use of supplements that contain ephedrine. In addition, the United States Olympic Committee and the National Collegiate Athletic Association prohibit the use of ephedrine. Taking ephedrine as a performance-enhancing or weight-loss supplement is not recommended.

Aristolochic Acid

The Food and Drug Administration is advising consumers to immediately discontinue use of any botanical products containing aristolochic acid. These products may have been sold as "traditional medicines" or as ingredients in dietary supplements. Aristolochic acid is found primarily in the plant *Aristolochia*, but may also be present in other botanicals. Consumption of products containing aristolochic acid has been associated with permanent kidney damage, sometimes resulting in kidney failure that has required kidney dialysis or kidney transplantation. In addition, some patients have developed certain types of cancers, most often occurring in the urinary tract.

Chaso

In August 2002, the FDA issued an alert regarding the Chinese weight-loss products Chaso (Jianfei) Diet Capsules and Chaso Genpi because they pose a potential public health risk. Several people in Japan became ill and some have died after consuming these diet products. Dr. Lester M. Crawford, FDA Deputy Commissioner, announced, "The FDA is taking this action as a precautionary measure to help assure that people are not exposed to this potentially dangerous product." The deaths in Japan linked to these Chinese weight-loss products may have resulted from the presence of such active drug ingredients as fenfluramine in the capsules.

These are only a few examples of potentially harmful weight-loss supplements on the market. The best way to lose fat is to restrict caloric consumption and exercise more frequently.

LOSING FAT: HIGH INTENSITY OR LOW INTENSITY?

In terms of weight management, there is often a debate over which level of intensity (or effort) is the most effective for losing fat. Specifically, the issue revolves around whether high-intensity activity is better for fat loss than low-intensity activity.

Energy Sources

During physical training, there are three possible sources of energy (or fuel) available for you to use: carbohydrates, fat, and protein. Of these three energy sources, your body does not like to use protein as a fuel. In fact, protein is used as a last resort. Remember, protein is located in your muscles and if you are in a situation where you must rely on it as an energy source, then you are literally cannibalizing yourself. So, that leaves you with carbohydrates and fat as your main energy sources.

Exactly which energy source is preferred during physical training is based upon the level of intensity that is required. Training with a relatively high level of intensity uses a greater percentage of carbohydrates as an energy source; training with relatively low level of intensity uses a greater percentage of fat as an energy source. (Carbohydrates are a more efficient source of energy. However, fat is used as an energy source because your body does not need to be efficient at lower levels of intensity.)

This is not to say that carbohydrates and fat are the sole sources of energy during activities of high and low intensity. Rather, they are both used, but to different degrees: During high-intensity activity, carbohydrates are the principal energy source, but fat is also used; during low-intensity activity, fat is the principal energy source, but carbohydrates are also used.

These physiological facts have led to the mistaken belief that low-intensity (or "fat-burning") activity is better than high-intensity (or "carbohydrate-burning") activity when it comes to "burning" fat as well as expending calories and losing weight. Furthermore, this misconception has spawned the hyped-up notion that people should train within their "fat-burning zones."

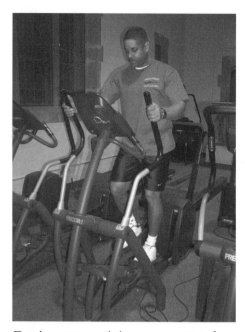

During any activity, your rate of caloric expenditure is directly related to your intensity of effort — the higher your intensity, the greater your rate of caloric expenditure.

Caloric Expenditure

The concept of training with a low level of intensity in order to mobilize and selectively utilize a higher percentage of fat may sound logical, but it does not hold up mathematically and has never been verified in a laboratory setting. In truth, even though a greater *percentage* of fat calories are used during low-intensity activity, a greater *number* of fat calories (and total calories) are used during high-intensity activity.

During any activity, your rate of caloric expenditure is directly related to your intensity of effort — the higher your intensity, the greater your rate of caloric expenditure. In the case of running, for example, your intensity is directly associated with your speed: The faster you run, the greater the rate of caloric expenditure. The time of your activity is also a factor: The longer you perform a given activity, the greater the total caloric expenditure.

As noted in Chapter 5, the American College of Sports Medicine offers equations for determining oxygen consumption and caloric expenditure during walking (an activity of relatively low intensity) and running (an activity of relatively high intensity). Based upon these equations, a 200-pound man who walks three miles in 60 minutes on a level surface will utilize roughly 5.25 calories per minute (cal/min). Over the course of his 60-minute walk, his total caloric usage would be about 315 calories [5.25 cal/min x 60 min]. If that same individual ran those three miles in 30 minutes on a level surface, he would use about 16.22 cal/min. (Note the higher rate of caloric expenditure.) During his 30-minute effort, he would have used about 487 total calories [16.22 cal/min x 30 min]. So, training with a higher level of intensity utilized significantly more calories than training with a lower level of intensity [487 cal compared to 315 cal]. This is true despite the fact that the activity of lower intensity was performed for twice as long as the activity of higher intensity [60 min compared to 30 min].

These calculations have been corroborated by research performed in the laboratory. In one study, a group of subjects walked on a treadmill at an average speed of 3.8 miles per hour (mph) for 30 minutes. In this instance, the subjects used an average of about 8 cal/min for a total caloric expenditure of 240 calories [8 cal/min x 30 min]. Of these 240 calories, 59% [144 cal] were from carbohydrates and 41% [96 cal] were from fat. As part of the study, the same group also ran on a treadmill at an average speed of 6.5 mph for 30 minutes. At this relatively higher level of intensity, the subjects used an average of about 15 cal/min for a total caloric expenditure of 450 calories [15 cal/min x 30 min]. Of these 450 calories, 76% [342 cal] were from carbohydrates and 24% [108 cal] were from fat. In other words, training with a higher level of intensity resulted in a greater total caloric expenditure than training with a lower level of intensity [450 cal compared to 240 cal] and also used a greater number of calories from fat in the same length of time [108 cal compared to 96 cal]. Additional studies have also demonstrated that more calories are expended when running a given distance than walking the same distance.

Appropriate Intensity

The intent behind advocating low-intensity activity of long duration is to enhance safety and improve compliance in the non-athletic population. However, low-intensity activity is not more effective for fat loss — or weight loss — than high-intensity activity. But suppose that low-intensity activity was better for losing fat and weight. Since activities of lowest intensity require the greatest percentage of fat as the energy source, this would suggest that the best activity for fat/weight loss would be sleeping.

In terms of losing weight, more calories must be expended than consumed in order to produce a caloric deficit. Whether you use carbohydrates or fat to produce this caloric shortfall is immaterial. A caloric deficit created by the selective use of fat as an energy source does not necessarily translate into greater fat loss compared to an equal caloric deficit created by the use of carbohydrate as an energy source. The main determinant of fat and weight loss is *calories*, not *composition*.

Researchers who perform studies and review the scientific literature in the area of exercise and weight management generally agree that it probably does not matter whether you use fat or carbohydrates while training in order to lose weight. Finally, it is unlikely that low-intensity activity would elevate your heart rate enough to improve your level of aerobic fitness.

So regardless of the type of physical training, you should use the highest possible level of effort. Make hard work a standard part of your athletic lifestyle and consider weight-management guidelines while implementing a proper nutritional program.

Chapter 19
Q & A

This chapter examines a number of frequently asked questions concerning the performance of your physical training. No doubt, many of you have the same or similar questions.

Q: What precautions should I take when training in hot, humid conditions?

A: The importance of safeguarding your body against heat-related injuries cannot be over-emphasized. Individuals who are overweight and/or unaccustomed to laboring in the heat are most susceptible to thermal disorders which include heat exhaustion, heat stroke, and heat cramps.

Under resting conditions, your core temperature is about 98.6 degrees Fahrenheit (or 37 degrees Celsius), and there is a balance between heat production and heat loss. When training, your core temperature increases and triggers several heat-loss mechanisms. Here, the primary mechanism for heat loss is the evaporation of sweat. Your blood carries internal body heat to the surface of your skin where sweat is secreted from an estimated 2.5 million sweat glands and evaporation occurs. As the sweat evaporates, it cools your skin; this, in turn, cools your blood. The cooled blood then returns to the warmer core and the cycle is repeated. This physiological process cools your internal body. (To illustrate the effects of evaporation, wet your finger and blow on it. You will quickly note a cooling sensation as the evaporative process withdraws heat from your skin.)

People constantly perspire. In cool, dry weather a relatively small amount of sweat is produced and the rate of evaporation can keep pace with the rate of perspiration. In this case, your skin is dry to the touch and you are not aware that you are sweating — even though this alone may involve about a quart of water per day. Unfortunately, this cooling mechanism does not work well when the heat and/or humidity is high. When the humidity is high, there is a large amount of moisture already in the air. At higher levels of humidity, the evaporation of your sweat is hindered because the air is highly saturated with water vapor and, as a result, there is little or no place for any extra moisture to go. This situation causes the body to overheat and may result in a heat-related injury. In fact, a temperature of only 80 degrees Fahrenheit becomes dangerous if the humidity reaches 90%.

You should gradually acclimatize to high heat and humidity. Initially, this may necessitate training outdoors during the cooler parts of the day such as the early morning and late evening. During anaerobic training, you should also adjust the length of your recovery intervals according to the environmental conditions. Most adverse reactions to heat and humidity occur during the first few days of training outdoors. As you adapt to hot, humid conditions, you will be able to train with greater levels of intensity while maintaining a safe body temperature. Another option is to move your physical training indoors to air-conditioned surroundings (if such an environment is readily available).

Rehydrating regularly with cold liquids as needed is important. You should measure your bodyweight each day before and after training. In this way, you can monitor your water loss to determine if adequate rehydration is taking place. You should consume about 16 ounces of water for every pound of bodyweight that you lose while training. Warning: If you deny yourself liquids under adverse conditions, you are putting yourself at risk for a heat disorder.

To promote heat loss, you should wear loose clothing that is lightweight and light-colored, or clothing made with microfibers to allow for the evaporation of sweat and the cooling of your body. (Lighter colors reflect the sun's rays; darker colors absorb them.) Under no circumstances should you train in rubberized clothing or a "sauna suit." Training with your body covered in this manner can be lethal since these garments trap perspiration and cause you to overheat rapidly.

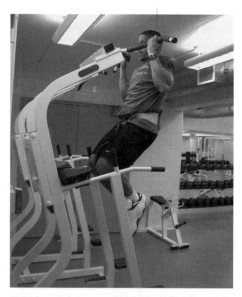

During intense activity, pain throughout a muscle is normal and indicates a high degree of effort; during intense activity, pain throughout a joint is abnormal and indicates a possible orthopedic problem.

Q: Is the adage "No pain, no gain" really true?

A: To a degree, yes. The most critical factor in achieving optimal results from physical training is your level of intensity (or effort). As an exercise or activity becomes more intense, it also becomes more uncomfortable . . . and more painful. The discomfort and pain are related to the high concentration of lactic acid in your blood. (The effects of lactic-acid accumulation are described in Chapter 4.) However, you must differentiate between muscular pain and orthopedic pain. During intense activity, pain throughout a muscle is normal and indicates a high degree of effort; during intense activity, pain throughout a joint is abnormal and indicates a possible orthopedic problem.

Q: How do I know if I am overtraining?

A: Overtraining is a result of overstressing your body. Generally speaking, the excessive stress is produced by excessive activity. Symptoms of overtraining include chronic fatigue, appetite disorders, insomnia, depression, anger, substantial weight loss or gain, prolonged muscular soreness, anemia, and an elevated resting heart rate.

The most obvious indicator of overtraining, however, is a lack of progress in your physical training. You can identify a lack of progress by keeping accurate records of your performances.

The best cure for overtraining is to obtain sufficient rest in order to allow your body the opportunity to recover. This may necessitate reducing the volume of activity that you perform (in terms of workouts, exercises, and/or sets). Taking some time off periodically from your physical training also helps to avoid overtraining.

Q: When I train, why do I sometimes wheeze and cough, and have a shortness of breath?

A: You may have "exercise-induced asthma" (EIA). Estimates show that as many as 80% of all asthmatic people experience this condition. As the name suggests, EIA is initiated by exercise (or physical training). This condition can occur within a few minutes before an activity or a few hours after an activity. Several factors contribute to EIA including the temperature and humidity of the air that you inhale. Breathing cold, dry air while training increases the likelihood of EIA. Certain intensities and durations of activity also contribute to EIA: The asthmatic attacks are more likely during efforts that are intense or prolonged.

Anyone suffering from EIA should seek the advice of a physician (who may prescribe medication as a preventive measure). If you must train outdoors in cold weather, you should cover your mouth with a scarf or facemask. Swimming is an excellent activity for those who have EIA because the air above the pool is warm and contains moisture. Finally, those suffering from EIA should adjust their levels of intensity and duration of their efforts accordingly.

Q: How can I change my body type?

A: Unfortunately, you cannot change your body type — or somatotype — to any significant degree. In the 1940s, Dr. William H. Sheldon — a physician and psychologist — proposed that there are three main body types: endomorph, mesomorph, and ectomorph. Endomorphs are characterized by softness and round physiques. They have high percentages of body fat and very little muscle tone. A sumo wrestler is a classic example of an endomorph. Mesomorphs are typified by heavily muscled physiques. They have athletic builds with broad shoulders, large chests, and slender waists. A competitive bodybuilder is a classic example of a mesomorph. Finally, ectomorphs are characterized by long limbs, leanness, and slender physiques. They have low percentages of body fat, but also little in the way of muscular size. A successful long-distance runner is a classic example of an ectomorph.

Since almost everyone has some degree of each component, various rating systems were developed in which an individual is given a "score" in each of the three areas. The system developed by Dr. Sheldon introduced a scale that ranged from 1 to 7, to designate the degree of each of the three components with 1 being the least amount and 7 being the greatest. In his system, a somatotype of 7-1-1 indicates extreme endomorphy (fatness), 1-7-1 extreme mesomorphy (muscularity), and 1-1-7 extreme ectomorphy (leanness). Relatively few people can be classified as being purely one body type or another. Although people have a tendency toward one body type, most are a combination of two types. For example, an individual who has a somatotype of 1-4-4 would have a slender physique, a low percentage of body fat, and a high degree of muscular development and be characterized as an ecto-mesomorph; an individual who has a somatotype of 4-4-1 would have a round physique, a high percentage of body fat, and a high degree of muscular development and be characterized as an endomesomorph.

Incidentally, a number of studies have related body type to physical performance. As you might suspect, the body type that has the greatest genetic potential for developing muscular size and strength is the mesomorph. In fact, one study concluded that world-class bodybuilders were the "prototype of pure extreme mesomorphs."

Q: How can I avoid getting shin splints?

A: "Shin splints" is a general term used to describe a variety of painful conditions on the anterior (front) part of the lower leg. The pain — often typified as a dull ache — is usually located on the lower two-thirds of the tibia (the shin bone), and is felt during dorsi flexion and plantar flexion.

Shin splints are considered to be an overuse injury and, for the most part, have two main causes. In some cases, there is a strength imbalance between the muscles of the lower leg. Specifically, the dorsi flexors on the anterior part of the lower leg are weaker than the calf muscles on the posterior part of the lower leg. In effect, the stronger calf muscles overpower the weaker dorsi flexors and produce an injury. This situation can be remedied by doing two things: performing exercises for your dorsi flexors and reducing exercises for your calves.

Shin splints can also result from high-impact forces that exceed the structural integrity of the lower leg. There are a number of ways to lessen this orthopedic stress. You should wear proper shoes that provide adequate support and shock-absorbing qualities. Decreasing the number of weightbearing activities that you perform and increasing the non-weightbearing ones is also important. If possible, you should perform weightbearing activities on softer, more yielding surfaces. If you have shin splints, you can alleviate the pain and swelling by applying ice to the inflamed area. The ice treatment should last about 20 minutes and be done as soon as possible after you have completed your physical training.

Q: Is there another formula for estimating an age-predicted maximum heart rate?

A: Yes. Researchers at the University of Colorado authored a study that was published in 2001, in which they determined new equations for estimating an individual's age-predicted maximum heart rate. The researchers collected data from 351 studies that involved 492 groups and 18,712 subjects. Based upon these data, they calculated an equation of 208 – (0.7 x age). This equation was cross-validated in a well-controlled, laboratory-based study that involved

AGE-PREDICTED MAXIMUM HEART RATE (bpm)			
AGE	**220 – age**	**208 – (0.7 x age)**	**209 – (0.7 x age)**
30	190.0	187.0	188.0
35	185.0	183.5	184.5
40	180.0	180.0	181.0
45	175.0	176.5	177.5
50	170.0	173.0	174.0
55	165.0	169.5	170.5

TABLE 19.1: ESTIMATES FOR AGE-PREDICTED MAXIMUM HEART RATES USING THREE EQUATIONS

514 subjects. In this study, they calculated an equation of 209 – (0.7 x age).

When comparing these equations to that which has been commonly used (220 – age), however, there is actually very little difference between them. When estimating the age-predicted maximum heart rate for a 40-year-old individual, for example, the three equations only differ by one beat per minute (which becomes an even smaller difference when multiplied by 60 - 90% to determine a heart-rate training zone). Table 19.1 gives estimates for age-predicted maximum heart rates for individuals of six different ages using the three equations.

Q: Can I really improve my muscular strength and aerobic fitness by doing strength training and aerobic training on the same day?

A: Absolutely. One study randomly assigned 30 subjects to one of three groups: a group that did strength training, a group that did aerobic training, and a group that did strength training and aerobic training. The latter group performed the same protocols as the former two groups, but their strength training and aerobic training were done in the same workout. All groups trained three times per week for 10 weeks. At the end of the training period, the subjects that did strength training and aerobic training in the same workout had significant increases in their muscular strength and aerobic fitness. Furthermore, their increases in muscular strength were comparable to the subjects who only did strength training and their increases in aerobic fitness were comparable to the subjects who only did aerobic training.

Essentially, you have two options for scheduling your strength training and aerobic (or anaerobic) training: You can perform both activities on the same day or on alternate days. The advantage of doing both activities on the same day is that it permits a more complete recovery. If strength training is performed on one day and aerobic (or anaerobic) training the next, your muscles will be constantly stressed and your body may not have adequate time to recover properly.

From a psychological standpoint, it may also be very difficult for you to perform intense training a number of days in a row with a high degree of enthusiasm. Therefore, the recommended way of scheduling your strength training and aerobic (or anaerobic) training is to do both activities on the same day. You can do the activities on alternate days, however, if you prefer or do not have enough time available to perform both activities on the same day.

Q: Is there a certain way that I should breathe when I lift weights?

A: Yes. Breathing properly when you perform a strenuous activity such as strength training is important — especially during intense efforts. Holding your breath during exertion creates an elevated pressure in your abdominal and thoracic cavities which is referred to as the "Valsalva maneuver." The elevated pressure interferes with the return of blood to your heart. This may deprive your brain of blood and can cause you to lose consciousness.

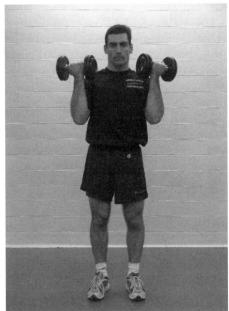

To emphasize correct breathing, exhale when you raise the resistance and inhale when you lower it.

To emphasize correct breathing, exhale when you raise the resistance and inhale when you lower it. Or simply remember EOE — Exhale On Effort. Inhaling and exhaling naturally usually results in correct breathing.

Q: If I stop lifting weights will my muscles turn to fat?

A: No. A common misconception is that muscle can turn into fat. In truth, muscle cannot be changed into fat — or vice versa — any more than gold can be changed into lead. Your muscle tissue consists of special contractile proteins that allow movement to occur. Muscle tissue is about 70% water, 22% protein, and 7% fat. (The remaining 1% or so includes inorganic salts such as calcium, potassium, and sodium.)

Conversely, your fatty (or adipose) tissue is composed of spherical cells that are specifically designed to store fat. Fatty tissue is about 22% water, 6% protein, and 72% fat. Since muscle and fat are two different and distinct types of biological tissue, a muscle cannot turn into fat if you stop lifting weights. Similarly, lifting weights — or doing any other type of physical training — will not change your fat into muscle. The fact is that muscles hypertrophy (or become larger) from physical activity and muscles atrophy (or become smaller) from physical inactivity.

Q: Will lifting weights make women less flexible and more bulky?

A: Not necessarily. One of the biggest misconceptions in strength training is the belief that women — and men, for that matter — who lift weights will lose flexibility. If anything, performing repetitions throughout a full range of motion against a resistance will maintain or even improve flexibility. Women — and men — who have residual fears about becoming less flexible can perform a series of flexibility movements both before and after their strength training. As an added measure, they can also stretch the muscles that were involved immediately after an exercise is completed. (Flexibility training is discussed in great detail in Chapter 3.)

Another popular misconception in strength training is the belief that women will develop large, unsightly muscles. Understand that increases in muscular strength are often accompanied by increases in muscular size. While this is true for both men and women, increases in muscular size are much less pronounced in women. Since the early 1960s, research has shown that most women can achieve significant improvements in their muscular strength without concomitant gains in their muscular size. One researcher, for example, found that a group of 47 women increased their strength in the leg press by nearly 30% after 10 weeks of training yet the largest increase in muscular size that was experienced by any of them was *less than one-quarter inch*. Clearly, strength training does not lead to excessive muscular bulk in the majority of women.

There are several physiological reasons that prevent or minimize the possibility that women will significantly increase the size of their muscles. First, most women are genetically bound by an unfavorable and unchangeable ratio of muscle to tendon (that is, short muscle bellies coupled with long tendinous attachments). In addition, most women have relatively low levels of serum testosterone. The low levels of this growth-promoting hormone restrict the degree to which women can increase their muscular size.

A final physiological factor that prevents or minimizes the possibility that women will significantly increase their muscular size is their percentage of body fat. Quite simply, women tend to inherit higher percentages of body fat than men. For example, the average 18- to 22-

year-old woman is about 22 - 26% body fat, whereas the average man of similar age is about 12 - 16%. The higher the percentage of body fat, the lower the percentage of muscle mass. This extra body fat also tends to soften or mask the effects of strength training. Women who possess very little body fat appear to be more muscular than they actually are because their muscles are more visible. Likewise, the appearance of more muscle mass may not be the result of muscular hypertrophy. Rather, a decrease in body fat may simply make the same amount of muscle mass become more noticeable.

If you are wondering about female bodybuilders, they have inherited a greater potential to increase the size of their muscles than the average woman. Highly competitive female bodybuilders have developed large muscles because of their genetic potential — not simply because they lifted weights. Keep in mind that female bodybuilders look much more muscular while posing on stage than they actually are in a relaxed state. Prior to a competition, female bodybuilders have restricted their caloric intakes — often severely — thereby reducing their body fat and body fluids. Immediately prior to posing on stage, they have also "pumped" their muscles. This engorges their muscles with blood and makes them temporarily bigger. Finally, the stage lighting as well as their tans and clothing — and even the oil that is rubbed on their bodies — all contribute to making female bodybuilders appear as if they have much more muscular size than they really do.

There are a relatively small number of women who have inherited the ingredients necessary to experience significant increases in their muscular size from lifting weights. However, the overwhelming majority of women can gain considerable muscular strength from lifting weights, yet have little or no change in their muscular size. Developing large muscles that are unsightly or unfeminine is physiologically improbable for the average woman.

Q: Does the composition and distribution of my muscle fibers influence my response to lifting weights?

A: Yes. Your predominant muscle-fiber type plays a major role in determining your potential for attaining muscular size and strength. The two main types of muscle fibers are fast twitch and slow twitch. Both of these fiber types have the potential to increase in muscular size or "hypertrophy." (A decrease in musclar size is known as "atrophy.") However, fast-twitch fibers have a much greater capacity for hypertrophy than slow-twitch fibers. This means that individuals who have inherited a high percentage of fast-twitch fibers have a greater potential to increase the size of their muscles than those who have inherited a high percentage of slow-twitch fibers. Moreover, fast-twitch fibers can produce greater force than slow-twitch fibers. This means that individuals who have inherited a high percentage of fast-twitch fibers have a greater potential to increase their muscular strength than those who have inherited a high percentage of slow-twitch fibers.

In addition, an increase in the number of muscle fibers — known as "hyperplasia" — is thought to take place by fiber splitting or "budding." Although hyperplasia has been demonstrated scientifically in many animals whose muscles were loaded with a resistance — including birds, cats, and rats — there is no definitive proof that it occurs in humans. Most likely, lifting weights results in the addition of contractile protein — namely, actin and myosin — not in the addition of muscle fibers.

Q: How often should I "max out" to check my progress in the weight room?

A: Workouts often morph into versions of a weightlifting contest with numerous sets leading to one-repetition maximum (1-RM) attempts. Unless you happen to be a competitive weightlifter, there is no need for you to "max out" to determine how much weight you can lift for one repetition. And even if you are a competitive weightlifter, you do not have to perform low-repetition sets until you get close to a contest.

One reservation with performing a 1-RM is that it is a highly specialized skill that requires proper warm-up, instruction, supervision, and practice. This time and effort could be used elsewhere such as perfecting your operational tactics and practicing your marksmanship skills. The main concern with doing a 1-RM, however, is an increased risk of musculoskeletal injury. Attempting a 1-RM with a maximal or near-maximal weight can place an inordinate and unreasonable amount of stress on the muscles, connective tissues, and bones. An injury occurs when this stress exceeds the structural integrity of those components. Any injury that occurs from attempting a 1-RM is simply inexcusable. Performing a 1-RM is not really necessary to monitor your progress. If you are recording your workout data — and you should — you can simply check your workout card or log to evaluate your levels of strength.

Over the years, a number of prediction equations have been developed and used to estimate a 1-RM based upon the relationship between muscular strength and muscular endurance. By using a prediction equation, you can estimate your 1-RM in a safe and practical — yet reasonably accurate — manner without having to "max out." The following equation can be used to predict a 1-RM based upon repetitions-to-fatigue (where "X" equals the number of repetitions performed):

$$\text{Predicted 1-RM} = \text{weight lifted} \div (1.0278 - 0.0278X)$$

To illustrate the equation, suppose you were able to perform 8 repetitions to the point of muscular fatigue with 150 pounds. Inserting these values into the equation yields a predicted 1-RM of about 186 pounds [0.0278 x 8 = 0.2224; 1.0278 – 0.2224 = 0.8054; 150 ÷ 0.8054 = 186.24]. In other words, you can perform 8 repetitions with about 80.54% (or 0.8054) of your predicted 1-RM. In a study that involved 48 subjects, researchers found that this equation had a high correlation for predicting a 1-RM bench press (r=0.99), and squat (r=0.96); in a study that involved 67 subjects, researchers showed that this equation had a high correlation for predicting a 1-RM in all three of the competitive powerlifts: the bench press (r=0.993), squat (r=0.969), and deadlift (r=0.956).

Note that this equation is most accurate for predicting a 1-RM when the number of repetitions-to-fatigue is 10 or less. In a study that involved 220 subjects, researchers compared six different equations and found that the aforementioned equation was the only one of the six in which the predicted bench press did not differ significantly from the actual bench press when 10 or fewer repetitions were completed (r=0.98; t=0.99).

A test of muscular endurance — though not a direct measure of pure maximal strength — is much safer than a 1-RM lift because it involves a submaximal load. (Because genetic factors — particularly your predominant muscle-fiber type — play a major role in your muscular endurance, prediction equations are not accurate for everyone. However, they are still very practical for much of the population.)

Q: Do higher repetitions build muscular endurance instead of muscular strength?
A: It has been believed that performing higher repetitions (with a lighter weight) builds

If you increase your muscular strength, you will also increase your muscular endurance.

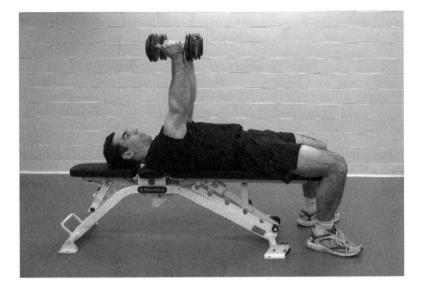

muscular endurance and doing lower repetitions (with a heavier weight) builds muscular strength. Actually, muscular endurance and muscular strength are directly related. If you increase your muscular endurance, you will also increase your muscular strength. Here is an example: Suppose that your one-repetition maximum (1-RM) in the bench press is 200 pounds and you can do 10 repetitions with 75% of it (150 pounds). And after several months of strength training with higher repetitions — within a range of about 8 - 12 — suppose that you have progressed to the point where you can do 180 pounds for 10 repetitions. Given that you increased the amount of weight that you could lift for 10 repetitions in the bench press by 20% — from 150 to 180 pounds — do you think that your 1-RM strength will now be greater than, less than, or equal to your previous 1-RM effort of 200 pounds? The odds are that it will be greater than your previous 1-RM. So even though you trained with higher repetitions, you increased your muscular strength.

By the way, it works the other way as well. If you increase your muscular strength, you will also increase your muscular endurance. Here is why: As you get stronger, you need fewer muscle fibers to sustain a sub-maximal effort (muscular endurance). This also means that you have a greater reserve of muscle fibers available to extend the sub-maximal effort.

Q: Should I perform higher repetitions to tone my muscles and lower repetitions to bulk them?

A: There is no scientific evidence that higher repetitions increase muscular definition or "tone" and lower repetitions increase muscular size or "bulk." In one 10-week study, there were no significant differences in muscular size (and strength) between a group who trained with sets of four repetitions and a group who trained with sets of 10 repetitions.

If you perform the same program — that is, the same exercises as well as the same number of sets and repetitions — as someone else for a period of time, it is highly unlikely that you will end up looking like physical clones of each other. The next time you are in the weight room, observe different pairs of training partners. You will see that people who train to-gether usually have different physiques — despite doing the same exercises while using the same number of sets and repetitions.

People respond differently to strength training because each person — except for monozy-gotic (identical) twins — is a unique genetic entity with a different genetic potential for achieving muscular size. Some people are predisposed toward developing heavily muscled physiques while others are predisposed toward developing highly defined physiques. Therefore, the belief that performing high repetitions with light weights will increase muscular definition and doing low repetitions with heavy weights will increase muscular size is entirely anecdotal with no factual basis whatsoever. Whether your sets consist of low repetitions, high repetitions, or intermediate repetitions, you are still going to develop according to your genetic (or inherited) blueprint — provided that you perform your sets with similar levels of intensity.

So, your response to strength training is not necessarily due to a particular program. Following the program of a successful bodybuilder does not mean that you will develop the same level of muscular size; likewise, following the program of a successful weightlifter does not mean that you will develop the same level of physical strength. If it were that simple, then millions of men and women would have award-winning physiques and awe-inspiring strength. Yet, millions of men and women make a terrible mistake by trying to heroically implement the programs of the current physique stars and strength athletes — programs that are usually impractical, inefficient and, in some cases, unsafe.

The truth is that heritability dictates trainability. The main determinant of your response to strength training is your genetics. The cumulative effect of your inherited muscular, mechanical, hormonal, and neural qualities is what determines your physical potential. An individual who has inherited a high percentage of fast-twitch fibers, long muscle bellies coupled with short tendinous attachments, high levels of testosterone, favorable lever lengths and body proportions, mesomorphic tendencies, low points of tendon insertions, and an efficient neurological system would prove to be incredibly strong as well as physically impressive.

Compared to the average person, this genetic marvel would be capable of almost unbelievable feats of strength. There are a few individuals like that, but most people are not so fortunate. However, this does not mean that you cannot get stronger or improve your physique. Indeed, you should be encouraged and challenged to progress as much as possible within your genetic profile.

Q: Should I perform high-velocity repetitions to recruit my fast-twitch fibers?

A: No. The selective recruitment of muscle fibers is physiologically impossible. Muscle fibers are recruited — or "innervated" — by the nervous system in an orderly fashion according to the intensity or force requirements and not by the speed of movement. Demands of low muscular intensity are met by slow-twitch fibers. Intermediate fibers are recruited once the slow-twitch fibers are no longer able to continue the task. The fast-twitch fibers are finally recruited only when the other fatigue-resistant fibers have severely depleted their energy stores and cannot meet the force requirements. All fibers are working when the fast-twitch fibers are being used. The orderly recruitment pattern remains the same regardless of whether the repetition speed was fast or slow.

This pattern is consistent with the "size principle" of recruitment that was proposed by Dr. Elwood Henneman in the 1950s. He described the experimental basis of his principle in 18 related articles that were published in the *Journal of Neurophysiology* over the course of 25 years. According to this principle — which is widely accepted by neurophysiologists and regarded by them as one of the most important advances ever in the field of motor control — motoneurons are recruited based upon increasing size: The motor unit with the smallest motoneuron is recruited first and the motor unit with the largest motoneuron is recruited last. (A motor unit consists of a motoneuron and all the muscle fibers that it innervates.) In general, the smallest motoneurons innervate slow-twitch fibers and the largest motoneurons innervate fast-twitch fibers. Therefore, slow-twitch fibers are recruited first and fast-twitch fibers are recruited last.

The orderly pattern of recruitment has another important training implication: If you want to engage as many fast-twitch fibers as possible, then it is critical that you train to the point of muscular fatigue.

Q: Is it true that lifting weights in an explosive manner will increase speed, power, and quickness?

A: No it is not. Lifting weights at rapid speeds of movement is only a *demonstration* of power — not an *adaptation*. There is absolutely no scientific evidence to suggest that "explosive" lifting leads to "explosive" performance. Keep in mind, too, that fast speeds of movement make an exercise less effective and more dangerous.

Q: Will plyometrics improve my speed, power, and explosiveness?

A: Since the mid 1960s, plyometrics have been romantically endorsed as a way to "bridge the gap" between strength and speed. In the United States, the first reference to these types of exercises in athletic literature appears to have been in 1966, by the Soviet author Yuri Verhoshanski (whose surname has also been spelled "Verkhoshansky"). The term "plyometrics," however, seems to have been coined in 1975 by Fred Wilt who was an American track and field coach.

Plyometrics apply to any exercise or jumping drill that uses the myotatic (or stretch) reflex of a muscle. This particular reflex is triggered when a muscle is pre-stretched prior to a muscular contraction, resulting in a more powerful movement than would otherwise be possible. Just before using a one-person ram, for example, a SWAT officer "cocks" the weight by pulling it backward. This "countermovement" pre-stretches the muscles which gives the officer the ability to generate more force with the ram than if the action was done without first cocking it. Plyometrics for the lower body include bounding, hopping, and various box drills such as depth jumping (in which an athlete steps off a box and, upon landing, immediately does a vertical jump); plyometrics for the upper body include ballistic (or "drop") push-ups and often incorporate medicine balls to induce the stretch reflex.

Understand that the use of plyometrics has been highly controversial for quite some time. Knowing that most of the support for plyometrics is based upon anecdotal — not scientific — evidence is important. The truth is that there is little unbiased research that convincingly and consistently proves plyometrics are effective. Although some research has shown that plyometrics are effective, roughly an equal amount of research has shown that they are no more effective than regular strength-training or jumping activities when it comes to improving strength, speed, power, explosiveness, or any other physiological function.

For instance, a study that involved 26 subjects found no significant improvement in the vertical jump in those who performed depth jumps two times per week. In a study that involved 38 subjects, researchers found no significant difference in the vertical jump between a group that trained with an isokinetic leg press and a group that trained with depth jumps. In a study that involved 44 subjects (in two different experiments), researchers concluded that depth jumps (of varying heights) are no more effective than "other more common training methods" for improving leg strength and the vertical jump. A study that involved 50 subjects found no significant differences in the 40-yard dash and vertical jump between one group that did strength training and two groups that did plyometrics. A study that involved 31 subjects showed no significant differences in dynamic leg strength and leg power between one group who performed maximum vertical jumps from ground level and two groups who performed depth jumps from different heights. And in a study that involved 24 subjects, researchers found no significant differences in the vertical jump, leg press, and peak power of the quadriceps between a group that performed a strength-training program and a group that performed a strength-training program and plyometrics.

One other piece of research deserves special note: In a study that involved 30 subjects, researchers found that as the height of the depth jump increased, the performance in the vertical jump and maximal vertical power output decreased in a linear fashion. Actually, the greatest performances were produced by depth jumping from a height of only *4.72 inches*. Given this information, there is difficulty in understanding why depth jumping is even done.

So while the mechanical output of a muscle is certainly increased by the pre-stretch mechanism, it does not necessarily follow that a physiological or neurological adaptation/alteration occurs. Even if there was indisputable evidence that plyometrics were an effective way to improve strength, speed, power, and explosiveness — or anything else — considering the risks is extremely important. Frankly, the potential for injury from plyometrics is enormous. A large number of strength and fitness professionals have questioned the safety of plyometrics for many years. When performing plyometrics, the musculoskeletal system is exposed to repetitive trauma and high-impact forces. The extreme biomechanical loading places an inordinate amount of stress on the muscles, bones, and connective tissues. Research has suggested that the stress from the impact forces increases the potential for injury. This is particularly true of plyometrics that have a large vertical component such as depth jumping.

The most common plyometric-related injuries in the lower body are patellar tendinitis ("jumper's knee"), stress fractures, shin splints, muscle strains, heel bruises, and sprains of the knee and ankle. Other potential injuries include compression fractures, ruptured tendons, and meniscal (cartilage) damage. Another area that is highly susceptible to injury from plyometrics is the lower back. Several studies have found that depth jumping results in "spinal shrinkage" — that is, a loss of stature — presumably from compression of the intervertebral discs. This makes it reasonable to think that decreases in the height of the discs increases the potential for injury to the spine. And performing depth jumps from greater heights or with added weight significantly increases the impact forces and spinal shrinkage. Doing so may also cause individuals to alter their landing strategies as a protective mechanism, thereby increasing the potential for other injuries.

When aerobic dancing was introduced years ago, most fitness enthusiasts eagerly accepted this activity with little or no reservation. Within a short period of time, untold numbers of participants suffered injuries that were directly attributable to the high-impact forces that were absorbed by their musculoskeletal systems. The concerns about these inherent dangers ushered in the development and acceptance of low-impact aerobics. If a multitude of injuries resulted from jumping up and down several *inches*, how many injuries can be expected from jumping up and down several *feet*? Also consider this: Most authorities recommend that athletes should stretch under control without any bouncing or ballistic movements to reduce their risk of injury. The fact that plyometrics are an extremely violent form of stretching is a blatant contradiction to these safety concerns.

Many individuals in the sports-medical community view plyometrics as "an injury waiting to happen." According to Dr. Ken Leistner — who has treated numerous injuries in his New York office — plyometrics "are not safe under any circumstances, nor for any particular athlete, no matter how 'advanced' he or she may be." Adds Dr. Leistner, " . . . plyometrics are dangerous stuff and it is not fair, right or ethical for a coach to impose plyometrics on his or her athletes. Plyometrics are dangerous in themselves and will also do things to the body that will increase the probability of injuries during future events."

Before plyometrics can be accepted as an appropriate method of training, research must show that they are effective and safe on a more convincing and consistent basis. At this point in time, a compelling number of scientific studies have found that plyometrics are no more effective than regular strength-training and jumping activities. Moreover, plyometrics carry an unreasonably — and unjustifiably — high risk of injury.

Understanding that many plyometric drills are actually nothing more than glorified agility drills that are intended to improve specific skills, kinesthetic awareness, and anaerobic conditioning is important. When these drills have a small vertical component and involve a low amount of impact forces, they are an effective and safe method of training. But when these drills have a large vertical component and involve a high amount of impact forces that aggressively pre-stretch muscles in an attempt to make the stretch reflex more responsive, they are an ineffective and dangerous method of training.

You can improve your strength, speed, power, and explosiveness in a much safer manner by simply practicing specific skills and techniques in the same way that they are used and by strengthening your major muscle groups, especially your hips and legs. Sooner or later, jumping off a plyometrics box will send you limping to a doctor's office. The bottom line: Look before you leap.

Q: When I perform a set, is it okay to stop and rest between every few repetitions until I reach my goal?

A: No. A recovery period between repetitions is virtually impossible to quantify. This makes it difficult for you to compare your performance in a set of an exercise to a set in the same exercise that is done at a later date. In addition, taking a recovery period between repetitions is less effective than not taking a recovery period between repetitions. In one study, 42 subjects were randomly assigned to a no-rest group, a rest group, and a control group. The two training groups — that is, the no-rest and rest groups — performed the same protocol three times per week for six weeks. The only difference was that the subjects in the no-rest group did their sets without any recovery between the repetitions while the subjects in the rest group did their sets with 30 seconds of recovery between each repetition. (The control group did not train.) After six weeks of training, the subjects in the no-rest group had a significantly greater improvement in their dynamic strength compared to the subjects in the rest group (56.3% compared to 41.2%). Although it was not statistically significant, the subjects in the no-rest group also had a greater improvement in their isometric strength compared to the subjects in the rest group (22.1% compared to 19.8%). The point is that you should not rest between repetitions.

Q: Is periodization the most effective way of scheduling workouts in the weight room?

A: Also referred to as "cycling," periodization is a theoretical schedule of pre-planned workouts that has been popularized by competitive weightlifters as their preferred method of training to peak for a one-repetition maximum (1-RM) during their contests. Essentially, the idea is to change or "cycle" program variables such as the number of sets and repetitions, the workloads (which are based upon percentages of a 1-RM), and the recovery intervals between the sets/exercises. These variables are manipulated during rigidly defined "phases" of training which usually are designated as "hypertrophy," "basic strength," "strength-power," "peaking," "maintenance," and "active rest." The belief is that by manipulating the variables, athletes can selectively target specific physiological functions.

Here is a relatively simple example of a classic (linear) model of periodization that is divided into two seven-week "cycles" or "periods" (to supposedly develop strength and power): During the first three weeks of each cycle, individuals are required to do 2 - 3 sets of 8 - 10 repetitions in each exercise with 50 - 70 percent of their 1-RMs; during the fourth and fifth weeks of each cycle, they must do 3 - 4 sets of 6 repetitions in each exercise with 70 - 85 percent of their 1-RMs; and during the sixth and seventh weeks of each cycle, they must do 3 - 5 sets of 1 - 4 repetitions in each exercise with 85 - 95 percent of their 1-RMs.

There are several issues and concerns relating to the use of periodization. Perhaps first and foremost is the fact that there is no legitimate scientific evidence to support the wild claim that doing different numbers of sets and repetitions with different percentages of a 1-RM while taking different intervals of recovery between sets will specifically influence hypertrophy, strength, strength-power, or anything else.

Second, periodization is overly — and unnecessarily — complicated and correspondingly confusing. The use of pseudoscientific terminology coupled with pre-planned workouts that specify inflexible instructions to vary the sets, repetitions, workloads, and recovery intervals in rigidly defined phases adds to the confusion. Equally confusing is the notion of "active rest" — a blatant contradiction in terms. Strength training is actually quite simple: Overload the muscles by increasing the resistance and/or repetitions from one workout to the next.

Third, periodization is far too inflexible because of the precise nature of pre-planned workouts. The reality is that individuals often get sick or injured, and are forced to miss workouts. In the event of a missed workout, do they renew their training according to their pre-planned schedule? If not, at what point in the pre-planned schedule do they resume? Essentially, "periodization" is another word for "variety." But incorporating variety into a program — which is certainly important — can be done as needed in a manner that is far less regimented and much more informal.

Fourth, periodization requires everyone to perform specific numbers of repetitions with certain percentages of their 1-RMs. For instance, individuals might be required to do 8 repetitions with 70% of their 1-RMs. Because of wide variations in muscular endurance, however, such a prescription might be far too easy for some and literally impossible for others. Therefore, pre-planned workouts that demand the same number of repetitions be done with a specific percentage of a maximal load are only effective for the relatively small segment of the population that has inherited a particular level of muscular endurance that corresponds exactly to the specifications and parameters of the training schedule.

Fifth, periodization makes some sense for competitive weightlifters since — for the most part — they only peak for two or three contests a year. But it makes little sense for other individuals — especially athletes who might have to peak once or twice a week for three or four months. Indeed, for what competitions do they peak? Every one is important. Imagine an athlete saying apologetically, "Sorry about my performance today, but I am not scheduled to peak in my Strength-Power Phase for two more weeks." Remember, too, that references to the training methods or techniques of competitive weightlifters are irrelevant and, therefore, do not apply to any athletes other than competitive weightlifters. The question that a SWAT officer must ask is, "Am I training to become a better officer or a better weightlifter?"

To summarize: Besides being confusing, trying to implement periodization with athletes other than competitive weightlifters is impractical, irrelevant, illogical, and unnecessary. There are other ways to address an individual's needs that are considerably less complicated as well as more practical, relevant, and logical.

Q: What are isometrics and can I get stronger by doing them?

A: Basically, isometrics are exercises in which you push or pull against an immovable resistance. Their popularity increased enormously in the middle of the 1900s primarily because of two events: First, Erich Müeller and Theodor Hettinger of Germany released their research findings in the 1950s that showed the benefits of isometrics. Second, Bob Hoffman — who was the president of the York Barbell Company and coach of the United States Olympic Weightlifting Team — authored an article in which he claimed that isometrics were largely responsible for the outstanding performances that were made by two of his weightlifters and declared that isometrics were "the greatest system of strength and muscle building the world has ever seen." (His claims were later discredited when it was determined that the two weightlifters had also taken anabolic steroids while performing isometrics.)

Can you get stronger by doing isometrics? Absolutely. But isometrics have several disadvantages. Isometrics increase your blood pressure beyond what would normally be encountered when strength training with conventional methods. In addition, isometrics do not involve full-range repetitions. As a result, any increases in strength are specific to the joint angle being worked plus or minus a small number of degrees. And since isometrics do not involve full-range repetitions, your muscles do not receive any stretch at all. So after a while of doing a program of isometrics, you will likely lose flexibility.

Q: What is ground-based training?

A: The notion of "ground-based training" has received a good bit of attention since the mid-1990s. Essentially, ground-based training is the belief that since many physical activities are done with your feet in contact with the ground then that is how you should lift weights. In other words, it is the belief that exercises should be done while standing on the ground. For instance, proponents of ground-based training contend that the barbell squat is more functional than the leg press because it is done in the standing position.

In response to the notion of ground-based training, Jeff Watson — the Strength and Conditioning Coach at Villanova University — once asked, "Does this mean that you cannot get stronger while sitting or lying down?" Obviously, you *can* get stronger in an exercise even though it is not done in the standing position. Many people know this from their personal experiences because they have improved their muscular strength in exercises that are not performed while standing such as the leg press, bench press, and lat pulldown — not to mention exercises that are done with their bodyweight in which their feet are not in contact with the floor such as dips and chins.

Q: How come my muscles are no longer sore the day after I lift weights?

A: There are two types of muscular soreness: acute and delayed-onset. Acute muscular soreness occurs during and immediately following an activity. One theory suggests that this soreness is associated with an occlusion of blood flow to your muscles (which is known as "ischemia"). Due to inadequate blood flow, metabolic waste products (such as lactic acid) cannot be removed and accumulate to the point of stimulating the pain receptors in your muscles. On the other hand, delayed-onset muscular soreness (DOMS) refers to the pain and discomfort that occurs 24 - 48 hours after an activity. The exact cause of DOMS is unknown. The most popular theory for DOMS is that cellular damage occurs to the muscle fibers and/or connective tissues (such as tendons). This theory would seem to be flawed, though, because doing physical activity when your muscles are sore tends to reduce some of the discomfort. If the soreness were due to cellular damage, then any subsequent training should *exacerbate* the pain, not *alleviate* it.

Regardless, just because you do not experience DOMS the day after you lift weights does not mean that your efforts were unproductive. If you accidentally bumped your shin bone on a tactical operation, the anterior (front) part of your lower leg may be sore next day . . . and perhaps for a few days afterward. This does not mean that the soreness was productive, however. So, muscular soreness — or lack thereof — is not necessarily indicative of your efforts. DOMS can result from several situations. You will experience DOMS if you have done an excessive amount of training. In this case, the soreness does not mean that your training was productive. It was certainly *excessive*, but not necessarily *productive*. You will also probably have DOMS if you do something unfamiliar in your workout. This could be changing the order of your exercises, the choice of your equipment (that is, using free weights instead of machines or vice versa), or the selection of your exercises (such as doing the incline press instead of the bench press). In all likelihood, you will also encounter DOMS if you increase your intensity to a level that is greater than usual or take a recovery interval between your exercises/sets that is shorter than usual.

But again, not having muscular soreness following a workout does not mean that it was unproductive (or that you did not do enough exercises/sets). Similarly, having muscular soreness following a workout does not mean that it was productive — it could simply indicate that you did something that was unfamiliar. For those individuals who are concerned with becoming sore, your potential for DOMS will be lower as you grow accustomed to the specific demands of an activity. A gradual progression in your intensity also helps to reduce the possibility of experiencing an excessive amount of muscular soreness.

Q: Should I avoid emphasizing the eccentric phase of a repetition since it is associated with excessive muscular damage and soreness?

A: Studies that have investigated eccentric contractions usually load the muscles with some type of eccentric-based activity such as running downhill, cycling backward, stepping down from heights, and lowering weights. The truth is that muscular damage and soreness can occur if a muscle is loaded in a concentric, static, or eccentric manner. And, in fact, some studies have shown that eccentric contractions do not induce a greater level of muscular soreness than concentric contractions. Research has suggested that the intensity of the activity — not the type of muscle contraction — may be the dependent factor in producing muscular soreness.

Interestingly, research has shown that an adaptive response occurs from doing eccentric contractions. In one study, subjects who only performed concentric contractions during their training "complained of severe muscle soreness" after completing post-training tests in which eccentric contractions were done. Meanwhile, subjects who performed a combination of concentric and eccentric contractions during their training did not report any muscle soreness after completing the same post-training tests.

The eccentric contractions that are most likely to produce an injury are those that occur during the braking of high-velocity movements. In terms of strength training, however, the eccentric phase of a repetition should be performed with a controlled speed of movement. Keep in mind, too, that the duration of the eccentric phase of a repetition involves a relatively brief period of loading. If a weight is lowered in about 3 - 4 seconds per repetition, for example, then the eccentric loading that occurs during a set of 15 repetitions only lasts about 45 - 60 seconds.

The eccentric phase of a repetition — and eccentric activity, for that matter — is safe and productive as long as it is not performed to an extreme. As your muscles become more familiar with eccentric loading, any amount of muscular soreness and tissue damage that you may experience will be reduced. Also note that oxygen consumption and energy expenditure are much lower during eccentric exercise than in comparable concentric exercise. In fact, the mechanical efficiency of eccentric exercise may be several times higher than that of pure concentric exercise. As an example, climbing stairs (which primarily involves concentric muscular contractions) will quickly elevate your heart rate and frequency of breathing, while going downstairs (which mainly involves eccentric muscular contractions) will have a much lower effect.

Q: Is there any significance that my muscles get pumped when I lift weights?

A: Not much — at least in terms of it being productive. During physical activity, blood flow is increased to your working muscles to deliver oxygen. Your muscles become larger — or "pumped" — from the pooled blood. This increase in muscular size is transient, however, and unrelated to the long-term, adaptive increases in muscular size that occur in response to progressive-resistance exercise.

Q: Do I need to perform any warm-up sets prior to a set in which I train to the point of muscular fatigue?

A: Just because you did not perform any warm-up sets does not mean that you are not warmed up. From a physiological perspective, an adequate warm-up is one in which your core temperature is increased by one degree. If you perform a relatively high number of repetitions and lift the weight in a deliberate, controlled fashion without any explosive or jerking movements, then you will actually warm-up as you do the exercise. Think about it: If you perform a set of 10 repetitions with a speed of movement that is roughly six seconds per repetition, you will have trained your muscles for about one minute before you reach muscular fatigue. After one minute of training, there is little doubt that you will be adequately warmed up and prepared — both physiologically and psychologically — to train to muscular fatigue.

An exception to this would be someone such as a competitive weightlifter who does low-repetition sets. In this case, one or more warm-up sets should be done prior to the low-repetition efforts to reduce the risk of injury.

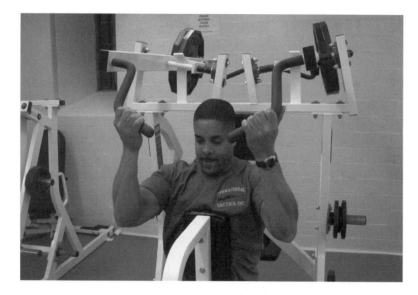

If you perform a relatively high number of repetitions and lift the weight in a deliberate, controlled fashion without any explosive or jerking movements, then you will actually warm-up as you do the exercise.

Q: Is the barbell squat the best exercise for training the lower body?

A: Everything else being equal, the best exercises for increasing muscular size and strength are those that involve the greatest amounts of muscle mass. Therefore, one of the most productive exercises for the lower body is the barbell squat.

But despite the all-important advantage of addressing an enormous amount of muscle mass, the barbell squat has an inherent disadvantage in that many individuals — because of their body type and/or physical condition — cannot perform the exercise in a safe manner. Indeed, the orthopedic concerns associated with the barbell squat have been voiced since at least the early 1960s. Since then, these concerns have been echoed by many strength coaches who are at the scholastic, collegiate, and professional levels.

One orthopedic concern is the knee. In order to maintain your balance during the descending phase of the barbell squat, you must move your knees forward of your ankles (from a horizontal perspective). The farther the knee moves forward, the greater the stretch of the joint and the greater the shear (side-to-side) force in the patellar tendon. As the length of the legs increases, so does the distance that the knees move forward of the ankles. Therefore, someone with long legs is more prone to the shearing or "grinding" effect in the knees than someone with short legs.

To minimize the shear force in the knees during a barbell squat, you would have to maintain a position in which your lower legs — that is, your shin bones — are as close to perpendicular to the floor as possible. Unfortunately, this position cannot be attained because your center of gravity would drop outside your base of support and you would fall backward. This problem can be avoided, however, by using what is known as a "safety squat bar." The bar has a heavily padded, "horse-collar" center yoke that — as oddly as it sounds — can balance itself on your shoulders. This frees your hands so that you can hold onto the sides of a power rack while squatting. When doing squats in this manner, you can keep your lower legs roughly perpendicular to the floor without losing your balance and falling backward.

A second area of orthopedic concern is the lower back. The fact is that some individuals might not be able to perform the barbell squat without experiencing low-back pain, especially if they have pre-existing low-back injuries or histories of low-back problems. Squatting with a barbell on the shoulders compresses the spinal column which, in extreme cases, could result in a herniated or ruptured disc. Compression is most evident when the lifter is in the bottom position of the barbell squat, where the anterior aspect of the lumbar vertebrae is compacted and the intervertebral discs are pushed in a posterior direction.

One study revealed that when performing the barbell squat with as little as 0.8 - 1.6 times bodyweight, the load in the low-back region is actually 6 - 10 times bodyweight. This means that if you weigh 200 pounds and do the barbell squat with 160 - 320 pounds, the compressive load on your lumbar area can be 1,200 - 2,000 pounds. The exact amount of loading is a function of how far the weight is from your lower back. Everything else being equal, someone with a long torso is subjected to higher compressive loads in the lower back than someone with a short torso.

Fortunately, there are safer ways of addressing the extensive musculature of your lower body without the inherent risk of injury to your knees and lower back. First, be aware of the general body type that has a higher risk of injury from the barbell squat, namely individuals with relatively long legs and torsos. An excellent alternative for those with this body type — and others who cannot squat in a safe manner — is the leg press which is essentially the squatting motion without any vertical compression of the spine. In addition, you have the freedom to position your lower legs so that there is minimal shear force in your knees.

Q: But what if I only have access to a barbell to train my hips?

A: If this is the case, your primary goal is to reduce the compressive loads and shear forces. You have at least two options for the barbell squat. One is to use a lighter weight and perform your repetitions with a speed of movement that is slower than what you normally use. This will decrease the orthopedic stress on your knees and lower back. A second option is to pre-fatigue your hips prior to performing the barbell squat. For example, you could do hip abduction using manual resistance with the aid of a partner. Once you finish this exercise, quickly move to the barbell squat. Because your hips are pre-fatigued, you will not be able to use as much weight as when they are not fatigued which will reduce the orthopedic stress on your knees and lower back.

If you choose to do the barbell squat, your technique is critical in decreasing your risk of injury. Here are some training tips:

- To reduce the compressive loads, minimize your trunk lean as much as possible. In other words, do not bend forward excessively at your waist when you perform your repetitions. Keeping the bar lower on your shoulders — rather than near or on the base of your neck — will help you reduce your forward lean.

- You should only squat to a point where your upper legs are approximately parallel to the floor. If you cannot squat to this depth, it may be because your stance is too narrow. Spread your feet slightly wider than shoulder-width apart. Also, keep your toes pointed slightly outward. These suggestions should help you to attain a proper depth. By the way, a narrow stance will also increase your trunk lean as you squat which will, in turn, increase the compressive load on your lower back.

- Do not "bounce" out of the bottom position of the barbell squat. Doing so produces higher compressive loads and shear forces.

- You should not "lock" or "snap" your knees in the top position of the barbell squat. This removes the load from the target muscles and may hyperextend your knees.

- Lastly, the benefits of using knee wraps to provide any significant advantage in safeguarding your knees against injury is unclear. By tightly wrapping your knees, you will get an artificial boost out of the bottom position of the squat which allows you to use much more weight than normal. This, however, relates more to *demonstrating* strength rather than to *developing* it. To build functional strength in your hips and legs, you would be better off not using knee wraps or other forms of synthetic support (such as a squat suit).

Q: How strong should my hamstrings be in relation to my quadriceps?

A: An imbalance of strength between the hamstrings and quadriceps has long been suspected to increase the likelihood of an injury. Specifically, the stronger quadriceps could overpower the weaker hamstrings and produce an injury. In the 1960s, Dr. Karl Klein measured the strength of the quadriceps and hamstrings using a crude tensiometer. He is credited with popularizing the notion that hamstring strength should be at least 60% of quadricep strength.

The resistance used for your hamstrings in the leg curl will likely differ from one machine to another. (The same is true for your quadriceps in the leg extension.) This is because mechanical differences in the design of a machine will affect your leverage and, therefore, the amount of resistance that you can lift. Factors that would affect your leverage include (1) the length and weight of the movement arm; (2) the weight of a counterbalance (if one is provided); (3) the distance between your knee and where you exert force against the pad; and (4) the mechanical friction of the machine.

Consider this example: When using a seated leg curl you might be able to do 12 repetitions with 100 pounds; when using a prone leg curl you might be able to do 12 repetitions with 120 pounds. If this is the case, which weight do you use for comparison with the leg extension? So, comparing the weight that you can lift on one machine to that of another — even those manufactured by the same company — would probably be inaccurate. The important thing is to make sure that your hamstrings are as strong as possible.

Q: Is it okay for me to raise my hips when I do the bench press?

A: No. By raising your hips, you are essentially shortening the distance that the bar must travel to and from your chest. While this may allow you to lift more weight, it does not mean that you increased your strength. In fact, look at it this way: Suppose that when you keep your hips flat on the back pad, you can lift 200 pounds a distance of 18 inches — or 3,600 inch-pounds of work [200 pounds x 18 inches]. If you raise your chest to the point where the bar now travels a distance of 15 inches, you would have to lift 240 pounds just to perform the same amount of work [3,600 inch-pounds ÷ 15 inches].

Q: Can I bounce the bar off my chest during the bench press?

A: Definitely not. Bouncing the bar off your chest means that you can *bounce* more weight, not *lift* more weight. Dropping a weighted bar onto your chest causes compression. When your musculoskeletal structure "rebounds" or returns to normal, it helps you raise the weight. The more you drop the weight, the more rebound you get; the more rebound you get, the less your muscles work; the less your muscles work, the less you increase your strength. Forcefully dropping a weighted bar onto your chest also increases the risk of injury to your sternum (or breastbone).

Q: Why is it better to use a narrow grip rather than a wide grip in exercises such as the bench press and lat pulldown?

A: Take an empty bar and hold it near the upper part of your chest (near your collarbones) with your hands spaced far apart. While standing in front of a mirror, press the bar overhead. Note the distance that the bar traveled vertically. Now, move your hands a bit closer together and try it again. You will find that the narrower grip allowed the bar to travel a greater distance. Being able to move the bar a greater distance means that you had a greater range of motion around your shoulder and elbow joints. The greater range of motion translates into a greater involvement of the targeted muscles. As a rule of thumb, your grip in the bench press and lat pulldown should be slightly wider than shoulder-width apart.

Q: Why is it easier to do a chin than it is to do a pull-up?

A: Regardless of how you position your hands, just about any type of pulling movement for your torso — whether it is rowing, chinning, or any pulling variation — targets the same muscles, namely your upper back, biceps, and forearms. However, there are differences in the leverage that you receive from your musculoskeletal system based upon the grip that you elect to use. For example, performing a chin with an underhand grip (your palms facing toward you) is more biomechanically efficient than doing a pull-up with an overhand grip (your palms facing away from you). With an underhand grip, the radius and ulna (the bones in your lower arms) run parallel to one another; with an overhand grip, the radius crosses over the ulna forming an "X". In this position, the bicep tendon gets wrapped around the lower portion of the radius, creating a biomechanical disadvantage and a loss in leverage.

This is also true when comparing an underhand and overhand grip during pulldown and rowing movements — the same muscles are used but with varying degrees of biomechanical leverage. (With a "parallel grip" — in which your palms face each other — the bones in your lower arms do not cross, either. This grip, then, is also more efficient than an overhand one.)

Q: Will I respond differently if I do the seated press with a machine rather than the seated press with a barbell?

A: Not really. In truth, any exercise that progressively applies a load on your muscles will stimulate improvements in muscular size and strength. The seated (or shoulder) press — whether it is done with a machine or a barbell — addresses the same major muscles, namely your anterior deltoid and triceps. Although balancing a barbell requires a greater involvement of synergistic muscles, it does not appear as if this results in a significantly greater response.

Indeed, studies have shown that there are no significant differences in the development of strength when comparing groups who used free weights and groups who used machines. The bottom line is that your muscles do not have eyes, brains, or cognitive ability. Therefore, they cannot possibly know whether the source of resistance is a barbell, dumbbells, a selectorized machine, a plate-loaded machine, or another human being. The sole factors that determine your response from strength training are your genetic profile and your level of effort — not the equipment that you used.

Q: What exercise can I do to develop a peak in my biceps?

A: Not everyone can develop a peak in the biceps by simply performing a certain exercise. Your potential to develop your muscles is based upon your genetic (or inherited) character-istics (which includes your predominant muscle-fiber type, the insertion points of your tendons, and so on). If you have the genetic potential to develop a peak in your biceps, then you will do so by performing any version of a bicep curl in a manner that provides a progressive overload.

Q: What is the best exercise for getting rid of the "spare tire" around my mid-section?

A: The abdominal area probably gets more attention than any other bodypart. Many people perform countless repetitions of sit-ups, knee-ups, and other abdominal exercises — sometimes more than once per day — with the belief that this will give them a highly prized set of "washboard abs." In exercise-physiology parlance, the belief that exercise causes a localized loss of body fat is known as "spot reduction."

A litmus test for evaluating the notion of spot reduction is to examine whether a significantly greater change occurs in an active or exercised bodypart compared to a relatively inactive or unexercised bodypart. In one study, researchers evaluated the effects of a 27-day sit-up program on the fat-cell diameter and body composition of 13 subjects. Over this four-week period, each subject performed a total of 5,004 sit-ups (with the legs bent at a 90-degree angle and no foot support). Fat biopsies from the abdominal, subscapular, and gluteal sites revealed that the sit-up program reduced the fat-cell diameter at all three sites to a similar degree. In other words, exercising the abdominal muscles did not preferentially affect the fat in the abdominal area more than the gluteal or subscapular areas.

Abdominal exercises certainly involve your abdominal muscles. However, the exercises have little effect on the subcutaneous fat that resides over the abdominal muscles (and below your skin). The reason why you cannot selectively lose fat from an isolated area is that when you exercise, fat (and carbohydrate) stores are drawn from throughout your body as a source of fuel — not just from one specific area. So, you can perform an endless amount of abdominal exercises, but these Olympian efforts will not automatically trim your mid-section. Quite simply, spot reduction is physiologically impossible.

Regarding sit-ups, the abdominals are primarily involved during the first 30 degrees or so of the exercise. Thereafter, the hip flexors accept most of the workload. For this reason, a partial sit-up — done with your bodyweight as described in Chapter 8 or with manual resistance as described in Chapter 10 — is more effective than a full sit-up. This limited-range exercise — sometimes referred to as a "crunch" or a "trunk curl" in weight-room jargon — will target your abdominals and reduce the involvement of your hip flexors.

Your abdominals should be treated like any other muscle. Once an activity for your abdominals exceeds about 70 seconds in duration, it becomes an increasingly greater test of aerobic (or muscular) endurance rather than muscular strength. Your abdominals can be targeted effectively in a time-efficient manner by training them to the point of concentric muscular fatigue within about 8 - 12 repetitions (or about 50 - 70 seconds).

Q: Is it okay for me to perform sit-ups and leg lifts with my legs straight?

A: No. Sit-ups and leg lifts should never be performed with straight legs. Lying flat on your back with your hips and legs in an extended position exaggerates the arch in your low-back area. When your legs are straight, the iliopsoas muscle located on the front of your hips is stretched and it tugs your lumbar spine into an exaggerated curve known as "lordosis." This position creates maximal peak compressive and shear forces in the lumbar region. But when your hips and legs are bent and supported, your iliopsoas muscle is relaxed. This flattens your lumbar curvature and decreases the load on your spine.

Research using computer simulation has shown that compressive and shear forces are dramatically reduced during the performance of a sit-up with the hips and legs bent at a 90-degree angle. When your hips and legs are in this position, your iliopsoas produces the least amount of tension. In brief, the compressive and shear forces in your lower back are *minimized* as the degree of hip flexion is *maximized*. Similarly, performing leg lifts with straight legs does little to involve your abdominal muscles. Rather, the iliopsoas is used more and tends to pull your lumbar spine into lordosis. Because of this, knee-ups should be performed instead of leg lifts with straight legs.

While on the subject of abdominal exercises, your repetitions should be done in a deliberate, controlled fashion. Rapid flexion of your spine can place excessive stress on the posterior structures of your lumbar area and may ultimately lead to its degeneration. And under no circumstances should you do "Roman Chair" sit-ups. This particular movement hyperextends the spine and places undue stress on the low-back area which has caused numerous injuries.

Q: Is there anything wrong with eating energy bars when I miss a meal?

A: First, keep in mind that use of the term "energy" can be misleading. Numerous products use the word "energy" in their name. This suggests that the product will improve your stamina or make you more energetic. In truth, calories provide you with energy and three nutrients provide you with calories: carbohydrates, protein, and fat. In short, you get energy from food. Technically, then, a can of soda is an "energy drink," a hot dog is an "energy roll," a pad of butter is an "energy square," a slice of bacon is an "energy strip," a chocolate-chip cookie is an "energy disc," and an ice-cream sandwich is an "energy bar." That being said, there is nothing inherently "wrong" with most of the products that have been dubbed "energy bars."

So, you can eat an energy bar — especially when it is more convenient for you because of time constraints or when on tactical operations in the field. Just do not make a habit of eating energy bars rather than regular foods and meals. Remember, there is nothing wrong with energy bars . . . but there is nothing magical about them, either. Check the list of ingredients on the packaging to determine which bar will be the most beneficial for you.

Q: Is it true that boron will increase muscular size and strength?

A: Because of gross exaggerations by the supplement industry, individuals have used boron thinking that it will increase their muscular size and strength. One study that was frequently cited by the supplement industry showed that boron increased serum testosterone concentration up to 300%. What the promoters did not mention was that the subjects in this study were postmenopausal women whose testosterone levels were quite low. In fact, these women had not received adequate boron intake for the previous 119 days prior to the supplementation. In a seven-week study that involved 19 male bodybuilders (aged 20 - 27), the researchers concluded that boron supplementation had little effect on total testosterone, lean-body mass, and muscular strength.

Q: What are ergolytic agents and are they really harmful?

A: Ergolytic agents are substances that impair physical, mental, or psychological performance. The main ergolytic agents that many individuals ingest are alcoholic beverages, tobacco products, and prescription and over-the-counter medications.

- Alcoholic beverages – SWAT officers and athletes should abstain from drinking alcohol. SWAT officers who have consumed alcoholic beverages should never deploy on a tactical operation. In addition to the obvious decision-making repercussions on tactical operations, in training, and during daily life, alcohol consumption can cause harmful side effects including dehydration and a decrease in the release of glucose from the liver which can lead to hypoglycemia. In addition, a severe decrease in performance can occur, even days after alcoholic beverages have been consumed.

- Tobacco products – Cigarette smoking and the use of smokeless tobacco cause an increased risk of cancer, heart attacks and strokes, and chronic lung disease. Aside from reduced lung and aerobic capacity, smokers as well as users of smokeless tobacco products become addicted to nicotine, the major ingredient of tobacco. Nicotine is a psychoactive drug that alters the normal functioning of the brain by stimulating the central nervous system. Contrary to this stimulation, improved reaction time has not been proven to occur, although there is some dispute among the medical community concerning this area. However, research clearly demonstrates that nicotine can cause tremors or convulsions depending upon the quantity and frequency it is used. Nicotine has both stimulant and depressive effects. Detrimental side effects include the tightening of blood vessels which raises blood pressure an average of 5 - 10 millimeters of mercury and an elevation of heart rate an average of 10 - 20 beats per minute, decreasing cardiac efficiency. Nicotine also elevates the level of blood glucose and increases insulin production.

- Prescription and over-the-counter medications – Any drug or medication can cause potentially detrimental effects on physical, mental, and psychological performance. Entire books have been dedicated to the analysis of potential effects of prescription and over-the-counter medications. What is most important for SWAT officers and athletes to understand is that unless these medications are prescribed by a medical professional to treat a specific health problem or injury, they should not be taken to enhance your performance and can cause severe health consequences. For example, anabolic steroids may make you more muscular and physically stronger in the short-term, but they will not directly improve your skill level and can cause serious long-term health problems.

Q: Does caffeine affect my performance?

A: Caffeine — a stimulant of the central nervous system — is perhaps the most widely used drug in the world. It is a component of tea, coffee, chocolate, and soft drinks as well as pills to lose weight and combat drowsiness. It has no significant nutritional value.

Interest in the use of caffeine as a performance enhancer — or "ergogenic aid" — was primarily inspired by two studies that were published in the late 1970s. In those studies, caffeine produced significant improvements in endurance (in cycling). To date, numerous studies done in a laboratory setting have shown that caffeine increases performance in cycling and running for efforts that last roughly 5 - 20 minutes. But studies done outside a laboratory have found mixed results. At this time, it does not appear as if caffeine improves sprint performance (inside or outside a laboratory).

In low doses, caffeine can improve perception, increase alertness, decrease reaction time, and lower anxiety levels. Keep in mind, though, that the effects are related to the dosage: Individual differences in the sensitivity and tolerance to caffeine certainly come into play.

When consumed in low doses, caffeine does not pose any serious risks for healthy individuals; when consumed in high doses, caffeine has the potential for many adverse side effects such as anxiety, jitters, tremors, inability to focus, gastrointestinal distress, diarrhea, insomnia, irritability, and "withdrawal headache." Obviously, these side effects would be problematic for SWAT officers. Since caffeine is a potent diuretic (which increases the production of urine), there has been some concern that it can increase the risk of dehydration — a major fear during physical activity, especially in a hot, humid environment. Although research has shown that caffeine does not pose any thermoregulatory risks, it is still an important consideration for SWAT officers. Megadoses of caffeine have the potential for heart arrhythmias and mild hallucinations. Additionally, note that individuals who have pre-existing ulcer conditions and those who are prone to stomach distress should avoid caffeine. Finally, be aware that the United States Olympic Committee restricts the use of caffeine.

Q: Does chromium melt fat or increase muscle mass?

A: Well, fat can certainly melt. But in order to do so, your body temperature would be so high that your brain would boil and your blood would probably coagulate. Chromium is an essential micromineral that functions in the metabolism of carbohydrates and fat, and helps to maintain blood-glucose levels (homeostasis). But to answer the first part of your question, chromium (picolinate) does not "melt" fat. Nor does it promote fat loss in any way. Numerous studies have shown that the short-term use of chromium does not decrease body fat. In a 16-week study that involved 95 healthy, active-duty Navy personnel, for example, a group that received chromium did not significantly reduce body fat more than a group that received a placebo.

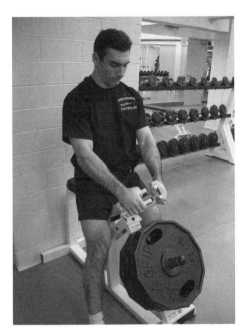

While on the subject, no known substance can "burn" fat or facilitate its metabolism. The only real method of using fat is physical activity. But what about its effect on muscle mass? As of 1999, all studies except one have reported that chromium does not increase muscle mass. And even in that study, muscle mass was estimated from anthropometric measurements which can be unreliable.

Incidentally, it appears as if chromium does not increase muscular strength, either. In a 12-week study, a group that received a placebo actually increased their strength more than a group that received chromium. (The researchers in this study also found that the subjects who received chromium had urinary chromium losses that were *nine times greater* than the subjects who were given a placebo.)

The only real method of using fat is physical activity.

Claims regarding the benefits of chromium are based upon two poorly controlled, unpublished studies that were referenced in a review article that was written by a chemist who was consulting for a supplement company. In 1996, the Federal Trade Commission ordered the company and (two others) to stop making unsubstantiated claims that chromium decreases body fat and increases muscle mass.

Q: *Will creatine improve my physical performance?*

A: Creatine is an amino acid that is made in the body by the liver and kidneys, and is derived from a diet of meat and animal products. It has received a great deal of attention in the athletic, scientific, and medical communities as well as the media. There are many anecdotal reports that creatine is effective as a strength- and performance- enhancing food supplement, but scientific research paints a different picture. Much of the research that has investigated creatine has been conducted in an extremely controlled environment, namely a laboratory. In a laboratory setting, the best evidence for performance enhancement from the use of creatine is in repeated maximal, short-term sprints on a stationary bicycle. And even then, some studies have shown no improvements. These data would be significant if your physical training — and tactical operations — involved repeated maximal, short-term sprints on a stationary bicycle. But they do not. Of the research that has been done outside a laboratory — or "in the field" — very few studies have shown that creatine had any beneficial effects during physical performances that are more apt to occur in realistic situations such as running and swimming.

As of 1998, a total of 14 different studies had investigated the effects of creatine on actual physical performance done outside a laboratory in efforts ranging from a handful of seconds to more than 150 seconds. In 12 of the 14 studies, creatine supplementation did not produce significant improvements in performance. For example, a study that used 24 U. S. Navy Special Warfare personnel (SEALs) determined that creatine did not significantly improve the time taken to complete an obstacle course. More recently, a study involving 16 military personnel concluded that "it is unlikely that creatine will enhance the overall readiness or performance of soldiers." (In some studies, creatine supplementation actually *worsened* physical performances.) Collectively, this research shows that any improved performance that may occur in laboratory settings does not translate into improved performance in realistic situations.

Promoters of creatine supplementation feverishly insist that there are no adverse side effects reported in the scientific literature when it is consumed in the recommended dosages (typically 20 - 25 grams per day for 4 - 7 days for "loading" and then 2 grams per day for "maintenance.") And for the most part, their contention is true. The fact is that there have not been any adverse side effects reported in studies using 20 - 30 grams of creatine per day for up to seven days. Nor have there been any adverse side effects reported in studies using smaller dosages of 2 - 3 grams of creatine per day for longer periods up to seven weeks. However, this is nowhere near the months — or years — that an individual might use creatine.

Countless scientific, medical, and nutritional authorities agree that the long-term effects of creatine supplementation are unknown. There is also a concern that many individuals typically exceed the recommended dosage — undoubtedly putting them at greater risk for incurring adverse side effects. One final consideration in this regard: Most of the scientific studies have not included any formal way of assessing adverse side effects from creatine.

And while there have been no adverse side effects reported in scientific studies conducted in a laboratory setting, there has been an endless exchange of anecdotal accounts from around the world concerning individuals who have taken creatine and experienced an abundance of adverse side effects. Although these observations are anecdotal, their sheer volume is such that they cannot be ignored. Considering a study that surveyed 52 collegiate athletes who voluntarily took creatine is also important. Of the 52 athletes, 14 (26.9%) did not report any adverse effects. Stated otherwise, 38 (73.1%) reported at least one adverse side effect.

Due to individual variability, some individuals may be more susceptible to adverse side effects than others. However, the following potential side effects are of greatest concern: water retention, muscle cramping, dehydration/heat-related illness, muscle strains/dysfunction, gastrointestinal distress (such as an upset stomach, gastrointestinal pain, flatulence, nausea, and vomiting), and liver and kidney dysfunction. Based upon the scientific information that is available at this point in time, it is not advisable to use creatine without the approval of a physician. When it comes to creatine supplementation, be *cautious*, not *careless*.

Q: Is it safe to use herbs and other nutritional supplements that are natural?

A: First, remember that the Food and Drug Administration does not regulate herbs and other nutritional supplements for safety, effectiveness, purity, or potency. Due to this lack of federal oversight, you really do not know exactly what is in the products. Independent researchers finding ingredients in the products that were not listed on the labels is not uncommon. In one study, researchers analyzed 75 different nutritional products and found that seven (9.33%) contained substances that were not shown on the labels. Moreover, the active ingredient may be higher or lower than the amount listed on the label.

Independent testing of 16 dehydroepiandrosterone (DHEA) products found that only eight (50%) contained the exact amount of DHEA that was stated on the labels and the actual levels varied *as much as 150%*. Amazingly, three (18.75%) of the 16 products did not contain any DHEA whatsoever. And some products may have ingredients that are truly bizarre. In a review of 311 advertisements for nutritional supplements, the researchers noted 235 unique ingredients including ecdysterone which is an insect hormone with no known use in humans. Herbs and other nutritional supplements may also contain contaminants — most likely from the manufacturing process — such as aluminum, lead, mercury, and tin.

Many herbs and other nutritional supplements are promoted as "natural." Because a product claims to be "natural" or have "natural" ingredients does not mean that it is necessarily safe. Dirt is "natural," but that does not mean it is safe to eat. The truth is that many "natural" substances can be quite harmful including high-potency doses of some vitamins, minerals, and certain herbs.

For instance, large doses of the natural stimulants found in ginseng can cause hypertension, insomnia, depression, and skin blemishes. In addition, the medical literature contains numerous reports of severe liver toxicity linked to such widely used herbs as chaparral, comfrey, and germander. There are similar safety concerns with high-potency enzymes, inert glandulars, and animal extracts. One final point is that it is difficult to predict how some herbs interact with prescription and over-the-counter medications (as well as other nutritional supplements).

Finally, remember that many herbs and other nutritional supplements come with express or implied disease-related claims, and are marketed for specific therapeutic purposes for which there may not be valid scientific proof. In one study, researchers reviewed all of the clinical trials that were published in 1966 - 1992 and compared the pertinent human and/or animal studies to that of the manufacturer's claims. It was found that 8 of the 19 products (42%) had no published scientific evidence to support the promotional claims. Another 6 of the 19 (32%) were judged as being marketed in a misleading manner. The fact is that the majority of herbs and other nutritional supplements have no recognized role in nutrition.

Q: Does whey protein increase muscle mass more than other proteins?

A: The supplement industry has claimed that whey protein promotes greater increases in muscle mass than other proteins. As support for this contention, the supplement industry has referenced a study in which the subjects significantly increased their bodyweight. What the promoters failed to mention was that the subjects in this study were starved rats. In the study, rats that were fed a whey-protein formula regained their lost weight faster than other rats that were fed a free-amino acid mixture. Obviously, it is difficult to extrapolate the influence of whey protein on starved rats to that of healthy humans.

Q: Does the Zone Diet work?

A: Invented and promoted by Dr. Barry Sears, the Zone Diet calls for a food intake that consists of 40% carbohydrates, 30% protein, and 30% fat. There is very little scientific evidence that the Zone Diet is more effective than other diets. In one study, subjects were randomly assigned to one of two diets that provided 1,200 calories per day. One group followed the Zone Diet and the other a "traditional" diet that consisted of 65% carbohydrates, 15% protein, and 25% fat. After six weeks, both groups had similar losses of bodyweight and body fat. The fact is that any weight loss experienced from the Zone Diet — or any other diet, for that matter — is the result of caloric restriction.

With that said, there are a number of concerns with the Zone Diet. Following the Zone Diet does not allow for the intake of a variety of foods that are required to meet nutritional needs. Rather, it calls for the consumption of a high amount of protein and fat. To achieve this, you must decrease your intake of carbohydrates. Doing so restricts the intake of healthy foods — such as fruits, vegetables, and whole-grain products — which may lead to vitamin and mineral deficiencies. Since fewer carbohydrates are available as a source of energy, you will also fatigue more quickly during physical activities.

More importantly, however, the Zone Diet poses significant health risks. The National Research Council recommends against consuming protein in amounts greater than twice the Recommended Dietary Allowances because high intakes are associated with certain cancers and heart disease. A high intake of fat is also associated with heart disease. Consider this: In the aforementioned study, the group that used the "traditional" diet had a decrease in triglycerides while the group that used the Zone Diet had an increase. (Elevated levels of triglycerides are associated with a greater risk of heart disease.) In addition, a high intake of protein increases the loss of calcium in the urine which may facilitate osteoporosis. A high intake of protein also increases the levels of uric acid which may cause gout in those who are susceptible. Excreting an excessive amount of protein stresses the liver and kidneys. There are additional concerns as well. Eating a well-balanced nutritional diet with a restricted caloric intake, combined with regular physical activity is the best way to lose weight.

Asking questions and continually educating yourself is the best way to achieve a healthy and physically fit body.

Chapter 20
Time to Deploy!

SWAT Fitness has provided you with a means to achieve an elite level of physical fitness. By understanding the importance of physical fitness, basic anatomy, muscular function, and exercise physiology you can determine your specific goals and objectives. Developing a comprehensive training program should include a cross-section of exercises designed to increase your strength, power, endurance, and flexibility, as well as your aerobic, anaerobic, and metabolic conditioning. If an injury occurs, then rehabilitative training will be critical to a rapid recovery. Understanding and utilizing the various formulas provided will allow you the ability to customize training and nutrition programs to meet your individual needs.

Proper nutrition and weight management will not only make you feel better, but will enhance the effectiveness of your training program. Whether your goal is to gain or lose weight, what and when you eat will have a direct impact on your ability to achieve the desired results. Eating high-quality foods instead of purchasing expensive nutritional supplements offers the opportunity to reach your physical potential in a much safer and more effective manner.

Operational fitness standards for SWAT team personnel set criteria for law enforcement agencies to follow. Each standard presented contains a detailed explanation of performance expectations along with the rationale and justification for compliance. Judicial decisions in this area now compel law enforcement agencies to enact non-discriminatory job-related standards. These standards reduce department liability, and increase the ability to select and maintain SWAT officers who are best suited to perform physically on critical incidents.

Sample workout programs are provided to meet a variety of training requirements. They can be customized for your specific goals and needs. Accurate documentation of your workouts will enable you to evaluate progress and to determine necessary adjustments. The Aerobic-, Anaerobic-, and Strength-Training Logs in Appendices A, B, and C provide an easy-to-use format to record information from all of your training sessions. Keeping these records will accelerate your progress.

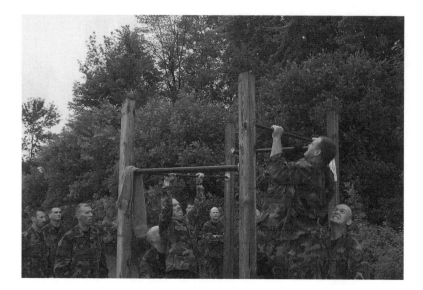

Whether you train by yourself, with a partner, or with a team, your level of intensity in training is critical to "game day" success.

Now it is up to you to provide the final ingredient for success: Intensity. A high level of intensity in every training session is fundamental to achieving your goals. Whether you are training for a future SWAT mission that could occur in a week or a month, or are training for a future competitive event, your intensity level in each workout is paramount. In other words, the precise moment when you are training is most important to your future success. Do not look past your workouts to "game day." Adopt a "Right Here – Right Now" training philosophy. Give everything you have in each training session. This will ensure success when your SWAT mission or competitive event is "Right Here – Right Now."

A SWAT call-out can occur at anytime, without warning. The following is a first-hand account of a 24-hour period in the life of one of the co-authors, as a SWAT Team member. To be able to participate in an average of 200 tactical operations per year, a high level of physical fitness was required to successfully complete the required objectives. During this 24-hour period, a series of critical incidents occurred where high stress levels were present, buildings were searched, multiple suspects were arrested, combative suspects were pursued and subdued, long hours were worked with minimal rest before the next mission, potentially incapacitating injuries occurred and were managed, and additional injuries were prevented; all relating to physical fitness.

To be an effective SWAT officer requires a high level of physical fitness achieved through hard work and dedication in the gym, as well as proficiency in tactical skills. During the following consecutive critical incidents, all of my physical fitness training would come into play in order to fulfill my responsibilities.

On December 10, 1992, after working a complete shift, our SWAT team was called back to work to execute a high-risk search warrant for crack cocaine at an apartment in Gaithersburg, Maryland. We were briefed by the narcotics investigators that multiple suspects were inside the apartment. The suspects had just sold crack cocaine to an informant. We formulated our tactical plans, assigning each officer on the team an area of responsibility. At 10:40pm we rammed the front door of the residence, breaking it off the frame and entered the apartment. I was assigned to the rear bedroom and with the assistance of my teammate, restrained and arrested three drug dealers who were in possession of crack cocaine inside of the bedroom. They were not cooperative and had to be forced to the ground and handcuffed. They were then turned over to the narcotics investigators for interrogation and processing. We finished the tactical operation at 11:20pm.

After returning home to sleep, we reported to our SWAT office the next morning, December 11, 1992, at 8:00am to prepare to execute high-risk search and arrest warrants at a house in Silver Spring, Maryland. Two suspects who were wanted for armed robbery were believed to be inside of the residence. At 10:20am, we entered the residence of the suspects by ramming the front door. Our team conducted a complete search of the location, however no one was found. After debriefing the operation, we went to the gym to continue our physical training. In the afternoon, we practiced SWAT tactics and finished our workday at 4:00pm.

Later that evening, at 9:15pm, we were called to execute a high-risk search warrant for crack cocaine at another apartment in Gaithersburg, Maryland. Physical fitness had always been a top priority. However, this particular evening it would be critical to the apprehension and arrest of a violent career criminal and several crack cocaine dealers. We received the briefing from the narcotics investigators and made our tactical assignments. Multiple armed drug dealers were inside the apartment. Narcotics officers had used informants to make two previous purchases of crack cocaine inside of the apartment.

The front door of the apartment was rammed and I proceeded down the hallway where I encountered one of the suspects. He attempted to run from the hallway to the master bedroom, but I was able to catch him just as he started to enter the room. He was forced to the ground and handcuffed. A search of the residence was then conducted. Three loaded handguns and one loaded shotgun were seized from the master bedroom. Eight ounces of crack cocaine, quantities of marijuana, and $13,000.00 in U.S currency were also seized in the raid. A total of four suspects were arrested inside of the apartment and charged with multiple crimes. One of the suspects received a mandatory five-year prison sentence under the Drug Kingpin statute.

After we made our entry and the apartment was secured, the front door was closed. On many occasions, additional people come to purchase drugs, not knowing the SWAT team and undercover narcotics officers are still inside. Once my initial assignment was complete, I took over responsibility of front door security. Within minutes there was a knock on the door. I prepared other SWAT officers inside of the apartment to take action and then opened the door.

As the 6'1", 190-pound male stepped into the apartment, I grabbed his jacket and turned him toward the inside wall. When I glanced down to see his two-year-old son standing next to him, he struck me full force in my face, with his elbow. Two bones in my face were instantly broken. He then ran out of the partially opened door, leaving his young son inside. My training and instincts took over when I tightened my grip on his jacket, causing him to pull me out of the apartment and down a flight of stairs. While we were descending the stairs, I was able to regain some control and tackle him when we reached the landing. A fight ensued, until he was finally restrained.

This suspect was on probation for narcotics offenses. He came to the apartment with one ounce of crack cocaine in his pocket and wanted to purchase more. Fighting with and subduing a slightly larger, very athletic, determined individual, after sustaining a devastating injury would not have been possible without a high level of physical fitness. This suspect was willing to leave his two-year-old child and fight to escape from the area. He was motivated not to return to prison. As a law enforcement officer, these are the people that should motivate you to train even harder. Intensity and preparation in the gym directly relates to intensity and success on tactical operations. Your life is dependant upon your level of physical fitness.

We responded to three tactical incidents within a 24-hour period, utilizing physical fitness throughout. Our SWAT team was successful because everyone on the team was prepared both mentally and *physically. Mental and physical preparation is applicable to athletes and people in all occupations; relating to not only work performance, but also everyday life.*

Approximately one month later, I underwent reconstructive facial surgery for 4½ hours. Micro-pulverized bone particles were inserted into my face to repair the damage. The surgery was performed on Thursday, January 21, 1993. On Monday, January 25, 1993, four days after surgery, I participated in the execution of a high-risk search and arrest warrant for a fugitive wanted for battery, and who was also a suspect in three armored car robberies. The suspect was successfully apprehended inside of his apartment. Again, the benefits of a high level of physical fitness were demonstrated by an accelerated recovery period from a serious debilitating injury.

Incidents such as these demonstrate the importance of physical fitness. However, it is up to you to realize the significance of fitness, and the role it plays in all aspects of a SWAT response to critical incidents and in your daily life. A comprehensive training program should be designed and implemented to meet your specific needs. These needs can include seeking an improved appearance or psychological benefits when you feel better about yourself. Every day a high level of physical fitness can improve your quality of life. And when you call upon your body and mind to perform under adverse conditions, the desired response will be obtainable.

The education that SWAT Fitness has provided, along with desire and intensity, are the necessary elements for you to reach a high level of physical fitness. Success will be hard earned, but will allow you the opportunity to achieve your goals in all areas of your personal and professional life. Regardless of your occupation, whether you are currently fit or are just starting a training program, take the next step down the path to improved fitness and put yourself in a position to be successful in life.

Excellence through superior preparation. Always train hard and with a purpose.

Appendix A: *SWAT FITNESS AEROBIC TRAINING LOG*

NAME:

DATE	BODY WEIGHT	ACTIVITY	TIME	DISTANCE	PACE	EXERCISE HEART RATE	RECOVERY HEART RATE

AGE-PREDICTED MAXIMUM HEART RATE: **HEART-RATE TRAINING ZONE:**   -

APPENDIX A: SAMPLE WORKOUT CARD FOR AEROBIC TRAINING

Appendix B: *SWAT FITNESS ANAEROBIC TRAINING LOG*

NAME:

DATE	BODY WEIGHT	ACTIVITY	REPS	DISTANCE	WORK INTERVAL	RECOVERY INTERVAL	WORKOUT DISTANCE

AGE-PREDICTED MAXIMUM HEART RATE:	HEART-RATE TRAINING ZONE:	-

APPENDIX B: SAMPLE WORKOUT CARD FOR ANAEROBIC TRAINING

Appendix C: *SWAT FITNESS STRENGTH TRAINING LOG*

NAME:			DATE:														
			BW:														
	EXERCISE	REPS	SEAT	wt / reps	wt / reps	wt / reps	wt / reps	wt / reps	wt / reps	wt / reps	wt / reps	wt / reps	wt / reps	wt / reps	wt / reps	wt / reps
Neck (2-4)																	
Hips (1)																	
Upper Leg (2)																	
Lower Leg (1)																	
Chest (2)																	
Upper Back (2)																	
Shoulders (2)																	
Upper Arm (2)																	
Lower Arm (1)																	
Abdominals (1-2)																	
Lower Back (1)																	
Other																	

APPENDIX C: SAMPLE WORKOUT CARD FOR SINGLE-SET TRAINING

Appendix D: *SWAT FITNESS STRENGTH TRAINING LOG*

NAME:			DATE:																	
			BW:																		
	EXERCISE	REPS	SEAT	wt/reps	wt/reps	wt/reps	wt/reps	wt/reps	wt/reps	wt/reps	wt/reps	wt/reps	wt/reps	wt/reps	wt/reps					
Neck (2-4)																				
Hips (1)																				
Upper Leg (2)																				
Lower Leg (1)																				
Chest (2)																				
Upper Back (2)																				
Shoulders (2)																				
Upper Arm (2)																				
Lower Arm (1)																				
Abdominals (1-2)																				
Lower Back (1)																				
Other																				

APPENDIX D: SAMPLE WORKOUT CARD FOR MULTIPLE-SET TRAINING

Appendix E: SUMMARY OF FREE-WEIGHT EXERCISES

EXERCISE	MUSCLE(S) INVOLVED	REPS
Deadlift (BB,DB,TB)	gluteus maximus, hamstrings, quadriceps, and erector spinae	15-20
Standing Calf Raise (DB)	gastrocnemius	10-15
Bench Press (BB,DB)	chest, anterior deltoid, and triceps	6-12
Incline Press (BB,DB)	chest (upper portion), anterior deltoid, and triceps	6-12
Decline Press (BB,DB)	chest (lower portion), anterior deltoid, and triceps	6-12
Dip (BW)	chest (lower portion), anterior deltoid, and triceps	6-12
Bent-Arm Fly (DB)	chest and anterior deltoid	6-12
Bent-Over Row (DB)	upper back ("lats"), biceps, and forearms	6-12
Chin (BW)	upper back ("lats"), biceps, and forearms	6-12
Pull-Up (BW)	upper back ("lats"), biceps, and forearms	6-12
Pullover (BB,DB)	upper back ("lats")	6-12
Seated Press (BB,DB)	anterior deltoid and triceps	6-12
Lateral Raise (DB)	middle deltoid and trapezius (upper portion)	6-12
Front Raise (DB)	anterior deltoid	6-12
Bent-Over Raise (DB)	posterior deltoid and trapezius (middle portion)	6-12
Internal Rotation (DB)	internal rotators	8-12
External Rotation (DB)	external rotators	8-12
Upright Row (BB,DB)	trapezius (upper portion), biceps, and forearms	6-12
Shoulder Shrug (BB,DB,TB)	trapezius (upper portion)	8-12
Bicep Curl (BB,DB)	biceps and forearms	6-12
Tricep Extension (BB,DB)	triceps	6-12
Wrist Flexion (BB,DB)	wrist flexors	8-12
Wrist Extension (DB)	wrist extensors	8-12
Finger Flexion (BB,DB)	finger flexors	8-12
Sit-Up (BW)	rectus abdominis and iliopsoas	8-12
Knee-Up (BW)	iliopsoas and rectus abdominis (lower portion)	8-12
Side Bend (DB)	obliques and erector spinae	8-12
Back Extension (BW)	erector spinae	10-15

EQUIPMENT CODES: BB = Barbell; BW = Bodyweight; DB = Dumbbells; TB = Trap Bar

NOTE: If more than one muscle is involved in an exercise, the first one listed is considered to be the prime mover. For example, the bench press involves the chest, anterior deltoid, and triceps. However, it is considered to be a chest exercise.

Appendix F: SUMMARY OF MACHINE EXERCISES

EXERCISE	MUSCLE(S) INVOLVED	REPS
Leg Press	gluteus maximus, quadriceps, and hamstrings	15-20
Hip Abduction	gluteus medius	10-15
Hip Adduction	hip adductors	10-15
Prone Leg Curl	hamstrings	10-15
Seated Leg Curl	hamstrings	10-15
Leg Extension	quadriceps	10-15
Standing Calf Raise	gastrocnemius	10-15
Seated Calf Raise	gastrocnemius and soleus	10-15
Dorsi Flexion	dorsi flexors	10-15
Chest Press	chest, anterior deltoid, and triceps	6-12
Pec Fly	chest and anterior deltoid	6-12
Seated Row	upper back ("lats"), biceps, and forearms	6-12
Underhand Lat Pulldown	upper back ("lats"), biceps, and forearms	6-12
Overhand Lat Pulldown	upper back ("lats"), biceps, and forearms	6-12
Pullover	upper back ("lats")	6-12
Shoulder Press	anterior deltoid and triceps	6-12
Lateral Raise	middle deltoid and trapezius (upper portion)	6-12
Internal Rotation	internal rotators	8-12
External Rotation	external rotators	8-12
Upright Row	trapezius (upper portion), biceps, and forearms	6-12
Scapulae Retraction	trapezius (middle portion)	8-12
Bicep Curl	biceps and forearms	6-12
Tricep Extension	triceps	6-12
Wrist Flexion	wrist flexors	8-12
Wrist Extension	wrist extensors	8-12
Abdominal	rectus abdominis and iliopsoas	8-12
Side Bend	obliques and erector spinae	8-12
Rotary Torso	obliques and erector spinae	8-12
Back Extension	erector spinae	10-15
Neck Flexion	sternocleidomastoideus	8-12
Neck Extension	neck extensors and trapezius (upper portion)	8-12
Neck Lateral Flexion	sternocleidomastoideus	8-12

NOTE: If more than one muscle is involved in an exercise, the first one listed is considered to be the prime mover. For example, the seated row involves the upper back ("lats"), biceps, and forearms. However, it is considered to be an upper-back exercise.

Appendix G:
SUMMARY OF MANUAL-RESISTANCE EXERCISES

EXERCISE	MUSCLE(S) INVOLVED	REPS
Hip Abduction	gluteus medius	10-15
Hip Adduction	hip adductors	10-15
Prone Leg Curl	hamstrings	10-15
Leg Extension	quadriceps	10-15
Dorsi Flexion	dorsi flexors	10-15
Push-up	chest, anterior deltoid, and triceps	6-12
Bent-Arm Fly	chest and anterior deltoid	6-12
Bent-Over Row	upper back ("lats")	6-12
Seated Row	upper back ("lats"), biceps, and forearms	6-12
Lat Pulldown	upper back ("lats")	6-12
Seated Press	anterior deltoid and triceps	6-12
Lateral Raise	middle deltoid and trapezius (upper portion)	6-12
Front Raise	anterior deltoid	6-12
Internal Rotation	internal rotators	8-12
External Rotation	external rotators	8-12
Bicep Curl	biceps and forearms	6-12
Tricep Extension	triceps	6-12
Sit-up	rectus abdominis	8-12
Neck Flexion	sternocleidomastoideus	8-12
Neck Extension	neck extensors and trapezius (upper portion)	8-12

NOTE: If more than one muscle is involved in an exercise, the first one listed is considered to be the prime mover. For example, the bicep curl involves the biceps and forearms. However, it is considered to be a biceps exercise.

Bibliography

Adams, J. A. 1987. Historical review and appraisal of research on the learning, retention and transfer of human motor skills. *Psychological Bulletin* 101 (1): 41-74.

Allison, D. B., and S. B. Heymsfield. 1998. "Natural" therapeutics for weight loss: garden of slender delights or dangerous alchemy? *Nutrition & the M. D.* 24 (1): 1-3.

American College of Sports Medicine [ACSM]. 2000. *ACSM's guidelines for graded exercise testing and exercise prescription. 6th ed.* Philadelphia, PA: Lippincott Williams & Wilkins.

American Council on Exercise [ACE]. 1991. *Personal trainer manual: the resource for fitness instructors.* San Diego, CA: ACE.

Anderson, O. 2002. You do have a "fat-burning zone," but do you really want to go there to "burn off" fat? *Running Research News* 18 (2): 7-10.

Andress, B. 1997. *Detroit Tigers off-season conditioning.* Detroit, MI: Detroit Tigers.

Andrews, J. G., J. G. Hay and C. L. Vaughan. 1983. Knee shear forces during a squat exercise using a barbell and a weight machine. In *Biomechanics VIII-B,* ed. H. Matsui and K. Kobayashi, 923-927. Champaign, IL: Human Kinetics Publishers, Inc.

Arendt, E. A. 1984. Strength development: a comparison of resistive exercise techniques. *Contemporary Orthopedics* 9 (3): 67-72.

Asimov, I. 1992. *The human body: its structure and operation. Revised ed.* New York, NY: Mentor.

Asmussen, E. 1952. Positive and negative muscular work. *Acta Physiologica Scandinavica* 28: 364-382.

Astrand, I. 1960. Aerobic work capacity in men and women with special reference to age. *Acta Physiologica Scandinavica* 49 (Supplementum 169): 1-92.

Astrand, P.-O., and K. Rodahl. 1977. *Textbook of work physiology. 2d ed.* New York, NY: McGraw-Hill Book Company.

Bachman, J. C. 1961. Specificity vs. generality in learning and performing two large muscle motor tasks. *Research Quarterly* 32: 3-11.

Barrette, E. P. 1998. Creatine supplementation for enhancement of athletic performance. *Alternative Medicine Alert* 1 (7): 73-84.

Barron, R. L., and G. J. Vanscoy. 1993. Natural products and the athlete: facts and folklore. *Annals of Pharmacotherapy* 27 (5): 607-615.

Bates, B., M. Wolf and J. Blunk. 1990. *Vanderbilt University strength and conditioning manual.* Nashville, TN: Vanderbilt University.

Ben-Ezra, V. 1992. Assessing physical fitness. In *The Stairmaster fitness handbook,* ed. J. A. Peterson and C. X. Bryant, 91-108. Indianapolis, IN: Masters Press.

Bennett, T., G. Bathalon, D. Armstrong III, B. Martin, R. Coll, R. Beck, T. Barkdull, K. O'Brien and P.A. Deuster. 2001. Effect of creatine on performance of militarily relevant tasks and soldier health. *Military Medicine* 166 (11): 996-1002.

Blakey, J. B., and D. Southard. 1987. The combined effects of weight training and plyometrics on dynamic leg strength and leg power. *Journal of Applied Sport Science Research* 1 (1): 14-16.

Blankenship, W. C. 1952. Transfer effects in neuro-muscular responses involving choice. Master of arts dissertation. University of California.

Blattner, S., and L. Noble. 1979. Relative effects of isokinetic and plyometric training on vertical jumping performance. *Research Quarterly* 50 (4): 583-588.

Bobbert, M. F., and A. J. van Soest. 1994. Effects of muscle strengthening on vertical jump height. *Medicine and Science in Sports and Exercise* 26 (8): 1012-1020.

Bolotte, C. P. 1998. Creatine supplementation in athletes: benefits and potential risks. *Journal of the Louisiana State Medical Society* 150 (July): 325-328.

Boocock, M. G., G. Garbutt, K. Linge, T. Reilly and J. D. Troup. 1990. Changes in stature following drop jumping and post-exercise gravity inversion. *Medicine and Science in Sports and Exercise* 22 (3): 385-390.

Borms, J., W. D. Ross, W. Duquet and J. E. L. Carter. 1986. Somatotypes of world class body builders. In *Perspectives in kinanthropometry,* ed. J. A. P. Day, 81-90. Champaign, IL: Human Kinetics Publishers, Inc.

Bouchard, C. 1983. Genetics of physiological fitness and motor performance. *Exercise and Sport Sciences Reviews* 11: 306-339.

Bouchard, C., and G. Lortie. 1984. Heredity and endurance performance. *Sports Medicine* 1: 38-64.

Bouchard, C., M. R. Boulay, J.-A. Simoneau, G. Lortie and L. Perusse. 1988. Heredity and trainability of aerobic and anaerobic performances: an update. *Sports Medicine* 5 (2): 69-73.

Brady, T. A., B. R. Cahill and L. M. Bodnar. 1982. Weight training-related injuries in the high school athlete. *The American Journal of Sports Medicine* 10 (1): 1-5.

Braith, R. W., J. E. Graves, M. L. Pollock, S. H. Leggett, D. M. Carpenter and A. B. Colvin. Comparison of 2 vs 3 days/week of variable resistance training during 10- and 18-week programs. *International Journal of Sports Medicine* 10 (6): 450-454.

Brand-Miller, J., S. Colagiuri, T. M. S. Wolever and K. Foster-Powell. 1999. *The glucose revolution.* New York, NY: Marlowe & Company.

Bryant, C. X., B. A. Franklin and J. M. Conviser. 2002. *Exercise testing and program design: a fitness professional's handbook.* Monterey, CA: Exercise Science Publishers.

Bryant, C. X. 1995. Understanding crossrobic training. In *The Stairmaster fitness handbook, 2d ed,* ed. J. A. Peterson and C. X. Bryant, 81-105. St. Louis, MO: Wellness Bookshelf.

Bryant, C. X. 1988. *How to develop muscular power.* Indianapolis, IN: Masters Press.

Bryant, C. X., and J. A. Peterson. 1992. Estimating aerobic fitness. *Fitness Management* 9 (August): 36-39.

Bryant, C. X., and J. A. Peterson. 1994. Strength training for the heart? *Fitness Management* 10 (February): 32-34.

Bryant, C.X., J. A. Peterson and R. J. Hagen. 1994. Weight loss: unfolding the truth. *Fitness Management* 10 (May): 42-44.

Bryant, C. X., and J. A. Peterson. 1996. All exercise is not equal. *Fitness Management* 12 (July): 32-34.

Brzycki, M. M. 1995. *A practical approach to strength training. 3d ed.* Indianapolis, IN: Masters Press.

_____. 1997. *Cross training for fitness.* Indianapolis, IN: Masters Press.

_____. 1986. Plyometrics: a giant step backwards. *Athletic Journal* 66 (April): 22-23.

_____. 1993. Strength testing — predicting a one-rep max from reps-to-fatigue. *The Journal of Physical Education, Recreation & Dance* 64 (1): 88-90.

_____. 1996. Improving skills: what the research says. *Wrestling USA* 35, no. 4 (November 15, 1999): 8-11.

_____. 1998. Fiber types and repetition ranges. *Wrestling USA* 33 (10): 9-10, 12.

_____. 1998. Quality REPS. *Fitness Management* 14 (June): 44-46.

_____. 1998. Strength training: what approach? *Coach and Athletic Director* 68 (November): 32-34.

_____. 1999. Free weights and machines. *Fitness Management* 15 (June): 36-37, 40.

_____. 1999. Losing fat: high or low intensity? *Wrestling USA* 35 (2): 14-15.

_____. 2000. Prescription for rehabilitative strength training. *Fitness Management* 16 (February): 40-41.

_____. 2000. Assessing strength. *Fitness Management* 16 (June): 34-37.

_____. 2000. Creatine supplementation: effective and safe? *Master Trainer* 10: 11-18.

_____. 2001. A practical approach to power training. *Strength and Health* 1 (4): 18-20.

_____. 2002. Tactical strength: the basics. *S.W.A.T.* 21 (5): 20-21, 70.

_____. 2002. Spicing up strength-training programs with variety. *Fitness Management* 18 (June): 40, 42, 44.

Bubb, W. J. 1992. Nutrition. In *Health fitness instructor's handbook, 2d ed*, by E. T. Howley and B. D. Franks, 95-114. Champaign, IL: Human Kinetics Publishers, Inc.

_____. 1992. Relative leanness. In *Health fitness instructor's handbook, 2d ed*, by E. T. Howley and B. D. Franks, 115-130. Champaign, IL: Human Kinetics Publishers, Inc.

Burke, L. M., G. R. Collier and M. Hargreaves. 1993. Muscle glycogen storage after prolonged exercise: effect of the glycemic index of carbohydrate feeding. *Journal of Applied Physiology* 75 (2): 1019-1023.

Butterfield, G. 1991. Amino acids and high protein diets. In *Perspectives in exercise science and sports medicine, volume 4*, ed. D. R. Lamb and M. Williams, 87-122. Indianapolis, IN: Brown & Benchmark.

Calder, A. W., P. D. Chilibeck, C. E. Webber and D. G. Sale. 1994. Comparison of whole and split weight training routines in young women. *Canadian Journal of Applied Physiology* 19 (2): 185-199.

Cappozzo, A., F. Felici, F. Figura and F. Gazzani. 1985. Lumbar spine loading during half-squat exercises. *Medicine and Science in Sports and Exercise* 17 (5): 613-620.

Carpinelli, R. N. 1999. Serious strength training. *High Intensity Training Newsletter* 9 (6): 9-10.

_____. 2001. The science of strength training. *Master Trainer* 11 (4): 10-17.

_____. 2002. Berger in retrospect: effect of varied weight training programmes on strength. *British Journal of Sports Medicine* 36 (5): 319-324.

Carpinelli, R. N., and B. Gutin. 1991. Effect of miometric and pliometric muscle actions on delayed muscle soreness. *Journal of Applied Sport Science Research* 5 (2): 66-70.

Carpinelli, R. N., and R. M. Otto. 1998. Strength training. Single versus multiple sets. *Sports Medicine* 26 (2): 73-84.

Carter, J. E. L. 1970. The somatotypes of athletes - a review. *Human Biology* 42 (4): 535-569.

Carter, J. E. L., and B. H. Heath. 1971. Somatotype methodology and kinesiology research. *Kinesiology Review* 1: 10-19.

Chapman, P. P., J. R. Whitehead and R. H. Binkert. 1998. The 225-lb reps-to-fatigue test as a submaximal estimate of 1-RM bench press performance in college football players. *Journal of Strength and Conditioning Research* 12 (4): 258-261.

Chestnut, J. L., and D. Docherty. 1999. The effects of 4 and 10 repetition maximum weight-training protocols on neuromuscular adaptations in untrained men. *Journal of Strength and Conditioning Research* 13 (4): 353-359.

Cheuvront, S. N. 1999. The Zone Diet and athletic performance. *Sports Medicine* 27 (4): 213-228.

Christenson, D., and S. Melville. 1988. The effects of depth jumps on university football players. *Journal of Applied Sport Science Research* 2 (3): 54.

City of New York Department of Consumer Affairs. 1992. *Magic muscle pills!! Health and fitness quackery in nutrition supplements*. New York, NY: Department of Consumer Affairs.

Clark, N. 1990. *Nancy Clark's sports nutrition guidebook*. Champaign, IL: Leisure Press.

Clarkson, P. M., and I. Tremblay. 1988. Rapid adaptation to exercise induced muscle damage. *Journal of Applied Physiology* 65 (1): 1-6.

Clarkson, P. M., and E. S. Rawson. 1999. Nutritional supplements to increase muscle mass. *Clinical Reviews in Food Science and Nutrition* 39 (4): 317-328.

Clausen, J. P. 1977. Effect of physical training on cardiovascular adjustments to exercise in man. *Physiological Reviews* 57 (4): 779-815.

Clutch, D., M. Wilton, C. McGown and G. R. Bryce. 1983. The effect of depth jumps and weight training on leg strength and vertical jump. *Research Quarterly for Exercise and Sport* 54 (1): 5-10.

Coleman, E. 1997. The chromium picolinate weight loss scam. *Sports Medicine Digest* 19 (1): 6-7.

_____. 2000. Does whey protein enhance performance? *Sports Medicine Digest* 22 (7): 80, 82.

_____. 2001. Being supplement savvy. *Sports Medicine Digest* 24 (4): 46-47.

Colliander, E. B., and P. A. Tesch. 1990. Effects of eccentric and concentric muscle actions in resistance training. *Acta Physiologica Scandinavica* 140 (1): 31-39.

Cook, S. D., G. Schultz, M. L. Omey, M. W. Wolfe and M. F. Brunet. 1993. Development of lower leg strength and flexibility with the strength shoe. *The American Journal of Sports Medicine* 21 (3): 445-448.

Costill, D. L., W. J. Fink and M. L. Pollock. 1976. Muscle fiber composition and enzyme activities of elite distance runners. *Medicine and Science in Sports* 8 (2): 96-100.

Costill, D. L., J. Daniels, W. Evans, W. F. Fink, G. S. Krahenbuhl and B. Saltin. 1976. Skeletal muscle enzymes and fiber composition in male and female track athletes. *Journal of Applied Physiology* 40 (2): 149-154.

Costill, D. L., G. P. Dalsky and W. J. Fink. 1978. Effects of caffeine ingestion on metabolism and exercise performance. *Medicine and Science in Sports and Exercise* 10 (3): 155-158.

Crouch, J. E. 1978. *Functional human anatomy. 3d ed*. Philadelphia, PA: Lea & Febiger.

Cummings, S., E. S. Parham and G. W. Strain. 2002. Position of the American Dietetic Association: weight management. *Journal of The American Dietetic Association* 102 (8): 1145-1155.

Daniels, J. 1989. Training distance runners — a primer. *Sports Science Exchange* 1 (11): 1-4.

DeLateur, B. J., J. F. Lehman and R. Giaconi. 1976. Mechanical work and fatigue: their roles in the development of muscle work capacity. *Archives of Physical Medicine and Rehabilitation* 57 (1): 319-324.

DeLorme, T. L. 1945. Restoration of muscle power by heavy resistance exercise. *Journal of Bone and Joint Surgery* 27 (October): 645-667.

DeLorme, T. L., and A. L. Watkins. 1948. Techniques of progressive resistance exercise. *Archives of Physical Medicine* 27 (October): 645-667.

Department of Health and Human Services. 2002. FDA warns public about Chinese diet pills containing fenfluramine. *FDA News* (August 13). <http://www.fda.gov/bbs/topics/NEWS/2002/NEW00826.html.

Department of Health and Human Services. 2003. HHS acts to reduce potential risks of dietary supplements containing ephedra. *FDA News* (February 28). <http://www.fda.gov/bbs/topics/NEWS/2003/NEW00875.html.

Desmedt, J. E., and E. Godaux. 1977. Fast motor units are not preferentially activated in rapid voluntary contractions in man. *Nature* 267 (5613): 717-719.

Deuster, P., A. Singh and P. Pelletier. 1994. *The Navy SEAL nutrition guide*. Bethesda, MD: Department of Military and Emergency Medicine Uniformed Services University of the Health Sciences F. Edward Hebert School of Medicine: 169-171.

deVries, H. A. 1974. *Physiology of exercise for physical education and athletics. 2d ed*. Dubuque, IA: William C. Brown.

van Dijk, M. J. 1994. Principles of physical training: implications for military training. *Annales Medicinne Militaris Belgicae* 8 (3): 18-25.

Dintiman, G. B. 1984. *How to run faster*. West Point, NY: Leisure Press.

Dons, B., K. Bollerup, F. Bonde-Petersen and S. Hancke. 1979. The effect of weight-lifting exercise related to muscle fiber composition and muscle cross-sectional area in humans. *European Journal of Applied Physiology* 40 (2): 95-106.

Drowatzky, J. N., and F. C. Zuccato. 1967. Interrelationships between selected measures of static and dynamic balance. *Research Quarterly* 38: 509-510.

Duda, M. 1988. Plyometrics: a legitimate form of power training? *The Physician and Sportsmedicine* 16 (3): 213-216, 218.

Dudley, G. A., P. A. Tesch, B. J. Miller and P. Buchanan. 1991. Importance of eccentric actions in performance adaptations to resistance training. *Aviation, Space, and Environmental Medicine* 62 (6): 543-550.

Dunn, J. R. 1989. Developing strength the L. A. Raiders way. *Strength and Fitness Quarterly* 1 (1): 7.

Durak, E. 1987. Physical performance responses to muscle lengthening and weight training exercises in young women. *Journal of Applied Sport Science Research* 1 (3): 60.

Enoka, R. M. 1994. *Neuromechanical basis of kinesiology. 2d ed*. Champaign, IL: Human Kinetics Publishers, Inc.

_____. 1988. Muscle strength and its development. *Sports Medicine* 6 (3): 146-168.

Ensign, W. Y., I. Jacobs, W. K. Prusaczyk, H. W. Goforth, P. B. Law and K. E. Schneider. 1998. Effects of creatine supplementation on short-term anaerobic exercise performance of U. S. Navy SEALs. *Medicine and Science in Sports and Exercise* 30 (5): S265.

Ernst, E. 1998. Harmless herbs? A review of the recent literature. *The American Journal of Medicine* 104 (February): 170-178.

Esbjornsson, M., C. Sylven, I. Holm and E. Jansson. 1993. Fast twitch fibres may predict anaerobic performance in both females and males. *International Journal of Sports Medicine* 14 (5): 257-263.

Fair, J. D. 1993. Isometrics or steroids? Exploring new frontiers of strength in the early 1960s. *Journal of Sport History* 20 (Spring): 1-24.

Falk, B., R. Burstein, I. Ashkanazi, O. Spilberg, J. Alter, E. Zylber-Katz, A. Rubenstein, N. Bashan and Y. Shapiro. 1989. The effects of caffeine ingestion on physical performance after prolonged exercise. *European Journal of Applied Physiology* 59 (3): 168-173.

Falk, B., R. Burstein, J. Rosenblum, Y. Shapiro, E. Zylber-Katz and N. Bashan. 1990. Effects of caffeine ingestion on body fluid balance and thermoregulation during exercise. *Canadian Journal of Physiology and Pharmacology* 68 (7): 889-892.

Farley, D. 1993. Dietary supplements: making sure hype doesn't overwhelm science. *FDA Consumer* 27 (November): 8-13.

Feigenbaum, M. S., and M. L. Pollock. 1997. Strength training: rationale for current guidelines for adult fitness programs. *The Physician and Sportsmedicine* 25 (2): 44-46, 49, 54-56, 63-64.

_____. 1999. Prescription of resistance training for health and disease. *Medicine and Science in Sports and Exercise* 31 (1): 38-45.

Fellingham, G. W., E. S. Roundy, A. G. Fisher and G. R. Bryce. 1978. Caloric cost of walking and running. *Medicine and Science in Sports and Exercise* 10 (2): 132-136.

Ferrando, A., and N. Green. 1993. The effect of boron supplementation on lean body mass, plasma testosterone levels and strength in bodybuilders. *International Journal of Sports Nutrition* 3 (2): 140-149.

Fincher II, G. 2000. Less is more in resistance training. *Biomechanics* 7 (11): 43-44,46,48,50,52.

_____. 2000. The effect of high intensity resistance training on peak upper and lower body power among collegiate football players. *Medicine and Science in Sports and Exercise* 32 (supplement): S152.

Fink, K. J., and B. Worthington-Roberts. 1995. Nutritional considerations for exercise. In *The Stairmaster fitness handbook, 2d ed*, ed. J. A. Peterson and C. X. Bryant, 205-228. St. Louis, MO: Wellness Bookshelf.

Fisher, E. 2003. Ephedra – weight loss and improved athletic performance. Over 100 deaths associated to the herbal drug. *The Washington Times* (February 18). <http://www.washingtontimes.com/sports.

Fitzgerald, G. K., J. M. Rothstein, T. P. Mayhew and R. L. Lamb. 1991. Exercise-induced muscle soreness after concentric and eccentric isokinetic contractions. *Physical Therapy* 71: 505-513.

Ford, Jr., H. T., J. R. Puckett, J. P. Drummond, K. Sawyer, K. Gantt and C. Fussell. 1983. Effects of three combinations of plyometric and weight training programs on selected physical fitness test items. *Perceptual and Motor Skills* 56 (3): 919-922.

Fowler, N. E., A. Lees and T. Reilly. 1994. Spinal shrinkage in unloaded and loaded drop-jumping. *Ergonomics* 37 (1): 133-139.

Fox, E. L., and D. K. Mathews. 1981. *The physiological basis of physical education and athletics. 3d ed*. Philadelphia, PA: Saunders College Publishing.

Fox, E. L. 1984. Physiology of exercise and physical fitness. In *Sports medicine*, ed. R. H. Strauss, 381-456. Philadelphia, PA: W. B. Saunders Company.

Frankel, V. H., and M. Nordin. 1980. *Basic biomechanics of the skeletal system*. Philadelphia, PA: Lea & Febiger.

Freedman, A. 1990. Specificity in exercise training. *Strength and Fitness Quarterly* 1 (3): 9.

Fukunaga, T., M. Miyatani, M. Tachi, M. Kouzaki, Y. Kawakami and H. Kanehisa. 2001. Muscle volume is a major determinant of joint torque in humans. *Acta Physiologica Scandinavica* 172 (4): 249-255.

Gannelli, S. 1997. *San Diego Padres 1997-98 off-season strength and conditioning manual*. San Diego, CA: San Diego Padres.

Garrett Jr., W. E., and T. R. Malone, eds. 1988. *Muscle development: nutritional alternatives to anabolic steroids*. Columbus, OH: Ross Laboratories.

Gettman, L. R., J.J. Ayres, M. L. Pollock and A. Jackson. 1978. The effect of circuit weight training on strength, cardiorespiratory function, and body composition of adult men. *Medicine and Science in Sports* 10 (3): 171-176.

Gettman, L. R., J.J. Ayres, M. L. Pollock, J. L. Durstine and W. Grantham. 1979. Physiologic effects on adult men of circuit strength training and jogging. *Archives of Physical Medicine and Rehabilitation* 60 (3): 115-120.

Gettman, L. R., P. Ward and R. D. Hagman. 1982. A comparison of combined running and weight training with circuit weight training. *Medicine and Science in Sports and Exercise* 14 (3): 229-234.

Gittleson, M. 1984. *Michigan football off-season conditioning*. Ann Arbor, MI: University of Michigan.

Goldberg, A. L., J. D. Etlinger, D. F. Goldspink and C. Jablecki. 1975. Mechanism of work-induced hypertrophy of skeletal muscle. *Medicine and Science in Sports* 7 (3): 248-261.

Goldman, R. M., and R. Klatz. 1992. *Death in the locker room: drugs & sports*. Chicago, IL: Elite Sports Medicine Publications, Inc.

Gollnick, P. D., B. F. Timson, R. L. Moore and M. Riedy. 1981 Muscular enlargement and number of fibers in skeletal muscles of rats. *Journal of Applied Physiology* 50 (5): 936-943.

Gonyea, W. J. 1980. Muscle fiber splitting in trained and untrained animals. *Exercise and Sport Sciences Reviews* 8: 19-39.

Gonyea, W. J., G. C. Ericson and F. Bonde-Petersen. 1977. Skeletal muscle fiber splitting induced by weight-lifting exercise in cats. *Acta Physiologica Scandinavica* 99 (1): 105-109.

Graham, A. S., and R. C. Hatton. 1999. Creatine: a review of efficacy and safety. *Journal of the American Pharmaceutical Association* 39 (6): 803-810.

Graham, T. E. 2001. Caffeine, coffee and ephedrine: impact on exercise performance and metabolism. *Canadian Journal of Applied Physiology* 26 (supplement): S103-S119.

Graham, T. E., and L. L. Spriet. 1996. Caffeine and exercise performance. *Sports Science Exchange* 9 (1): 1-5.

Graves, J. E., and M. L. Pollock. 1995. Understanding the physiological basis of muscular fitness. In *The Stairmaster fitness handbook, 2d ed*, ed. J. A. Peterson and C. X. Bryant, 67-80. St. Louis, MO: Wellness Bookshelf.

Graves, J. E., M. L. Pollock, S. H. Leggett, R. W. Braith, D. M. Carpenter and L. E. Bishop. 1988. Effect of reduced training frequency on muscular strength. *International Journal of Sports Medicine* 9 (5): 316-319.

Graves, J. E., M. L. Pollock, A. E. Jones, A. B. Colvin and S. H. Leggett. 1989. Specificity of limited range of motion variable resistance training. *Medicine and Science in Sports and Exercise* 21 (1): 84-89.

Graves, J. E., M. L. Pollock, D. Foster, S. H. Leggett, D. M. Carpenter, R. Vuoso and A. Jones. 1990. Effect of training frequency and specificity on isometric lumbar extension strength. *Spine* 15 (6): 504-509.

Guthrie, H. A. 1983. *Introductory nutrition. 5th ed*. St. Louis, MO: The C. V. Mosby Company.

Hakkinen, K., A. Pakarinen and M. Kallinen. 1992. Neuromuscular adaptations and serum hormones in women during short-term intensive strength training. *European Journal of Applied Physiology* 64 (2): 106-111.

Hallmark, M. A., T. H. Reynolds, C. A. DeSousa, C. O. Dotson, R. A. Anderson and M. A. Rogers. 1993. Effects of chromium supplementation and resistive training on muscle strength and lean body mass in untrained men. Abstract presented at the American College of Sports Medicine 40th Annual Meeting. Seattle, WA.

_____. 1996. Effects of chromium and resistive training on muscle strength and body composition. *Medicine and Science in Sports and Exercise* 28 (1): 139-144.

Hamel, P., J. A. Simoneau, G. Lortie, M. R. Boulay and C. Bouchard. 1986. Heredity and muscle adaptation to endurance training. *Medicine and Science in Sports and Exercise* 18 (6): 690-696.

van Handel, P. 1983. Caffeine. In *Ergogenic aids in sport*, ed. M. L. Williams, 128-163. Champaign, IL: Human Kinetics Publishers.

Harvard School of Public Health. 2002. Food pyramids. What should you really eat? <http://www.hsph.harvard.edu/nutritionsource/pyramids.html.

Hass, C. J., L. Garzarella, D. De Hoyos and M. L. Pollock. 2000. Single versus multiple sets in long-term recreational weightlifters. *Medicine and Science in Sports and Exercise* 32 (1): 235-242.

Hather, B. M., P. A. Tesch, P. Buchanan and G. A. Dudley. 1991. Influence of eccentric actions on skeletal muscle adaptations to resistance training. *Acta Physiologica Scandinavica* 143 (2): 177-185.

Hay, J. G., and J. G. Reid. 1988. *Anatomy, mechanics, and human motion. 2d ed*. Englewood Cliffs, NJ: Prentice-Hall, Inc.

Hellebrandt, F. A. 1958. Special review: application of the overload principle to muscle training in man. *American Journal of Physical Medicine* 37 (5): 278-283.

Hellebrandt, F. A., and S. J. Houtz. 1956. Mechanisms of muscle training in man: experimental demonstration of the overload principle. *Physical Therapy Review* 36 (6): 371-383.

Hempel, L. S., and C. L. Wells. 1985. Cardiorespiratory cost of the Nautilus express circuit. *The Physician and Sportsmedicine* 13 (4): 86-86, 91-97.

Henneman, E. 1957. Relation between size of neurons and their susceptibility to discharge. *Science* 126: 1345-1347.

Henry, F. M. 1961. Reaction time - movement time correlations. *Perceptual and Motor Skills* 12: 63-66.

_____. 1968. Specificity vs. generality in learning motor skill. In *Classical studies on physical activity*, ed. R. C. Brown and G. S. Kenyon. Englewood Cliffs, NJ: Prentice-Hall.

Herbert, V., and G. J. Subak-Sharpe, eds. 1990. *The Mount Sinai school of medicine complete book of nutrition*. New York, NY: St. Martin's Press.

Hickson, R. C., C. Kanakis, J. R. Davis, A. M. Moore and S. Rich. 1982. Reduced training duration effects on aerobic power, endurance and cardiac growth. *Journal of Applied Physiology* 53 (1): 225-229.

Higbie, E. J., K. J. Cureton, G. L. Warren III and B. M. Prior. 1996. Effects of concentric and eccentric training on muscle strength, cross-sectional area, and neural activation. *Journal of Applied Physiology* 81 (5): 2173-2181.

Hill, A. V. 1922. The maximum work and mechanical efficiency in human muscles, and their most economical speed. *Journal of Physiology* 56: 19-41.

Hirt, S. 1967. Historical bases for therapeutic exercise. *American Journal of Physical Medicine* 46 (1): 32-38.

Hoeger, W. W. K. 1988. *Principles and labs for physical fitness and wellness*. Englewood, CO: Morton Publishing Co.

Hoffman, B. 1939. *Weight lifting*. York, PA: Strength & Health Publishing Co.

Horrigan, J., and D. Shaw. 1990. Plyometrics: the dangers of depth jumps. *High Intensity Training Newsletter* 2 (4): 15-21.

Houston, M. E. 1999. Gaining weight: the scientific basis of increasing skeletal muscle mass. *Canadian Journal of Applied Physiology* 24 (4): 305-316.

Howley, E. T., and B. D. Franks. 1992. *Health fitness instructor's handbook. 2d ed*. Champaign, IL: Human Kinetics Publishers, Inc.

Howley, E. T., and M. Glover. 1974. The caloric costs of running and walking one mile for men and women. *Medicine and Science in Sports and Exercise* 6 (4): 235-237.

Humphries, B. J., R. U. Newton and G. J. Wilson. 1995. The effect of a braking device in reducing the ground impact forces inherent in plyometric training. *International Journal of Sports Medicine* 16 (2): 129-133.

Hurley, B. F., D. R. Seals, A. A. Ehsani, L.-J. Cartier, G. P. Dalsky, J. M. Hagberg and J. O. Holloszy. 1984. Effects of high-intensity strength training on cardiovascular function. *Medicine and Science in Sports and Exercise* 16 (5): 483-488.

Hutchins, K. 1992. *Super Slow: the ultimate exercise protocol. 2d ed*. Casselberry, FL: Super Slow Systems.

Huxley, H. E. 1958. The contraction of muscle. *Scientific American* 199 (5): 66-82.

Ikai, M., and T. Fukunaga. 1968. Calculation of muscle strength per unit cross-sectional area of human muscle by means of ultrasonic measurement. *Internationale Zeitschrift fur angewandte Physiologie einschliesslich Arbeitphysiologie* 26: 26-32.

_____. 1965. The mechanism of muscular contraction. *Scientific American* 213 (6): 18-27.

Ivy, J. L. 1991. Muscle glycogen synthesis before and after exercise. *Sports Medicine* 11 (1): 6-19.

_____. 2001. Dietary strategies to promote glycogen synthesis after exercise. *Canadian Journal of Applied Physiology* 26 (supplement): S236-S245.

Ivy, J. L., D. L. Costill, W. J. Fink and R. W. Lower. 1979. Influence of caffeine and carbohydrate feedings on endurance performance. *Medicine and Science in Sports and Exercise* 11 (1): 6-11.

Jakicic, J. M., K. Clark, E. Coleman, J. E. Donnelly, J. Foreyt, E. Melanson, J. Volek and S. L. Volpe. 2001. ACSM position stand on the appropriate intervention strategies for weight loss and prevention of weight regain for adults. *Medicine and Science in Sports and Exercise* 33 (12): 2145-2156.

Johnson, C., and J. G. Reid. 1991. Lumbar compressive and shear forces during various trunk curl-up exercises. *Clinical Biomechanics* 6: 97-104.

Jones, A. 1970. *Nautilus training principles, bulletin #1*. DeLand, FL: Arthur Jones Productions.

_____. 1971. *Nautilus training principles, bulletin #2*. DeLand, FL: Arthur Jones Productions.

_____. 1993. *The lumbar spine, the cervical spine and the knee: testing and rehabilitation*. Ocala, FL: MedX Corporation.

Jones, A., M. L. Pollock, J. E. Graves, M. Fulton, W. Jones, M. MacMillan. D. D. Baldwin and J. Cirulli. 1988. *Safe, specific testing and rehabilitative exercise of the muscles of the lumbar spine*. Santa Barbara, CA: Sequoia Communications.

Jones, N. L., N. McCartney and A. J. McComas, eds. 1986. *Human muscle power*. Champaign, IL: Human Kinetics Publishers, Inc.

Juhn, M. S., J. W. O'Kane and D. M. Vinci. 1999. Oral creatine supplementation in male collegiate athletes: a survey of dosing habits and side effects. *Journal of the American Dietetic Association* 99 (5): 593-595.

Juhn, M. S., and M. Tarnopolsky. 1998. Potential side effects of oral creatine supplementation: a critical review. *Clinical Journal of Sports Medicine* 8 (4): 298-304.

Kalamen, J. 1968. Measurement of maximum muscle power in man. Doctoral dissertation. Columbus, OH: The Ohio State University.

Kamber, M., N. Baume, M. Savgy and L. River. 2001. Nutritional supplements as a source for positive doping cases? *International Journal of Sport Nutrition and Exercise Metabolism* 11 (2): 258-263.

Kaneko, M., P. V. Komi and O. Aura. 1984. Mechanical efficiency of concentric and eccentric exercises performed with medium to fast contraction rates. *Scandinavian Journal of Sport Science* 6: 15-20.

Karlsson, J., P. V. Komi and J. H. T. Viitasalo. 1979. Muscle strength and muscle characteristics in monozygous and dizygous twins. *Acta Physiologica Scandinavica* 106 (3): 319-325.

Katch, F. I., P. M. Clarkson, W. A. Kroll and T. McBride. 1984. Effects of sit up exercise training on adipose cell size and adiposity. *Research Quarterly for Exercise and Sport* 55 (3): 242-247

Katzmarzyk, P. T., R. M. Malina, L. Perusse, T. Rice, M. A. Province, D. C. Rao and C. Bouchard. 2000. Familial resemblance for physique: heritabilities for somatotype components. *Annals of Human Biology* 27 (5): 467-477.

Kaczkowski, W., D. L. Montgomery, A. W. Taylor and V. Klissouras. 1982. The relationship between muscle fiber composition and maximal anaerobic power and capacity. *Journal of Sports Medicine* 22 (4): 407-413.

Kennedy, P. M. 1986. Setting the record straight about negative exercise. *Scholastic Coach* 56 (November): 22-23, 69.

Klein, K. K. 1962. Squats right. *Scholastic Coach* 32 (2): 36-38, 70-71.

Klissouras, V. 1971. Heritability of adaptive variation. *Journal of Applied Physiology* 31 (3): 338-344.

_____. 1973. Genetic aspects of physical fitness. *Journal of Sports Medicine* 13: 164-170.

_____. 1997. Heritability of adaptive variation: an old problem revisited. *The Journal of Sports Medicine and Physical Fitness* 37 (1): 1-6.

Komi, P. V., J. H. T. Viitasalo, M. Havu, A. Thorstensson, B. Sjodin and J. Karlsson. 1977. Skeletal muscle fibres and muscle enzyme activities in monozygous and dizygous twins of both sexes. *Acta Physiologica Scandinavica* 100 (4): 385-392.

Komi, P. V., and J. Karlsson. 1979. Physical performance, skeletal muscle enzyme activities and fiber types in monozygous and dizygous twins of both sexes. *Acta Physiologica Scandinavica* (Supplementum 462): 1-28.

Koshy, K. M., E. Griswold and E. E. Schneeberger. 1999. Interstitial nephritis in patient taking creatine. *New England Journal of Medicine* 340 (10): 814-815.

Kraemer, W. J. 1992. Involvement of eccentric muscle action may optimize adaptations to resistance training. *Sports Science Exchange* 4 (6): 1-4.

Kramer, J. F., A. Morrow and A. Leger. 1993. Changes in rowing ergometer, weight lifting, vertical jump and isokinetic performance in response to standard and standard plus plyometric training programs. *International Journal of Sports Medicine* 14 (8): 449-454.

Kreider, R. B. 1999. Dietary supplements and the promotion of muscle growth with resistance exercise. *Sports Medicine* 27 (2): 97-110.

Krieder, R. B., V. Miriel and E. Bertun. 1993. Amino acid supplementation and exercise performance: analysis of the proposed ergogenic value. *Sports Medicine* 16 (3): 190-209.

Kris-Etherton, P. M. 1989. The facts and fallacies of nutritional supplements for athletes. *Sports Science Exchange* 2 (8): 1-4.

Kuehl, K., L. Goldberg and D. Elliot. 1998. Renal insufficiency after creatine supplementation in a college football athlete. *Medicine and Science in Sports and Exercise* 30 (5): S235.

Lamb, D. R. 1984. *Physiology of exercise: responses & adaptations. 2d ed.* New York, NY: MacMillan Publishing Company.

Lambert, M.D., J. G. 2002. Tobacco use – smoking and smokeless tobacco. *A.D.A.M. Editorial* (September 19). <http:www.umm.edu.

Lambrinides, T. 1990. High intensity training and overtraining. *High Intensity Training Newsletter* 2 (2): 9-10.

Lees, A., and E. Fahmi. 1990. Playing the percentages: is it a good or bad idea? *High Intensity Training Newsletter* 2 (4): 12-13.

_____. 1994. Optimal drop heights for plyometric training. *Ergonomics* 37 (1): 141-148.

Leistner, K. E. 1986. The quality repetition. *The Steel Tip* 2 (June): 6-7.

_____. 1987. More from Ken Leistner. *Powerlifting USA* 10 (April): 17.

_____. 1989. Explosive training: not necessary. *High Intensity Training Newsletter* 1 (2): 3-5.

Lesmes, G. R., D. W. Benham, D. L. Costill and W. J. Fink. 1983. Glycogen utilization in fast and slow twitch muscle fibers during maximal isokinetic exercise. *Annals of Sports Medicine* 1 (3): 105-108.

LeSuer, D. A., and J. H. McCormick. 1993. Prediction of a 1-RM bench press and 1-RM squat from repetitions to fatigue using the Brzycki formula. Abstract presented at the National Strength and Conditioning Association 16th National Conference. Las Vegas, NV.

LeSuer, D. A., J. H. McCormick, J. L. Mayhew, R. L. Wasserstein and M. D. Arnold. 1997. The accuracy of prediction equations for estimating 1-RM performance in the bench press, squat and deadlift. *Journal of Strength and Conditioning Research* 11 (4): 211-213.

Lewis, D. 1862. The new gymnastics. *Atlantic Monthly* 10 (August): 129-148.

Lieber, D. C., R. L. Lieber and W. C. Adams. 1989. Effects of run-training and swim-training at similar absolute intensities on treadmill VO$_2$ max. *Medicine and Science in Sports and Exercise* 21 (6): 655-661.

Lindeburg, F. A. 1949. A study of the degree of transfer between quickening exercises and other movements. *Research Quarterly* 20: 180-189.

Lindh, M. 1980. Biomechanics of the lumbar spine. In *Basic biomechanics of the skeletal system*, by V. H. Frankel and M. Nordin, 255-290. Philadelphia, PA: Lea & Febiger.

Lillegard, W. A., and J. D. Terrio. 1994. Appropriate strength training. *Sports Medicine* 78 (2): 457-477.

Lomangino, K. 2002. More doubt cast on value of pre-exercise stretching. *Sports Medicine Digest* 24 (10): 109, 111-112.

Londeree, B. R., and M. L. Moeschberger. 1982. Effect of age and other factors on maximal heart rate. *Research Quarterly for Exercise and Sport* 53 (4): 297-304.

Lowenthal, D. T., and Y. Karni. 1990. The nutritional needs of athletes. In *The Mount Sinai School of Medicine complete book of nutrition*, ed. V. Herbert and G. J. Subak-Sharpe, 396-414. New York, NY: St. Martin's Press.

Lukaski, H. C. 1995. Micronutrients (magnesium, zinc, and copper): are mineral supplements needed for athletes? *International Journal of Sports Nutrition* 5 (supplement): S74-S83.

Lukaski, H. C., W. W. Bolonchuk, W. A. Siders and D. B. Milne. 1996. Chromium supplementation and resistance training: effects on body composition, strength, and trace element status of men. *American Journal of Clinical Nutrition* 63 (6): 954-965.

MacDougall, D., and D. G. Sale. 1981. Continuous vs. interval training: a review for the athlete and coach. *Canadian Journal of Applied Sport Sciences* 6 (2): 87-92.

Mannie, K. 2001. *Michigan State summer manual.* East Lansing, MI: Michigan State University.

————. 1988. Key factors in program organization. *High Intensity Training Newsletter* 1 (1): 4-5.

————. 1990. Strength training follies: the all-P.U.B. team. *High Intensity Training Newsletter* 2 (2): 11-12.

————. 1992. Athletic skill development: an open and closed case. *High Intensity Training Newsletter* 3 (4): 4-6.

————. 1993. Lift risks are a weighty matter. *NCAA News* 30 (January 27): 4-5.

————. 1994. Some thoughts on explosive weight training. *High Intensity Training Newsletter* 5 (1 & 2): 13-18.

Manore, M. M., S.I. Barr and G. E. Butterfield. 2000. Joint position statement by the American College of Sports Medicine, American Dietetic Association and Dieticians of Canada on nutrition and athletic performance. *Medicine and Science in Sports and Exercise* 32 (12): 2130-2145.

Margaria, R., P. Aghemo and E. Rovelli. 1966. Measurement of muscular power (anaerobic) in man. *Journal of Applied Physiology* 21: 1662-1664.

Marsden, C. D., J. A. Obeso and J. C. Rothwell. 1984. The function of the antagonist muscle during fast limb movements in man. *Journal of Physiology* (London) 335: 1-13.

Mayhew, J. L., J. L. Prinster, J. S. Ware, D. L. Zimmer, J. R. Arabas and M. G. Bemben. 1995. Muscular endurance repetitions to predict bench press strength in men of different training levels. *The Journal of Sports Medicine and Physical Fitness* 35 (2): 108-113.

McArdle, W. D., F. I. Katch and V. L. Katch. 1986. *Exercise physiology: energy, nutrition and human performance. 2d ed.* Philadelphia, PA: Lea & Febiger.

McArdle, W. D., J. R. Margel, D. J. Delio, M. Toner and J. M. Chase. 1978. Specificity of run training on VO_2 max and heart rate changes during running and swimming. *Medicine and Science in Sports and Exercise* 10 (1): 16-20.

McCarthy, J. P., J. C. Agre, B. K. Graf, M. A. Pozniak and A. C. Vailas. 1995. Compatibility of adaptive responses with combining strength and endurance training. *Medicine and Science in Sports and Exercise* 27 (3): 429-436.

McCarthy, P. 1989. How much protein do athletes really need? *The Physician and Sportsmedicine* 17 (5): 170-175.

McGuine, T. A., J. C. Sullivan and D. T. Bernhardt. 2001. Creatine supplementation in high school football players. *Clinical Journal of Sports Medicine* 11 (4): 247-253.

Mentzer, M. 1993. *Heavy duty.* Venice, CA: Mike Mentzer.

Messier, S. P., and M. Dill. 1985. Alterations in strength and maximal oxygen uptake consequent to Nautilus circuit weight training. *Research Quarterly for Exercise and Sport* 56 (4): 345-351.

Meyers, S. A. 2001. *A guide to police sniping – revised edition.* Gaithersburg, MD: Operational Tactics, Inc.: 30, 34, 62, 157, 177, 220.

————. 2002. Operational Tactics, Inc. Operational Fitness Requirements For SWAT Officers. Gaithersburg, MD: Operational Tactics, Inc.

_____. 2003. SWAT fitness. presented at the Operational Tactics, Inc. National SWAT/Sniper Symposium. Gaithersburg, MD: Operational Tactics, Inc.

Montgomery County Department of Police. 1992. Search warrant service. *Tactical Section Incident Report – Gaithersburg* (December 10).

_____. 1992. Search warrant/arrest warrant service. *Tactical Section Incident Report – Silver Spring* (December 11).

_____. 1992. Search warrant service. *Tactical Section Incident Report – Gaithersburg* (December 11).

_____. 1993. Search warrant service. *Tactical Section Incident Report – Gaithersburg* (January 25).

Moritani, T., and H. A. deVries. 1979. Neural factors vs hypertrophy in the course of muscle strength gain. *American Journal of Physical Medicine and Rehabilitation* 58 (3): 115-130.

Morton, C. 1990. The relationship between sprint training and conditioning: a time for quality and a time for quantity. *High Intensity Training Newsletter* 2 (3): 9-11.

Mujika, I., and S. Padilla. 1997. Creatine supplementation as an ergogenic aid for sports performance in highly trained athletes: a critical review. *International Journal of Sports Medicine* 18 (7): 491-496.

National Collegiate Athletic Association [NCAA]. 1991. No miracles found in many "natural potions." *NCAA News* 28 (July 17): 7.

NCAA Committee on Competitive Safeguards and Medical Aspects of Sports. 1992. Ergogenic aids and nutrition. Overland Park, KS: NCAA memorandum (August 6).

National Research Council, Committee on Diet and Health, Food and Nutrition Board. 1989. *Diet and health: implications for reducing chronic disease risk.* Washington, D. C.: National Academy Press.

Nelson, R. C., and M. R. Nofsinger. 1965. Effect of overload on speed of elbow flexion and the associated aftereffects. *Research Quarterly* 36: 174-182.

Nielson, F. 1992. Facts and fallacies about boron. *Nutrition Today* 27 (May/June): 6-12.

Parascrampuria, J., K. Schwartz and R. Petesch. 1998. Quality control of dehydroepiandrosterone dietary supplements. *Journal of the American Medical Association* 280 (8): 1565.

Paton, C. D., W. G. Hopkins and L. Vollebregt. 2001. Little effect of caffeine ingestion on repeated sprints in team-sport athletes. *Medicine and Science in Sports and Exercise* 33 (5): 822-825.

Pecci, M. A., and J. A. Lombardo. 2000. Performance-enhancing supplements. *Physical Medicine and Rehabilitation Clinics of North America* 11 (4): 949-960.

Peterson, J. A., ed. 1978. *Total fitness: the Nautilus way.* West Point, NY: Leisure Press.

_____. 1975. Total conditioning: a case study. *Athletic Journal* 56 (September): 40-55.

Peterson, J. A., and C. X. Bryant, eds. 1992. *The Stairmaster fitness handbook.* Indianapolis, IN: Masters Press.

Peterson, J. A., and C. X. Bryant, eds. 1995. *The Stairmaster fitness handbook. 2d ed.* St. Louis, MO: Wellness Bookshelf.

Peterson, J. A., and W. L. Westcott. 1990. Stronger by the minute. *Fitness Management* 6 (June): 22-24.

Pezzullo, D., S. Whitney and J. Irrgang. 1993. A comparison of vertical jump enhancement using plyometrics and strength footwear shoes versus plyometrics alone. *Journal of Orthopedic and Sports Physical Therapy* 17: 68.

Philen, R. M., D. I. Ortiz, S. B. Auerbach and H. Falk. 1992. Survey of advertising for nutritional supplements in health and bodybuilding magazines. *Journal of the American Medical Association* 268 (8): 1008-1011.

Piehl, K. 1974. Glycogen storage and depletion in human skeletal muscle fibers. *Acta Physiologica Scandinavica* (Supplementum 402): 1-32.

Pipes, T. V. 1989. *The steroid alternative.* Placerville, CA: Sierra Gold Graphics.

_____. 1977. Physiological responses of fire fighting recruits to high intensity training. *Journal of Occupational Medicine* 19 (2): 129-132.

_____. 1978. Variable resistance versus constant resistance strength training in adult males. *European Journal of Applied Physiology* 39 (1): 27-35.

_____. 1979. High intensity, not high speed. *Athletic Journal* 59 (December): 60, 62.

_____. 1988. A.C.T. - The steroid alternative. *Scholastic Coach* 57 (January): 106, 108-109, 112.

_____. 1994. Strength training & fiber types. *Scholastic Coach* 63 (March): 67-70.

Pitts, E. H. 1992. Pills, powders, potions and persuasions. *Fitness Management* 9 (November): 34-35.

Pollock, M. L. 1973. The quantification of endurance training programs. In *Exercise and sport sciences reviews*, ed. J. H. Wilmore: 155-188. New York, NY: Academic Press.

Pollock, M. L., J. Dimmick, H. S. Miller, Z. Kendrick and A. C. Linnerud. 1975. Effects of mode of training on cardiovascular function and body composition of middle-aged men. *Medicine and Science in Sports and Exercise* 7 (2): 139-145.

Pollock, M. L., G. A. Gaesser, J. D. Butcher, J.-P. Despres, R. K. Dishman, B. A. Franklin and C. E. Garber. 1998. ACSM position on the recommended quantity and quality of exercise for developing and maintaining cardiorespiratory and muscular fitness, and flexibility in healthy adults. *Medicine and Science in Sports and Exercise* 30 (6): 975-991.

Porcari, J. P. 1994. Fat-burning exercise: fit or farce. *Fitness Management* 10 (July): 40-41.

Porcari, J., and J. Curtis. 1996. Can you work strength and aerobics at the same time? *Fitness Management* 12 (June): 26-29.

Poulton, E. C. 1957. On prediction in skilled movements. *Psychological Bulletin* 54:467-478.

Pritchard, N. R., and P. A. Kalra. 1998. Renal dysfunction accompanying oral creatine supplements. *Lancet* 351: 1252-1253.

Rasch, P. J. 1989. *Kinesiology and applied anatomy. 7th ed*. Philadelphia, PA: Lea & Febiger.

Rasch, P. J., and C. E. Morehouse. 1957. Effect of static and dynamic exercises on muscular strength and hypertrophy. *Journal of Applied Physiology* 11: 29-34.

Rasmussen, B. B., K. D. Tipton, S. L. Miller, S. E. Wolf and R. R. Wolfe. 2000. An oral essential amino acid-carbohydrate supplement enhances muscle protein anabolism after resistance exercise. *Journal of Applied Physiology* 88: 386-392.

Reid, C. M., R. A. Yeater and I. H. Ullrich. 1987. Weight training and strength, cardiorespiratory functioning and body composition in men. *British Journal of Sports Medicine* 21 (1): 40-44.

Reinebold, J. 1993. H.I.T. in the CFL British Columbia style. *High Intensity Training Newsletter* 4 (4): 7-8.

Reston, J. 1982. Strength training philosophies come to trial. *Coach & Athlete* (March): 42-43.

Riley, D. P. 1982. *Strength training by the experts. 2d ed*. West Point, NY: Leisure Press.

_____. 1982. *Maximum muscular fitness: strength training without equipment*. West Point, NY: Leisure Press.

_____. 1979. Speed of exercise versus speed of movement. *Scholastic Coach* 48 (May/June): 90, 92-93, 97-98.

_____. 1980. Time and intensity: keys to maximum strength gains. *Scholastic Coach* 50 (November): 65-66, 74-75.

_____. 1982. Guidelines for strength program. *Scholastic Coach* 51 (May/June): 64-65, 80.

Riley, D. P., and J. Arapoff. 2000. *Washington Redskins strength & conditioning guide*. Ashburn, VA: Washington Redskins.

Riley, D. P., and R. Wright. 2002. *Houston Texans strength & conditioning program*. Houston, TX: Houston Texans.

Roberts, D. F. 1984. Genetic determinants of sports performance. In *Sport and human genetics*, ed. R. M. Malina and C. Bouchard, 105-121. Champaign, IL: Human Kinetics Publishers, Inc.

Rogucki, B. 1997. *Arizona Cardinals strength/conditioning program.* Phoenix, AZ: Arizona Cardinals.

Rooney, K. J., R. D. Herbert and R. J. Balnave. 1994. Fatigue contributes to the strength training stimulus. *Medicine and Science in Sports and Exercise* 26 (9): 1160-1164.

Sage, G. H. 1977. *Introduction to motor behavior: a neuropsychological approach.* 2d ed. Reading, MA: Addison-Wesley Publishing Company.

Sale, D. G. 1988. Neural adaptation to resistance training. *Medicine and Science in Sports and Exercise* 20 (5): S135-S145.

Sale, D. G., and D. MacDougall. 1981. Specificity in strength training: a review for the coach and athlete. *Canadian Journal of Applied Sport Sciences* 6 (2): 87-92.

Saltin, B., J. Henriksson, E. Nygaard and P. Andersen. 1977. Fiber types and metabolic potentials of skeletal muscles in sedentary men and endurance runners. In *The marathon,* ed. P. Milvy. New York, NY: New York Academy of Sciences.

Sargent, V. J. 1921. The physical test of man. *American Physical Education Review* 26 (April): 188-194.

Schantz, P., E. Randall-Fox, W. Hutchison, A. Tyden and P.-O. Astrand. 1983. Muscle fiber type distribution, muscle cross-sectional area and maximal voluntary strength in humans. *Acta Physiologica Scandinavica* 117 (2): 219-226.

Schmidt, R. A. 1975. *Motor skills.* New York, NY: Harper & Row.

————. 1991. *Motor learning and performance: from principles to practice.* Champaign, IL: Human Kinetics Books.

Scoles, G. 1978. Depth jumping! Does it really work? *Athletic Journal* 58 (January): 48-50, 74-76.

Scrimshaw, N. S., and V. R. Young. 1976. The requirements of human nutrition. *Scientific American* 235 (3): 50-64.

Seliger, V., L. Dolejs and V. Karas. 1980. A dynamometric comparison of maximum eccentric, concentric and isometric contractions using EMG and energy expenditure measurements. *European Journal of Applied Physiology* 45 (2-3): 235-244.

Selye, H. 1956. *The stress of life.* New York, NY: McGraw-Hill.

Sharkey, B. J. 1975. *Physiology and physical activity.* New York, NY: Harper & Row.

————. 1984. *Physiology of fitness.* Champaign, IL: Human Kinetics Publishers, Inc.

Silver, M. D. 2001. Use of ergogenic aids by athletes. *Journal of the American Academy of Orthopedic Surgeons* 9 (1): 61-70.

Singh, A., F. M. Moses and P. A. Deuster. 1992. Chronic multivitamin-mineral supplementation does not enhance physical performance. *Medicine and Science in Sports and Exercise* 24 (6): 726-732.

Skinner, J. S. 1995. Understanding the physiological basis of cardiorespiratory fitness. In *The Stairmaster fitness handbook, 2d ed,* ed. J. A. Peterson and C. X. Bryant, 57-65. St. Louis, MO: Wellness Bookshelf.

Skinner, J. S., and T. McLellan. 1980. The transition from aerobic to anaerobic metabolism. *Research Quarterly for Exercise and Sport* 51 (1): 234-248.

Smith, N. J. 1984. Nutrition. In *Sports medicine,* ed. R. H. Strauss, 468-480. Philadelphia, PA: W. B. Saunders Company.

Song, T. M., L. Perusse, R. M. Malina and C. Bouchard. 1994. Twin resemblance in somatotype and comparisons with other twin studies. *Human Biology* 66 (3): 453-464.

Sorani, R. 1966. *Circuit training.* Dubuque, IA: Wm. C. Brown Company Publishers.

Sparling, P., R. Recker and T. Lambrinides. 1994. Position statement to football players from Cincinnati Bengals Training Staff and nutrition consultant.

Spriet, L. L. 1995. Caffeine and performance. *International Journal of Sports Nutrition* 5 (supplement): S84-S99.

St. Jeor, S. T., B. V. Howard, T. E. Prewitt, V. Bovee, T. Bazzarre and R. H. Eckel. 2001. Dietary protein and weight reduction. *Circulation* 104 (15): 1869-1874.

Steinhaus, A. H. 1933. Chronic effects of exercise. *Physiological Reviews* 13 (1): 103-147.

Stockholm, A. J., and R. C. Nelson. 1965. The immediate aftereffects of increased resistance upon physical performance. *Research Quarterly* 36: 337-341.

Strauss, R. H., ed. 1984. *Sports medicine*. Philadelphia, PA: W. B. Saunders Company.

Stromme, S. B., and H. Skard. 1980. *Physical fitness and fitness testing*. Sandnes, Norway: Jonas Oglaend A.s.

Swanger, T., M. Bradley and S. Murray. 1996. *Army strength & conditioning manual*. West Point, NY: United States Military Academy.

Tanaka, H., K. D. Monahan and D. R Seals. 2001. Age-predicted maximal heart rate revisited. *Journal of the American College of Cardiology* 37 (1): 153-156.

Taylor, G. H. 1860. *An exposition of the Swedish movement-cure*. New York, NY: Fowler and Wells.

Taylor, M. R. 1993. *The dietary supplement debate of 1993: an FDA perspective*. Presented at the Federation of American Societies for Experimental Biology Annual Meeting. New Orleans, LA.

Telford, R., E. Catchpole, V. Deakin, A. Hahn and A. Plank. 1992. The effect of 7 to 8 months of vitamin/mineral supplementation on athletic performance. *International Journal of Sports Nutrition* 2 (2): 135-153.

Terjung, R. L., P. Clarkson, E. R. Eichner, P. L. Greenhaff, P. J. Hespel, R. G. Israel, W. J. Kraemer, R. A. Meyer, L. L. Spriet, M. A. Tarnopolsky, A. J. M. Wagenmakers and M. H. Williams. 2000. The ACSM roundtable on the physiological and health effects of oral creatine supplementation. *Medicine and Science in Sports and Exercise* 32 (3): 706-717.

Thomas, J. 2001. *Penn State football strength and conditioning*. University Park, PA: Penn State University.

Thomas v. City of Evanston 610 F.Supp. 422, 42 Fair Empl.Prac.Cas. (BNA) 1795 (N.D.Ill., Feb 26, 1985) (NO. 80 C 4803).

Thompson, C. W. 1985. *Manual of structural kinesiology. 10th ed*. St. Louis, MO: Times Mirror/Mosby College Publishing.

Thorstensson, A. 1976. Muscle strength, fiber types and enzyme activities in man. *Acta Physiologica Scandinavica* (Supplementum 443): 1-44.

Thrash, K., and B. Kelly. 1987. Flexibility and strength training. *The Journal of Applied Sport Science Research* 1 (4): 74-75.

Todd, T. 1986. A brief history of resistance exercise. In *Getting stronger*, revised ed, by B. Pearl and G. T. Moran, 413-431. Bolinas, CA: Shelter Publications, Inc.

Trent, L. K., and D. Thieding-Cancel. 1995. Effects of chromium picolinate on body composition. *The Journal of Sports Medicine and Physical Fitness* 35 (4): 273-280.

U.S. Food and Drug Administration. 2001. FDA warns consumers to discontinue use of botanical products that contain aristolochic acid. *Consumer Advisory, Center for Food Safety and Applied Nutrition* (April 11). <http://www.cfsan.fda.gov/~dms/addsbot.html>.

Vander, A. J., J. H. Sherman and D. S. Luciano. 1975. *Human physiology: the mechanisms of body function. 2d ed*. New York, NY: McGraw-Hill, Inc.

Vanderburgh, P. M., and W. J. Considine. 1995. Assessing health-related & functional fitness. In *The Stairmaster fitness handbook, 2d ed*, ed. J. A. Peterson and C. X. Bryant, 131-156. St. Louis, MO: Wellness Bookshelf.

Verhoshanski, Y. 1966. Perspectives in the improvement of speed and strength preparation of jumpers. *Track and Field* 9: 11-12.

Wateska, M., and M. Bradley. 1998. *Cardinal conditioning*. Palo Alto, CA: Stanford University.

Weight, L. M., T. D. Noakes, D. Labadorios, J. Graves, D. Haem, P. Jacobs and P. Berman. 1988. Vitamin and mineral status of trained athletes including the effects of supplementation. *American Journal of Clinical Nutrition* 47 (2): 186-191.

Wenger, H. A., and G. J. Bell. 1986. The interactions of intensity, frequency and duration of exercise training in altering cardiorespiratory fitness. *Sports Medicine* 3 (5): 346-356.

Westcott, W. L. 1983. *Strength fitness: physiological principles and training techniques*. Expanded ed. Boston: Allyn and Bacon, Inc.

_____. 1996. *Building strength and stamina: new Nautilus training for total fitness*. Champaign, IL: Human Kinetics.

_____. 1986. Integration of strength, endurance and skill training. *Scholastic Coach* 55 (May/June): 74.

_____. 1987. Individualized strength training for girl high school runners. *Scholastic Coach* 57 (December): 71-72.

_____. 1989. Strength training research: sets and repetitions. *Scholastic Coach* 58 (May/June): 98-100.

Westcott, W. L., and J. R. Parziale. 1997. Golf power. *Fitness Management* 13 (December): 39-41.

Westcott, W. L., R. A. Winett, E. S. Anderson, J. R. Wojcik, R. L. R. Loud, E. Cleggett and S. Glover. 2001. Effects of regular and slow speed resistance training on muscle strength. *The Journal of Sports Medicine and Physical Fitness* 41 (2): 154-158.

Wilcox, A. R. 1990. Caffeine and endurance performance. *Sports Science Exchange* 3 (26): 1-4.

Wikgren, S. 1988. The plyometrics debate. *Coaching Women's Basketball* 1 (May/June): 10-13.

Willett, W. C., and M. J. Stampfer. 2003. Rebuilding the food pyramid. *Scientific American* 288 (1): 64-71.

Williams, M. H. 1992. *Nutrition for fitness and sport*. Dubuque, IA: Brown & Benchmark.

Williams, M. H., and J. D. Branch. 1998. Creatine supplementation and exercise performance: an update. *Journal of the American College of Nutrition* 17 (3): 216-234.

Willis, T., and K. A. Beals. 2000. The Zone Diet vs. traditional weight loss diet: effects on weight loss and blood lipid levels. *Journal of the American Dietetic Association* (supplement) 100 (9): A-74.

Wilmore, J. H. 1982. *Training for sport and activity: the physiological basis of the conditioning process*. 2d ed. Boston, MA: Allyn and Bacon, Inc.

_____. 1974. Alterations in strength, body composition and anthropometric measurements consequent to a 10-week weight training program. *Medicine and Science in Sports* 6 (2): 133-138.

Wilmore, J. H., R. B. Parr, R. N. Girandola, P. Ward, P. A. Vodak T. J. Barstow, T. V. Pipes, G. T. Romero and P. Leslie. 1978. Physiological alterations consequent to circuit weight training. *Medicine and Science in Sports* 10 (2): 79-84.

Wilt, F. 1975. Plyometrics: what it is — how it works. *Athletic Journal* 55 (May): 76, 89-90.

Winett, R. A. 1996. Dose-response. *Master Trainer* 6 (June): 1-2.

Winter, D. A. 1990. *The biomechanics of human movement*. New York, NY: Wiley & Sons.

Wirhed, R. 1984. *Athletic ability: the anatomy of winning*. New York: Harmony Books.

Wolf, M. D. 1982. Muscles: structure, function and control. In *Strength training by the experts, 2d ed*, by D. P. Riley, 27-40. West Point, NY: Leisure Press.

Wood, K. 1991. Cincinnati Bengals' strength training program. *American Fitness Quarterly* 10 (July): 38, 40.

About the Authors

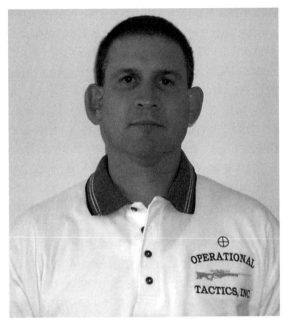

Stuart A. Meyers

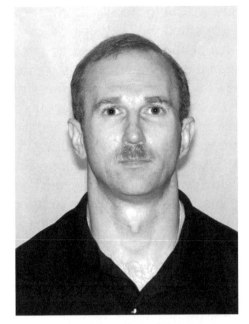

Matt Brzycki

Mr. Stuart A. Meyers is the founder and President of Operational Tactics, Inc. He is the author of the books, *A Guide To Police Sniping* and *Police Sniper Administrative Policy & Training*, with sales worldwide. Mr. Meyers has taught courses throughout the world on SWAT operations, hostage rescue, domestic and international terrorism, tactical command, operational fitness requirements for SWAT team personnel, sniper operations, undercover and narcotics operations, patrol response, weapons training, breaching, and law enforcement/military instructor certification. Agencies he has trained include U.S. Navy Seals, U.S. Army Special Forces instructors, international counter-terrorist teams, in addition to U.S. and foreign law enforcement agencies. Mr. Meyers is the creator and Executive Director of the Operational Tactics National SWAT/Sniper Symposium and the *World Sniper Championship™*. He has a Bachelor of Arts degree from the University of Maryland in Criminal Justice/Law Enforcement. Mr. Meyers has received counter-terrorism training at Georgetown University in Washington, D.C., and chemical and biological terrorism training at the Navy Medical Center in Bethesda, Maryland. He was a member of the Montgomery County, Maryland, Department of Police from 1982 to 1998, participating in hundreds of high-risk tactical operations. As a member of the full-time Special Weapons and Tactics team, Mr. Meyers competed in the 1996 H&K Invitational Counter-Sniper Team Competition at Fort Meade, Maryland, where he placed first in the team competition, as well as first in the individual competition. He speaks fluent Spanish and is a consultant for the U.S. Department of State Anti-Terrorism Assistance Program. He has had articles published in periodicals throughout the United States on a variety of law enforcement related topics. Mr. Meyers has provided expert commentary on television programs to include: Connie Chung Tonight, Larry King Live, the O'Reilly Factor, CNN, Fox News, MSNBC, Court TV, and the BBC.

Mr. Matt Brzycki enlisted in the United States Marine Corps in June

1975. In May 1978, he entered Drill Instructor (DI) School at the Marine Corps Recruit Depot in San Diego, California. When Mr. Brzycki completed his basic training in November 1975, he was presented the Leatherneck Award for achieving the highest score in rifle marksmanship in his platoon. When he graduated from the school in August 1978 at the age of 21, he was one of the youngest DIs in the entire Marine Corps. Among his many responsibilities as a DI was the physical preparedness of Marine recruits. In August 1979, Mr. Brzycki was awarded a Certificate of Merit for successfully completing a tour of duty as a DI. During his four-year enlistment, he also earned a Good Conduct Ribbon and qualified as a rifle expert three times. In May 1983, Mr. Brzycki earned a Bachelor of Science degree in Health and Physical Education from Penn State University. He represented the university for two years in the Pennsylvania State Collegiate Powerlifting Championships (1981 and 1982) and placed third in his first bodybuilding competition (1981). In September 1984, he was named the Assistant Strength and Conditioning Coach at Rutgers University and remained in that position until July 1990. In August 1990, he became the Strength Coach and Health Fitness Coordinator at Princeton University. In March 2001, he was named the Coordinator of Recreational Fitness and Wellness Programming. Mr. Brzycki taught academic courses in strength training at the collegiate level for more than ten years. He developed the Strength Training Theory and Applications course for Exercise Science and Sports Studies majors at Rutgers University and taught the program from March 1990 – July 2000 as a member of the Faculty of Arts and Sciences (Department of Exercise Science and Sport Studies). He also taught the same course to Health and Physical Education majors at The College of New Jersey from January 1996 – March 1999 as a member of the Health and Physical Education Faculty. All told, more than 600 university students in fitness-related majors received academic credit in his strength-training courses. Since September 1990, Mr. Brzycki has taught non-credit physical-education courses at Princeton University including all of those that pertain to weight training. Mr. Brzycki has been a featured speaker at local, regional, state and national conferences and clinics throughout the United States and Canada. Since November 1984, he has authored more than 225 articles on strength and fitness that have been featured in 39 different publications. Mr. Brzycki has written five books: *A Practical Approach to Strength Training* (1995), *Youth Strength and Conditioning* (1995), *Cross Training for Fitness* (1997), *Wrestling Strength: The Competitive Edge* (2002) and *Wrestling Strength: Prepare to Win* (2002). He also co-authored *Conditioning for Basketball* (1993) with Shaun Brown (currently the Strength and Conditioning Coach for the Boston Celtics). In addition, Mr. Brzycki served as the editor of *Maximize your Training: Insights from Leading Strength and Fitness Professionals* (1999). In 1997, he developed a correspondence course in strength training for Desert Southwest Fitness (Tucson, Arizona) that is used by strength and fitness professionals to update their certifications. The course has been approved and accepted for continuing education credits by 19 international organizations including the American Council on Exercise, the Australian Fitness Advisory Council, the International Fitness Professionals Association, the International Weightlifting Association and the National Federation of Professional Trainers. In January 2001, Mr. Brzycki was named a Fellow at Forbes College (Princeton University). In April 2001, he was selected to serve on the Alumni Society Board of Directors for the College of Health & Human Development (Penn State). He and his wife, Alicia, reside in Lawrenceville, New Jersey, with their son, Ryan.